WORKBOOK TO ACCOMPANY

MOSBY'S
PARAMEDIC
TEXTBOOK

About the Authors

Kim D. McKenna, RN, CEN, EMT-P, has practiced in intensive care, emergency nursing, and prehospital education since her graduation in 1977 from nursing school in Ottawa, Canada. For the past 7 years, she has been involved in prehospital education, including 4 years as the primary instructor of a paramedic training program. Ms. McKenna is currently an education coordinator in the Office of Paramedic Education and a staff nurse in the Emergency Department at St. John's Mercy Medical Center in St. Louis, Missouri.

Mick J. Sanders received his paramedic training in 1978 from St. Louis University Hospitals. He earned a Bachelor of Science degree in 1982 and a Master of Science degree in 1983 from Lindenwood College in St. Charles, Missouri. For the past 15 years, he has worked in various health care systems as a field paramedic, emergency department paramedic, and EMS instructor. For 12 years, Mr. Sanders served as a training specialist with the Bureau of Emergency Medical Services, Missouri Department of Health.

WORKBOOK TO ACCOMPANY

Mosby's Paramedic Textbook

KIM D. McKENNA, RN, CEN, EMT-P
Education Coordinator
Office of Paramedic Education
Staff Nurse, Emergency Department
St. John's Mercy Medical Center
St. Louis, Missouri

MICK J. SANDERS, MSA, EMT-P
EMS Training Specialist
St. Charles, Missouri

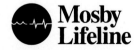

Mosby Lifeline

St. Louis   Baltimore   Berlin   Boston   Carlsbad   Chicago   London   Madrid
Naples   New York   Philadelphia   Sydney   Tokyo   Toronto

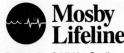

Executive Editor: Claire Merrick
Developmental Editor: Nancy J. Peterson
Assistant Editor: Carla Goldberg
Project Manager: Carol Sullivan Wiseman
Senior Production Editor: Pat Joiner
Designer: Betty Schulz
Cover Design: GW Graphics & Publishing
Manufacturing Supervisor: Theresa Fuchs

Credits for illustrations appear on p. 326.

Printed in the United States of America
Composition by Top Graphics
Printing/binding by Plus Communications

Mosby–Year Book, Inc.
11830 Westline Industrial Drive
St. Louis, MO 63146

ISBN   0-8016-4314-7

94 95 96 97 98 / 9 8 7 6 5 4 3 2 1

To my pony girls, Ginny, Becky, and Maggie; to my husband Don, who shared their time so I could write this book; and to my parents

K.M.

PREFACE

The *Workbook to accompany Mosby's Paramedic Textbook* has been written to enhance the paramedic student's understanding and retention of the material presented in the textbook. This has been accomplished using a variety of questions designed to encourage the various levels of learning necessary in this field, from recall and memorization to application of concepts. Some of the features of this workbook include:

- A special section on studying and test-taking skills (see p. viii) so that good habits can begin early in the program
- Format that follows *Mosby's Paramedic Textbook* chapter by chapter, with *answers referenced to the appropriate page number* in the text
- *Matching questions* that reinforce key terms or content within the chapters
- *True/false questions* that require an explanation of false answers to ensure understanding
- Extensive use of *scenario-based questions* to help visualize the "real-life" application of information
- Self-evaluation sections that offer the opportunity to review material using multiple-choice questions, a testing format often used by instructors for examinations
- Complete rationale for all answers (even false) that ensures understanding of material
- A programmed review of basic math skills that precedes the drug dose calculation section
- Illustrations for student identification of anatomy, patient management techniques, and special equipment
- Five multiple-choice division tests that review a larger body of material and help identify areas in which additional study would be helpful
- Paramedic career options section (see p. 256) that introduces some of the choices in the paramedic profession

ECG and drug flashcards at the end of the book can be removed for easy reference and study purposes. Flashcards are completed by the students and are keyed to questions in the workbook. The electrocardiogram flashcards show actual patient rhythms, and the drug flashcards are based on patient-care scenarios. Three blank drug flashcards will allow students to create cards for regional drugs.

Before completing each chapter of the workbook, the student should read the accompanying chapter in *Mosby's Paramedic Textbook* and review the learning objectives. When areas of difficulty are encountered while completing the questions, reread the text and attempt the questions again. We hope that this workbook, when used effectively, will facilitate mastery of the complex knowledge necessary to become a paramedic. Enjoy!

● ACKNOWLEDGMENTS

This workbook would, of course, never have been possible without the wonderful manuscript of *Mosby's Paramedic Textbook* , written by Mick J. Sanders. His commitment to detail and excellence is reflected throughout the text, and his encouragement and suggestions made the completion of the workbook possible.

A debt of gratitude goes to to my fellow instructors in the Office of Paramedic Education: Julie Long, EMT-P; Christine Neal, EMT-P; Mindy McCoy, EMP-T; Molly Barry, RN, EMP-T; and Mark Lockhart, EMT-P. They listened to many ideas and scenarios during the process. Many thanks to Catherine Parvensky, who wrote the studying and test-taking tips and the paramedic career options sections of the workbook.

Thanks to Mark Wieber for his illustrations and Don McKenna for the photographs included in this text. For the original patient electrocardiogram strips, I am indebted to the staff of the intensive care unit and especially to my colleagues in the emergency department at St. John's Mercy Medical Center.

To all of my paramedic students, past and present, I sincerely appreciate all that you have taught me and your suggestions for the content of this workbook.

And to my friends (the fellow paramedics) I have ridden with in the field, thanks for showing me where the textbook ends and reality begins.

I am also grateful to the reviewers, Bob Nixon, BA, EMT-P; Monroe Yancie, NREMT-P; and Janet Fitts, RN, EMT-P for their suggestions and fresh ideas.

Thanks to the staff at Mosby, especially Nancy Peterson, my conscience, adviser, cheerleader, and gentle critic; Claire Merrick for bringing together resources when we needed them; Pat Joiner in production editing (who is still looking for the address of my former English teachers); Derril Trakalo in marketing; and Betty Schulz in art and design for such a great presentation of this book.

Kim D. McKenna
Mick J. Sanders

STUDY TIPS

For all the emphasis placed on furthering one's education, little guidance is given for how to be a good student. Learning the following studying and test-taking tips can help you get the most out of your paramedic course and other classes in the future.

● STUDY SESSIONS

The way that an individual studies may determine the likelihood of successful completion of a training program. It is important to develop a routine pattern for studying and then stick to it. The following are various methods to increase the effectiveness of study sessions:

- Set a regular time for studying each day.
- Pace yourself by scheduling a specific amount of time for each subject or chapter.
- Take periodic breaks to prevent burnout.
- Read lesson information before each session and review notes immediately after the class.
- Do not wait until the last minute and expect to cram information and do well. Instead pace yourself throughout the course.
- Be aware of distractions, both internal and external.
  - Internal distractors include hunger, tension, fatigue, illness, glucose levels, day-dreaming, and getting side-tracked.
  - External distractors include room temperature (hot or cold), noise levels, and lighting.
- Make a game of it; drill the information by using:
  - Flash cards for memorizing facts
  - Jeopardy cards
  - Trivial Pursuit cards
- When frustration sets in:
  - Take a break
  - Have a snack (sugar helps).
  - Take a walk (increased cardiovascular activity increases blood flow to the brain).
  - Take a few deep breaths and relax.

● WHERE AND WHEN DO YOU STUDY BEST?

Everyone has a particular time and place in which they are most productive. For some it is late at night, and for others it is early in the morning. Determine when you are at your peak and study daily at that time.

- Where do you do the best work?
  - At a desk or table?
  - In front of the television? (Some people need background noise to focus.)

- Decide if you work better studying alone or in work groups. Sometimes, work sessions are a great motivation for studying.

Decide what form of studying works best for you:
  - Writing notes from the book
  - Highlighting information in the book
  - Taking copious notes
  - Listening to the instructor and asking questions

● INCREASING RETENTION

There are many ways to increase retention of material, including association, mnemonics, imagery, and recitation. Try them all and see what works best for you.

Association: Relate information to something you understand. Build new information on what is already known.

Mnemonics: Use letters or words to remember facts. For example *AVPU* to determine a patients level of consciousness: *A*lert, *V*erbal, *P*ainful stimuli, or *U*nconscious.

Imagery: Visualize a picture of the information. Memorize a chart or picture of the body and associated organs; then remember that picture for questions on anatomy.

Recitation: Read notes loud or discuss the information with peers. Hearing information repeatedly helps retention.

● TEST TAKING TIPS

Test taking is a skill that can be learned. Most state examinations are multiple-choice questions and are graded solely on the number of correct answers. Because there is no penalty for guessing, it is best not to leave any questions unanswered, since they will be marked incorrect.

Multiple-choice questions are made up of two parts, the stem (question) and possible answers. These type questions can be factual or situational in format:

Factual: During one-person CPR, the ratio of compressions to ventilations is:
  a. 15 to 2
  b. 5 to 1
  c. 12/min
  d. 20/min

Situational: A 55-year-old man was shoveling his driveway when he developed shortness of breath and pain in the middle of his chest. He is most likely suffering from:

    a. Myocardial infarction
    b. Congestive heart failure
    c. Emphysema
    d. Angina pectoris

It is important when answering a question to thoroughly analyze it. To do this:

- Read the stem without looking at the answers. Evaluate the question looking for key words such as *not, except, first,* or *final*.
- Identify key content words such as *one rescuer, adult victim, radiating pain, slurred speech,* or *conscious victim*.
- Think of a correct answer; then look at all the choices to see if your answer is there. If not, find the next *best answer*.
- Do not read into the question.
- Eliminate obviously wrong answers and select from those remaining.
- Do not change answers. Your first hunch is usually correct.

● PREPARING FOR TESTS

You can take some simple steps to prepare yourself for a test:

- Get a good night sleep before the examination.
- Avoid milk products because they tend to induce sleep.
- Eat a good meal but not too much before the examination. (Blood flow is forced to the digestive tract the first hour after eating a large meal, which tends to induce sleep.)
- Exercise moderately to increase blood supply to the brain.
- Layer clothes so that you can add or remove layers as necessary to be comfortable during the examination.
- Use a wristwatch to pace yourself.
- Sit away from friends or other distractions.
- Be prepared and be positive. If you have studied properly, you know the material and will do well on the examination.

● STRATEGIES FOR INCREASING TESTING PERFORMANCE

If you use the following strategies, you are sure to improve your performance during tests:

- Pace yourself to make certain that you have enough time to answer all questions.
- Use scrap paper to work through questions.
- At the end, make certain you have answered *all* questions. Do not change answers unless you initially misread the question.
- Make sure that you complete the answer sheet correctly. Fill in circles completely, and do not leave stray marks. Make certain that you check the number on the answer sheet against the number on the test every 10 questions to avoid the unnecessary stress of finding yourself on the wrong line.

CONTENTS

QUESTIONS

DIVISION ONE
THE PREHOSPITAL ENVIRONMENT

CHAPTER 1
ROLES AND RESPONSIBILITIES

● **READING ASSIGNMENT**

Chapter 1, pp. 2-9, in *Mosby's Paramedic Textbook*

● **OBJECTIVES**

As a paramedic, you should be able to:

1. Outline key historical events that influenced the development of the EMS profession.
2. Differentiate among the four nationally recognized levels of EMS licensure and certification: EMT-B, EMT-I, EMT-D, and EMT-P.
3. Apply to a patient care situation the seven components of the paramedic's role as defined by the Department of Transportation.
4. List paramedic relicensure and recertification requirements in your state.
5. Describe the benefits of continuing education.
6. Differentiate between professionalism and professional licensure and certification.
7. Distinguish ethical from legal issues.
8. List the benefits of membership in a professional association.

● **REVIEW QUESTIONS**

Match the description in Column 1 with the appropriate level of licensure listed in Column 2.

Column 1	Column 2
_____ 1. Trained in basic life support, including pneumatic antishock garments	a. EMT-B
_____ 2. Trained in all aspects of basic and advanced life support	b. EMT-D
_____ 3. Trained in basic life support and defibrillation	c. EMT-I
_____ 4. Trained in basic life support, including intravenous therapy	d. EMT-P

5. The study of medical ethics is known as *bioethics*. True/false. If this answer

   is false, what is the correct term? _____

6. List seven components of the role of the paramedic as defined by the Department of Transportation and describe how each would be applied when caring for the seriously injured victim of a motor vehicle collision.

   a.

   b.

   c.

   d.

    e.

    f.

    g.

7. List three possible requirements for relicensure or recertification of the paramedic.

    a.

    b.

    c.

8. Identify two benefits of continuing education for the paramedic.

    a.

    b.

9. *On successful completion of course and state requirements for paramedic licensure and certification, you begin practicing your trade.* Describe two or more ways in which you will demonstrate your *professional* commitment, surpassing the minimum requirements for licensure.

---

10. *You are called to the home of a comatose patient you have transported many times. He is chronically ill and dying of cancer. The family states that he has a living will expressing his wish that no lifesaving measures be initiated if he ceases breathing or if his heart stops. You cannot legally recognize the family's assertion that there is a living will. The patient goes into cardiac arrest.* What are you legally required to do, and is this ethical?

---

11. List two benefits of membership in a national professional association.

    a.

    b.

● **STUDENT SELF-EVALUATION**

12. Which of the following is *not* a role of the paramedic as defined by the Department of Transportation?
    - **a.** Documenting and communicating patient care
    - **b.** Assessing and providing emergency patient care
    - **c.** Ensuring that an adequate stock of supplies is on the ambulance
    - **d.** Coordinating collection of outstanding patient bills

13. Relicensure and recertification requirements vary from state to state and may include all of the following, *except:*
    - **a.** Attendance at an initial EMT-P training program
    - **b.** Continuing education as mandated by state
    - **c.** Verification of skills required by medical control
    - **d.** Reexamination by written or practical testing

14. In which of the following activities should paramedics participate to ensure adherence to current standards of care in emergency practice?
    - **a.** Conferences and seminars
    - **b.** Certification programs
    - **c.** Journal studies

4

    d. Quality-improvement reviews

    e. All of the above

15. Which of the following situations involves ethical patient care issues?

    a. Multiple-victim shooting in which the gunman is the most seriously injured

    b. Do-not-resuscitate order on a person who says that he or she wants everything done

    c. Unconscious patient unable to give consent for care

    d. Minor auto collision in which a conscious adult refuses care

CHAPTER 2
THE EMS SYSTEM

● READING ASSIGNMENT
Chapter 2, pp. 10-19, in *Mosby's Paramedic Textbook*

● OBJECTIVES
As a paramedic, you should be able to:
 1. Describe citizen involvement in the EMS system.
 2. Identify how the public can gain access to the EMS system.
 3. Distinguish between patient groups who need brief scene care and those who need extended scene care.
 4. Describe the benefits of each aspect of off-line and on-line medical direction.
 5. Discuss the appropriate transfer of responsibility for patient care in the receiving emergency department.
 6. Discuss the benefits of prehospital call reviews.
 7. List standards that influence ambulance design and equipment requirements.
 8. Outline the factors that must be considered when determining effective ambulance placement in the community.
 9. Describe the advantages and disadvantages of air medical transport.
 10. Identify the components of an EMS system that may interact in a patient care situation.

● REVIEW QUESTIONS
 1. The American College of Surgeons' system for trauma center designation identifies the readiness and capability of a hospital and its staff to provide the best treatment for trauma patients. True/false. If this is false, why is it false?

_____

_____

 2. Air medical patient transport is always preferable to ground transport for critically ill patients. True/false. If this is false, why is it false?

_____

_____

 3. Identify two ways in which the public is directly involved in EMS?
    a.
    b.
 4. Which of the following patients would likely require rapid transport to a medical facility without prolonged care on the scene?
    a. A multiple-trauma patient with a rigid abdomen and low blood pressure
    b. A patient in cardiac arrest of medical origin
 5. Explain the reasons for your choice in Question 4.

_____

_____

6. Describe the role of off-line medical direction.

_____

_____

_____

7. Describe the purpose of on-line medical direction.

_____

_____

_____

8. What are two advantages of patient care protocols?

   a.

   b.

9. Identify two benefits of EMT-P follow-up of patient condition and diagnosis during the course of hospitalization.

   a.

   b.

10. At what point does the paramedic transfer responsibility for the care of the patient to the emergency department staff?

_____

_____

11. _Your crew was involved in the care and transport of a critically ill patient during which numerous problems were encountered and patient care was compromised. Describe the benefits you anticipate as a result of a call critique in this situation._

_____

_____

_____

12. Cite two standards that define ambulance design and equipment requirements.

   a.

   b.

13. EMS and community planners must consider a number of factors when determining ambulance placement to provide acceptable availability and response times. List four of these factors.

   a.

   b.

   c.

   d.

14. _A 56 year-old man collapses in his office after suffering a cardiac arrest._ Identify the missing components of the EMS system in Figure 2-1 that are necessary to effectively resuscitate this victim and return him to society.

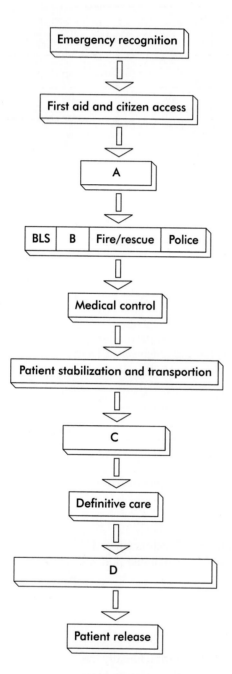

Figure 2-1

15. The EMS physician medical director is responsible for:
    a. Providing patient care in the field on advanced life-support units
    b. Negotiating staff salary and benefit disputes
    c. Ensuring the direction and quality of EMS care
    d. Ensuring maintenance of ambulances and equipment

16. Which of the following is *not* a component of the EMS system?
    a. Paramedic training   c. Intensive care units
    b. Disaster planning   d. Insurance providers

17. Call critiques should routinely serve all of the following purposes, *except:*
    a. Documenting problems that need disciplinary action
    b. Identifying future training and education needs
    c. Decreasing personnel stress from difficult calls
    d. Preparing for future calls of a similar nature

18. Emergency vehicle placement should be determined by:
    a. Number of paying patients per area
    b. Availability of EMS personnel
    c. Average scene response times
    d. Receiving hospitals in the region

19. In which of the following situations would the use of air medical transport by an advanced life-support unit be justified?
    a. Possible fractured tibia with good pulses
    b. Possible aneurysm with absent pedal pulses
    c. Home delivery with both patients stable
    d. Adult asthma patient with a pulse of 100 and respiration rate of 20

20. A person who claims to be an emergency department physician is attempting to direct care in an inappropriate manner on a cardiac arrest call. You should:
    a. Immediately ask the police to arrest him.
    b. Follow his orders because he has appropriate credentials.
    c. Ignore him and carry on as you see appropriate.
    d. Contact medical control for instructions.

MEDICAL-LEGAL CONSIDERATIONS

● READING ASSIGNMENT
Chapter 3, pp. 20-29, in *Mosby's Paramedic Textbook*

● OBJECTIVES
As a paramedic, you should be able to:
1. Describe the four elements involved in a claim of negligence.
2. Define common medical-legal terms that apply to prehospital situations involving patient care.
3. Describe measures that paramedics may take to protect themselves from claims of negligence.
4. List situations that the paramedic is legally required to report in most states.
5. Describe the paramedic's responsibilities with regard to patient confidentiality.
6. Describe the process for obtaining expressed, informed, and implied consent.
7. Describe actions to be taken in a refusal-of-care situation.
8. List uses of the prehospital care report.
9. Detail the components of the narrative report.
10. Discuss the implications of Good Samaritan legislation.

● REVIEW QUESTIONS
Match the legal term in Column 2 with its definition in Column 1. Use each answer only once.

Column 1	Column 2
_C_ 1. Forcefully restraining the arm of an alert competent patient while an intravenous line is being placed	a. Abandonment
_H_ 2. Advising the emergency department staff that the patient is a prostitute because of her clothing	b. Assault
	c. Battery
_____ 3. Telling a friend that you treated a nurse you both know for a drug overdose	d. False imprisonment
	e. Invasion of privacy
_____ 4. Restraining an alert, conscious adult with an obvious fracture and transporting him or her by ambulance against his or her will	f. Libel
	g. Malpractice
_____ 5. Documenting on the patient care report that the patient is homosexual based on your observations at his or her home	h. Slander
_____ 6. Leaving a patient in the emergency department to go on another call before you have an opportunity to give a report to the nurse or physician on duty	

7. Violations of state motor vehicle codes by a paramedic can result in civil lawsuits only. True/false. If this answer is false, why is it false?

_____

8. Good Samaritan legislation may protect off-duty EMS providers from litigation, provided that there was no negligence or reckless disregard. True/false. If this answer is false, why is it false?

_____

9. Group insurance policies will protect EMS providers from lawsuits arising from negligent acts. True/false. If this answer if false, why is it false?

_____

10. Describe three functions of a regulatory agency such as a state EMS bureau.
   a.
   b.
   c.
11. Name three effective means by which the paramedic may avoid claims of liability when providing patient care.
   a.
   b.
   c.
12. List four situations that most states require a paramedic to report to the authorities.
   a.
   b.
   c.
   d.
13. List the four elements necessary to prove negligence.
   a.
   b.
   c.
   d.
14. *A 40-year-old patient involved in a motor vehicle collision is complaining of mild neck pain and tingling in her fingers. She is quickly assessed and signs a refusal-of-care form at the urging of the paramedic crew. Later that day, she loses sensation and movement in all extremities, ceases breathing, and dies. Which, if any, of the four elements in Question 13 could be used to prove negligence in this situation and why?*

_____

_____

_____

15. Fill in the blanks with the types of consent that best apply to the situation. *You are called to treat an alert, 72-year-old patient who is experiencing chest pain. The patient exhibits classic signs and symptoms of myocardial infarction. You explain to him that he needs to go to the hospital because you feel that his symptoms could be those of a heart attack and proper medicine could be given to aid his condition. He states that he wishes his wife to drive him instead of going by ambulance. You advise him that, if his condition worsens in the car, his wife would be unable to help him and he might die. You again urge him to come with you.* The patient

can now make a(n) _____ consent. *He indicates verbally that he has decided to go in the ambulance.* This constitutes a(n)

_____ consent. If he had lost consciousness before agreeing to ambulance transport, his consent is said to be a(n)

_____ consent, and treatment could be rendered.

16. List four uses of the patient care report.
   a.
   b.
   c.
   d.

17. *You respond to the scene of an automobile collision, where you find an awake, alert, 24-year-old man complaining of neck pain and tingling in his right arm. Vital signs are stable. The patient's vehicle was struck from behind and sustained considerable damage. The patient is refusing transport to the hospital.* What five things should be done or explained to this patient and documented on the patient care report regarding his refusal of care?
   a.
   b.
   c.
   d.
   e.

● **STUDENT SELF-EVALUATION**

18. Which of the following is necessary to successfully prosecute a criminal law case?
   a. Criminal intent must be proved.
   b. Injury must be demonstrated.
   c. A patient must sue for financial gain.
   d. A statute must be violated.

19. In which of the following situations may abandonment be alleged when a paramedic relinquishes care to an EMT?
   a. A patient with asthma who has been given epinephrine
   b. A patient going from nursing home to hospital for a wrist injury
   c. A hysterical, uninjured patient from a mass casualty situation
   d. A dialysis patient being transported for routine care

20. Paramedics may protect themselves from claims of negligence by doing all of the following, *except:*
   a. Thorough documentation   c. Frequent education updates
   b. Following standards of care   d. Buying malpractice insurance

21. Patient confidentiality would be breached in most states if a paramedic discussed the patient's comments and care with:
   a. Lawyers in court
   b. Emergency department personnel
   c. Personal friends
   d. A quality-assurance committee

22. When a patient agrees verbally or in writing to treatment, it is known as:
   a. Expressed consent   **c.** Informed consent
   b. Implied consent   **d.** Referred consent
23. Which of the following should be included in the narrative portion of the patient care report?
   a. Care rendered   **c.** Physical findings
   b. History   **d.** All of the above

CHAPTER 4
EMS COMMUNICATIONS

● READING ASSIGNMENT
Chapter 4, pp. 30-43 in *Mosby's Paramedic Textbook*

● OBJECTIVES
As a paramedic, you should be able to:
1. Outline the chain of EMS communications.
2. Define common EMS communication terms.
3. Differentiate simple and complex communication systems.
4. Define the functions of key structural and equipment components in an EMS communication system.
5. Discuss how frequency selection influences radio coverage.
6. Describe the role of the Federal Communications Commission (FCC) in EMS communications.
7. Indicate measures for maintaining optimal function of communication equipment.
8. Describe the role of dispatching as it applies to prehospital emergency medical care.
9. Outline techniques for relaying EMS communications clearly and effectively.
10. List various types of documentation and record-keeping that may be required by an EMS agency.

● REVIEW QUESTIONS
Match the communication term in Column 2 with the appropriate definition in Column 1. Use each answer only once.

Column 1	Column 2
_____ 1. A unit of frequency equal to one cycle per second	**a.** Base station
_____ 2. The ability to transmit or receive in one direction at a time	**b.** Duplex
_____ 3. A grouping of radio equipment that includes a transmitter and receiver	**c.** Hertz
_____ 4. Radio frequencies between 300 and 3000 MHz	**d.** Kilohertz
_____ 5. The ability to transmit and receive simultaneously through two different frequencies	**e.** Megahertz
	f. Mobile station
_____ 6. A unit of frequency equal to 1,000,000 cycles per second	**g.** Remote console
_____ 7. Radio frequencies between 30 and 300 MHz	**h.** Repeater
_____ 8. A unit that receives transmissions from a mobile radio and retransmits them at higher power on another frequency	**i.** Simplex
	j. UHF
	k. VHF

9. A nonrepeater system would offer a greater advantage in a service area covering a large geographical area. True/false. If this statement is false, why is it false?

10. Satellite receivers are used to ensure that low-power units will always be within communication range. True/false. If this statement is false, why is it false?

_____

11. Dispatch services located away from base stations or hospital terminals that facilitate communications with field personnel and receive and display

    telemetry transmissions are known as_____.

12. The HEAR network uses a radio resembling a telephone dial or pad to receive radio transmissions. The unit that opens the audio circuits to receive on

    the HEAR system is a(n) _____.

13. List three common causes of interference with radio transmissions.
    a.
    b.
    c.

14. Identify three ways in which the Federal Communications Commission directly influences EMS.
    a.
    b.
    c.

15. Briefly describe four responsibilities of an EMS dispatcher.
    a.
    b.
    c.
    d.

16. *A man is seriously injured at a rural site.* Describe the communication process from the time of his injury until the EMS crew returns to service.

_____

_____

_____

_____

_____

17. List three essential pieces of information that the dispatcher must obtain from the bystander in the incident described in Question 16.
    a.
    b.
    c.

18. Describe six actions the paramedic may take that will ensure clear, understandable radio transmissions.
    a.
    b.
    c.

d.

e.

f.

Questions 19 and 20 pertain to the following case scenario: *Johnny Smith, a paramedic who works on City Unit 7, is called to an industrial site. He finds a 30-year-old patient lying on his back on the grass, where he landed after falling 20 feet from a painting platform. On arrival at 1:00 PM, the patient's vital signs are blood pressure 120/80, pulse 116, and respiration 20. He states he got dizzy and fell. The patient complains of pain in the lumbar region of the back and on both heels. Distal pulses, sensation, and movement are present in all extremities. Lung sounds are clear and equal bilaterally. He gives you his name and knows the date and time. His skin is warm and dry. The patient weighs approximately 100 kg and takes ibuprofen prescribed by Dr. Jones for back pain. You place him on 100% oxygen and on a backboard with cervical collar and notify Dr. Kane, the on-line medical physician, of the patient's condition and your 15-minute estimated arrival time to City Hospital. Vital signs at 1:25 PM are unchanged. The patient's condition remains the same en route.*

19. Write a concise, complete radio report to communicate the appropriate information regarding this patient to your base hospital.

_____

_____

_____

_____

_____

_____

_____

_____

_____

_____

_____

_____

20. Write a narrative documenting your findings on this patient as you would on your state patient care report.

_____

_____

_____

_____

_____

_____

_____

_____

_____

_____

_____

_____

_____

_____

● STUDENT SELF-EVALUATION

21. A radio receiver circuit used for suppressing the audio portion of unwanted radio noises or signals is the:
   a. Decibel
   b. Frequency modulation
   c. Squelch
   d. Tone

22. The number of repetitive cycles per second completed by a radio wave is the:
   a. Amplitude modulation
   b. Frequency
   c. Range
   d. Wattage

23. Transmission and reception of electrocardiograms over the radio or telephone is called:
   a. Coverage
   b. Hot line
   c. Patch
   d. Telemetry

24. Which of the following is a component of a simple communication system?
   a. Remote console
   b. Microwave links
   c. Mobile unit
   d. Satellite receivers

25. The HEAR and EACOM radios used to tie hospitals together and receive and transmit tone pulses are known as:
   a. Cellular telephones
   b. Decoders and encoders
   c. Microwave transmitters
   d. Satellite dishes

26. All of the following are responsibilities of the dispatcher, *except:*
   a. Dispatching EMS resources
   b. Coordinating with public safety
   c. Receiving calls for assistance
   d. Providing off-line medical control

27. If the respiratory rate section is left blank on the ambulance reporting form, it will be assumed that respirations were:
   a. Within normal limits for this patient age group
   b. Not specifically assessed by the paramedic
   c. Not pertinent in this patient situation
   d. Not an important vital sign assessment

RESCUE MANAGEMENT

● **READING ASSIGNMENT**

Chapter 5, pp. 44-53, in *Mosby's Paramedic Textbook*

● **OBJECTIVES**

As a paramedic, you should be able to:

1. Compare the various types of EMS rescue systems found throughout the United States.
2. Describe hazards that may be encountered during rescue situations.
3. List protective clothing and equipment that should be used by EMS personnel during rescue operations.
4. Describe adjuncts that may be used to ensure patient safety during rescue operations.
5. Identify fuel supply hazards.
6. Identify heat source hazards.
7. Discuss safe EMS approach and rescue techniques to be used when an electrical hazard exists.
8. List helpful equipment for vehicle stabilization during rescue operations.
9. Discuss the three elements of the assessment phase.
10. Given a patient care situation, describe the role of EMS in each phase of a rescue operation.

● **REVIEW QUESTIONS**

1. Fuel supply hazards include combustible solids, combustible gases, and chemicals. True/false. If this is false, why is it false?

_____

_____

2. Class ABC, all-purpose extinguishers can be used to suppress fires from combustible metals. True/false. If this is false, why is it false?

_____

_____

3. List the minimum protective clothing necessary for EMS personnel assisting with rescue operations as recommended by the National Institute of Occupational Safety and Health.

_____

_____

4. List six hazards that may be encountered when responding on rescue operations.

   a.
   b.
   c.
   d.
   e.
   f.

Questions 5 to 12 pertain to the following scenario: *You are called to the scene of a motor vehicle collision at a busy urban shopping center. On arrival at the scene, you find that a large sedan has hit the side of a compact car, wedging it between the sedan and a storefront. A large crowd of spectators has gathered and is impeding your access to the patient. No other equipment or law enforcement has been dispatched.*

5. List the three elements of the assessment phase as defined by the EMT-P National Standard Curriculum.

    a.

    b.

    c.

6. Describe how you will apply each of the three elements in Question 5 to this situation.

    a.

    b.

    c.

7. What steps should you take to gain control of the crowd?

_____

_____

_____

One patient was pulled from the sedan by bystanders before your arrival. He is pale and complaining of abdominal pain. Your partner begins care. A second patient in the compact car is unconscious. He is trapped and inaccessible.

8. List the additional equipment and assistance you should request at this time.

_____

A rescue truck arrives and breaks a window, which provides limited access to the patient while rescue operations proceed.

9. What can you do for your patient at this time?

_____

10. How can you ensure patient safety during the rescue?

_____

A brief primary survey reveals an unconscious patient with gurgling respirations and a strong radial pulse of 70 beats/min. There is a large ecchymotic area on the temporal region of the patient's head.

11. You have limited time and access to the patient. What are your first priorities of care?

_____

_____

12. Describe the disentanglement and packaging and removal segments of the rescue operation and your responsibilities to the patient during these phases.

_____

_____

_____

_____

_____

_____

_____

_____

13. Discuss safety measures that should be taken at the scene of an accident when there is an energized wire in contact with an involved auto for:
    a. The rescuers

_____

_____

    b. The persons trapped in the involved automobile

_____

_____

14. Give two examples of equipment that may be used to disentangle a person who is trapped inside a vehicle.
    a.
    b.

● STUDENT SELF-EVALUATION

15. Safety of the _____ should be the *first* priority at the scene of any rescue.
    a. Bystanders   c. Injured
    b. Crew   d. Trapped
16. According to OSHA standards, EMS rescue personnel should have access to all of the following personal protective equipment, *except:*
    a. Ear plugs   c. Rubber boots
    b. Protective helmet   d. Waterproof gloves
17. Ordinary combustible gases, liquids, solids, and chemicals are classified as:
    a. Combustion hazards   c. Heat source hazards
    b. Fuel supply hazards   d. Ignition source hazards
18. Which of the following energy sources can generate heat?
    a. Chemical   c. Mechanical
    b. Electrical   d. All of the above
19. To decrease the risk of fire at the scene of a motor vehicle collision in which gasoline is leaking, a paramedic should *always:*
    a. Disconnect the battery cable
    b. Douse the vehicle with foam
    c. Place a tarp over the spilled fuel
    d. Turn off the automobile ignition
20. Equipment that is helpful for vehicle stabilization during rescue includes:
    a. Chain saws   c. Hurst tools
    b. Cribbing   d. Pry bars

CHAPTER 6
MAJOR INCIDENT RESPONSE

● **READING ASSIGNMENT**

Chapter 6, pp. 54-65, in *Mosby's Paramedic Textbook*

● **OBJECTIVES**

As a paramedic, you should be able to:
1. Describe situations that may be classified as major incidents.
2. Describe how federal agencies and legislation have played a role in the development of the incident command system.
3. Define common terms of the incident command system.
4. Describe critical elements of the incident command system that must be incorporated in the preplanning process.
5. List command responsibilities during a major incident response.
6. Given a major incident, describe sectors that would need to be established and the responsibilities of each.
7. Describe how effective communications can be maintained during a major incident.
8. List common errors of incident command systems.
9. Outline two methods of patient categorization.
10. Describe the process for safely deploying air medical rescue.

● **REVIEW QUESTIONS**

Match the terms in Column 2 with their definitions in Column 1. Use each term only once.

Column 1	Column 2
_____ 1. Contracts agreeing to interagency exchange of resources when necessary	a. Apparatus
	b. Command
_____ 2. Pumpers, ladder trucks, rescue trucks	c. Command post
	d. Communication center
_____ 3. Rendezvous location for all arriving EMS fire and rescue equipment	e. Mutual aid
_____ 4. Responsible for coordination of major incident situation	f. Sector
	g. Staging area

5. A *major incident* is defined as any incident necessitating that additional equipment be brought in. True/false. If this is false, why is it false?

_____

_____

6. What four activities are essential during the preplanning phase of an incident command system to ensure success of the plan?
   a.
   b.
   c.
   d.

7. Identify three key components of the incident command system structure necessary for successful implementation of the plan.

   a.

   b.

   c.

8. List five special resources that may be necessary in a major incident.

   a.

   b.

   c.

   d.

   e.

9. Two systems are used to categorize patients at a mass casualty incident: METTAG cards and the START Field Guide. List the patient classifications for the METTAG system, beginning with the category that requires immediate care and ending with the category that is the last priority for care.

_____

_____

10. List the patient classifications for the START system.

_____

_____

Questions 11 to 15 pertain to the following scenario: *Dispatch radios your crew to respond to a local sports stadium for a bleacher collapse at a college football game. During your initial size-up, you determine that 50 to 100 people are injured, with a substantial number of victims still trapped under the fallen concrete seats. It is rush hour, and traffic conditions will be heavy for at least 2 more hours.*

11. How will command be determined?

_____

_____

12. List nine command responsibilities during this incident.

   a.

   b.

   c.

   d.

   e.

   f.

   g.

   h.

   i.

13. Briefly describe the responsibilities of each of the following sectors:

   a. Support:

_____

_____

   b. Staging:

_____

_____

  c. Extrication:

_____

_____

  d. Treatment:

_____

_____

  e. Transportation:

_____

_____

14. Explain how communications can be initiated in an effective manner in this situation.

_____

_____

_____

15. What special resources will be necessary during this incident?

_____

_____

16. Describe site selection and preparation for an air medical rescue.

_____

_____

_____

● STUDENT SELF-EVALUATION

17. Which of the following situations would be *least* likely to be declared a major incident?
  a. Rural EMS service, motor vehicle collision requiring four EMS units
  b. City EMS service, train derailment, possible hazardous materials leak
  c. Rural EMS service, two-patient incident with high-angle rescue
  d. City EMS service, two-person motor vehicle collision, no patient trapped

18. Which of the following agencies or associations was largely responsible for the development of the incident command system?
  a. Firefighting Resources of California for Potential Emergencies
  b. National Association of Emergency Medical Technicians
  c. National Fire Protection Association
  d. American College of Emergency Physicians

19. Except in unusual circumstances, patient care and stabilization should be provided by the _____ sector.
  a. Extrication   **c.** Treatment
  b. Support   **d.** Triage

20. The most appropriate *radio* communication during a mass casualty incident would be between:

  a. Command and sector officers
  b. Individuals within each sector
  c. Treatment sector and hospital
  d. Public information officer and press

21. Patient classification during mass casualty incidents should be based on:

  a. Physiological signs, mechanism of injury, and anatomical injury
  b. Mechanism of injury, anatomical injury, and patient age
  c. Chief complaint, physiological signs, and anatomical injury
  d. Physiological signs, anatomical injury, and concurrent disease

22. Your patient has a gunshot wound to the chest, is conscious, and has a respiratory rate of 36. Which of the following would be the appropriate triage category using the triage systems discussed in the text.

  a. Nonsalvageable or dead, yellow   **c.** Delayed, black
  b. Immediate, red   **d.** Immediate, green

23. When approaching the helicopter to load patients, which of the following safety measures should be used?

  a. The most people available should help to load.
  b. The aircraft should be approached from the rear.
  c. The aircraft should be approached in a crouched position.
  d. The paramedic should carry long objects vertically to maintain control.

HAZARDOUS MATERIALS

● **READING ASSIGNMENT**

Chapter 7, pp. 66-85, in *Mosby's Paramedic Textbook*

● **OBJECTIVES**

As a paramedic, you should be able to:

1. Define *hazardous materials.*
2. Identify major legislation regarding hazardous materials that influences emergency health care workers.
3. Describe informal and formal means of identifying hazardous materials.
4. List resources for identifying and managing hazardous materials situations.
5. Identify protective clothing and equipment necessary for rescuers responding to various hazardous materials incidents.
6. Describe potential internal damage caused by exposure to hazardous materials.
7. Describe symptoms of exposure to hazardous materials that require intervention.
8. Recognize external symptoms that may present after exposure to corrosive hazardous materials.
9. Outline management techniques for external exposure to corrosive hazardous materials.
10. Describe how radiation causes its harmful effects.
11. Describe emergency care for victims of radiation exposure.
12. Outline the response to a hazardous materials emergency.
13. Describe the three safety zones for a hazardous materials response.
14. Discuss the paramedic's role in medical monitoring at a hazardous materials incident.
15. Describe the emergency management of patients who have been contaminated with hazardous materials.

● **REVIEW QUESTIONS**

Match each of the hazardous chemicals listed in Column 1 with *all* of the health hazards in Column 2 that they pose. You may use answers more than once.

Column 1	Column 2
_____ 1. Arsenic	a. Asphyxiant
	b. Anesthetic
_____ 2. Halogenated hydrocarbons	c. Carcinogen
	d. Cardiotoxin
_____ 3. Hydrochloric acid	e. Hemotoxin
	f. Hepatotoxin
_____ 4. Hydrogen cyanide	g. Irritant
	h. Nephrotoxin
_____ 5. Lead	i. Nerve poison
	j. Neurotoxin
_____ 6. Malathion	
_____ 7. Mercury	

8. Hazardous materials are substances and materials capable of posing an unreasonable risk to health, safety, and property. True/False. If this is false, why is it false?

_____

_____

9. Hazardous materials are encountered primarily in industrial settings. True/False. If this is false, why is it false?

_____

_____

10. The legislation that established requirements for federal, state, and local governments and industry regarding emergency planning and the reporting

of hazardous materials in 1986 was known as _____.

11. Briefly describe each of the five categories of emergency response personnel who may respond to a hazardous materials situation:
   a. First responder awareness:

_____

_____

   b. First responder operations:

_____

_____

   c. Hazardous material technician:

_____

_____

   d. Hazardous material specialist:

_____

_____

   e. On-scene incident commander:

_____

12. *You arrive on the scene of a motor vehicle collision involving an overturned tanker truck. You note a cloud of white vapor escaping from a relief valve on top of the truck.* Describe the formal and informal means of identifying hazardous materials that may be involved in this situation.
   a. Formal:

_____

_____

   b. Informal:

_____

13. After a hazardous material has been identified, what other resources can help the emergency response crew in determining hazards and management of the scene?

_____

_____

14. Describe the protective clothing that will be necessary in the following hazardous materials response situations:

   a. *The hazardous materials crew provides emergency care to a seriously injured worker who is lying in an area contaminated with a liquid acidic chemical. There is no contaminated gas present from the spill.*

   _____

   b. *Your fire rescue team must enter a burning building to extricate trapped victims. No known hazardous materials are reported on the scene.*

   _____

   _____

   c. *An equipment malfunction inside a chemical manufacturing plant has resulted in the release of toxic gases. Hazardous materials specialists must enter to attempt to locate a victim known to be just inside the hot zone.*

   _____

   _____

15. Describe the health problems that can be encountered when an individual sustains exposure to the following agents:

   a. Irritants:

   _____

   b. Asphyxiants:

   _____

   c. Nerve poisons, anesthetics, and narcotics:

   _____

   d. Hepatotoxins:

   _____

   e. Cardiotoxins:

   _____

   f. Neurotoxins:

   _____

   g. Hemotoxins:

   _____

   h. Carcinogens:

   _____

16. *You respond to the scene of a fire in which hazardous materials of unknown origin are involved.* Describe the signs and symptoms that scene workers may exhibit, causing you to suspect exposure to hazardous materials.

_____

17. External exposure to corrosive chemicals will generally cause _____.

18. *Your crew arrives at an industrial chemical manufacturing plant where a worker has sustained a splash exposure of a corrosive chemical to the eyes.* Describe patient management in this situation.

_____

_____

19. Describe the characteristics of the following three types of radiation particles:
    a. Alpha:

_____

_____

    b. Beta:

_____

_____

    c. Gamma:

_____

_____

20. What effects can be expected at the following levels of radiation exposure?
    a. Less than 100 rem:

_____

    b. 100 to 200 rem:

_____

    c. Greater than 450 rem:

_____

Questions 21 to 23 pertain to the following scenario: *You arrive at the scene of a clinical laboratory, where it has been reported that a significant amount of radioactive material was released when a worker fell 15 feet from a platform.*

21. Describe your approach to the emergency scene.

_____

_____

_____

22. It has been determined that the victim must be accessed. Describe how radiation exposure can be minimized to the crew designated to perform the rescue.

_____

23. Describe any special measures that you should use in the care of this victim after access has been obtained.

_____

_____

_____

24. Label Fig. 7-1 and briefly describe each of the three safety zones for a hazardous materials situation response that has been established by hazardous materials specialists.

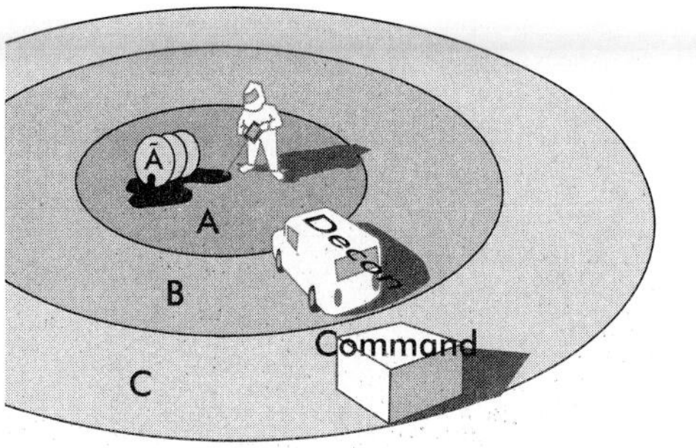

Figure 7-1

a.

_____

b.

_____

c.

_____

Questions 25 to 27 pertain to the following scenario: _You are the first team dispatched to the scene of a train derailment where there are three victims still trapped. The bystanders who called in the incident report that placards indicating the presence of hazardous materials are present on several of the involved train cars._

25. Describe any actions you should take during your initial response to this situation.

_____

_____

_____

_____

_____

_____

26. Describe special considerations in the prehospital management of contaminated patients.

_____

_____

_____

_____

_____

27. The incident commander on this scene delegates your EMS crew to establish a medical monitoring station. Describe the responsibilities of this role.

_____

_____

_____

● STUDENT SELF-EVALUATION

28. A hazardous material is any substance or material capable of:
  a. Posing an unreasonable risk to health, safety, and property
  b. Causing corrosive damage to humans when skin is exposed
  c. Initiating a mass casualty incident when an accident occurs
  d. Exploding when in the presence of an ignition source

29. The five categories of individuals who may respond to an emergency involving hazardous materials according to the HAZWOPER rules include all of the following, _except:_
  a. First responder operations   **c.** Hazardous material specialist
  b. Hazardous material technician   **d.** Rescue operation technician

30. Which of the following is a formal means of identifying hazardous products?
  a. Container characteristics   **c.** Patient signs and symptoms
  b. Incident location   **d.** United Nations Labeling System

31. Which agency requires Material Safety Data Sheets when chemicals are stored, handled, or used in the workplace?
  a. International Air Transport Association
  b. National Fire Protection Association
  c. U.S. Department of Labor
  d. U.S. Department of Transportation

32. Which of the following signs or symptoms should prompt a rescuer to seek immediate medical attention at the site of a hazardous materials incident?
  a. Confusion and lightheadedness   **d.** Nausea and vomiting
  b. Shortness of breath and coughing   **e.** All of the above
  c. Tingling of the extremities

33. When responding to the scene of a hazardous material incident, the EMS crew should approach from:
  a. Downhill and downwind   **c.** Uphill and downwind
  b. Downhill and upwind   **d.** Uphill and upwind

34. The "pre-suit" medical monitoring of an individual who will be entering a hazardous material situation should include all of the following, _except:_
  a. Cardiac rhythm   **c.** Temperature
  b. Reflexes   **d.** Weight

35. General recommendations for emergency management of contaminated patients include all of the following, *except:*
    a. Emergency patient care overrides all safety considerations.
    b. All patients in the hot zone are considered contaminated.
    c. Intravenous therapy should be initiated only with a physician's order.
    d. The patient's clothing should be completely cut off.
36. If a rescue must be made in an area with possible radioactive contamination, risk to the rescuers can be minimized by:
    a. Having one rescuer remain with the patient at all times
    b. Rendering patient care from behind the radioactive source
    c. Placing a face mask on the contaminated patient
    d. Waiting behind a concrete wall between rescue attempts

CHAPTER 8
STRESS MANAGEMENT

● READING ASSIGNMENT
Chapter 8, pp. 86-97, in *Mosby's Paramedic Textbook*

● OBJECTIVES
As a paramedic, you should be able to:
1. Define *stress* and outline the three phases of the stress response.
2. Define *anxiety.*
3. Differentiate between normal and detrimental reactions to anxiety and stress.
4. Describe the paramedic's management of patients, family members, and by-standers who are encountering a stressful situation.
5. List situations that may provoke job stress for the paramedic.
6. List stress-management techniques.
7. Identify various defense mechanisms.
8. Recognize the five stages of grief that a patient or significant other may experience during death or dying, as described by Dr. Elizabeth Kübler-Ross.
9. Describe appropriate ways to help the patient, family, or significant other deal with a situation in which death is imminent or has occurred.
10. Describe the special needs of children related to their understanding of death and dying.

● REVIEW QUESTIONS
Match the defense mechanism in Column 2 with its appropriate example in Column 1. Use each defense mechanism only once.

Column 1	Column 2
_____ 1. A rape victim who cannot recall anything from the time she was abducted until the police find her	a. Compensation
	b. Denial
	c. Isolation
_____ 2. A paramedic who, when passed over for a promotion, states that the boss always plays favorites	d. Projection
	e. Rationalization
	f. Reaction formation
_____ 3. A paramedic who is upset by a violent death and washes all of the vehicles in the garage	g. Regression
	h. Repression
	i. Substitution
_____ 4. An automobile accident victim refuses to acknowledge that he cannot move his legs	
_____ 5. An EMT who complains about the poor care that a patient received at a hospital when his own care was inadequate	
_____ 6. A 10-year-old who begins to suck his thumb en route to the hospital after sustaining a fracture from a fall	

7. Anxiety is always a negative response. True/false. If this is false, why is it false?

_____

_____

8. A preschooler does not understand that death is permanent and irreversible. True/false. If this is false, why is it false?

_____

9. Define *stress.*

_____

_____

10. List five causes of stress that are job-related and non-job-related
    a. Job-related stress:

_____

_____

    b. Non-job-related stress:

_____

_____

11. Briefly explain how each of the areas of the body labeled in Fig. 8-1 respond to stress during the alarm reaction.

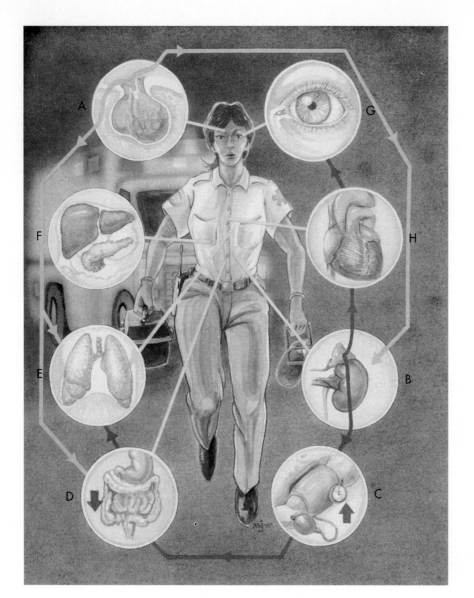

Figure 8-1

a.

b.

c.

d.

e.

f.

g.

_____

h.

_____

12. List four potential symptoms of decompensation from the effects of stress.
    a.
    b.
    c.
    d.

13. Name five effective stress-management techniques that can minimize the effects of EMS job-related stress.
    a.
    b.
    c.
    d.
    e.

14. Describe five services that can be provided by a critical incident stress debriefing team.
    a.
    b.
    c.
    d.
    e.

15. List the five stages of death and dying as identified by Elizabeth Kübler-Ross.
    a.
    b.
    c.
    d.
    e.

Questions 16 and 17 pertain to the following case scenario: _You arrive at a family gathering where you find a 46-year-old man in full cardiopulmonary arrest. His mother is crying and begging, "Please, Lord, don't take him, take me." His wife is distraught, pacing and saying, "It's going to be OK; it's not as bad as it seems." The brother yells at you as you enter, "What took you so long? Hurry up. What are you waiting for?"_

16. Identify which of the stages of grief listed in Question 15 each family member is exhibiting.
    a. Mother:
    b. Wife:
    c. Brother:

17. How should you deal with the family members?

_____

_____

_____

18. How can EMS personnel deal with the pent-up emotions they must suppress while caring for dying patients?

_____

_____

19. *You are called to a scene to take over care from a rescue unit. You immediately recognize the paramedic who is caring for the patient as an individual who you consistently disagree with over patient care issues.* What type of stress is this call likely to produce?
    a. Environmental
    c. Personality
    b. Managerial
    d. Psychosocial

20. Generalized feelings of apprehension are known as:
    a. Anxiety
    c. Reaction formation
    b. Phobias
    d. Stress

21. All of the following are physical effects that may accompany chronic anxiety, *except:*
    a. Dry mouth
    c. Hypoglycemia
    b. Gastric upset
    d. Palpitations

22. All of the following are measures that can effectively decrease work-related stress for the paramedic, *except:*
    a. A few drinks to unwind after every shift
    b. Proper diet, sleep, and rest
    c. Pursuing a hobby outside the field of EMS
    d. Frequent age-appropriate exercise

23. Critical incident stress debriefing is most helpful for:
    a. New employees after every critical patient situation
    b. Selected high-risk employees with psychological problems
    c. Mass casualty incidents involving more than 10 patients
    d. Situations in which a high degree of stress is perceived

24. A paramedic student has just failed his practical examination station because of improper airway-management technique and states, "Well, I would have done it, but we never practiced it in class this way." This is an example of which defense mechanism?
    a. Projection
    c. Regression
    b. Rationalization
    d. Sublimation

25. When dealing with the family of a patient who is dying, the paramedic can best interact with them by:
    a. Reassuring them that no one you ever care for dies
    b. Changing the subject every time someone brings up death
    c. Allowing the family to remain with the patient if possible
    d. Avoiding direct communication with the immediate family

26. School-age children (7 to 12 years) feel that death:
    a. Is temporary and reversible
    b. Happens to others, not themselves
    c. Is punishment for their bad thoughts
    d. Is the same as severe illness

DIVISION ONE REVIEW TEST

1. At which of the following nationally recognized levels of EMT licensure is the emergency medical technician responsible for administration of a large number of emergency drugs?
   a. EMT-B
   b. EMT-D
   c. EMT-I
   d. EMT-P

2. Which of the following patients will benefit most from rapid transportation to a receiving hospital rather than prolonged care on the scene of the emergency by a paramedic?
   a. A shooting victim who is bleeding profusely from the chest
   b. A psychiatric patient who is paranoid and frightened
   c. A person in cardiac arrest with good citizen cardiopulmonary resuscitation
   d. A patient who is experiencing wheezing after a sting

3. Training, skill evaluation, and the development of protocols for prehospital services are known as _____ medical direction.
   a. Direct
   b. Indirect
   c. Off-line
   d. On-line

4. Which of the following are elements necessary to prove negligence?
   a. Duty to act, criminal intent, and damage to the patient
   b. Breach of statute, duty to act, and breach of duty
   c. Duty to act, criminal intent, and breach of duty
   d. Duty to act, breach of duty, and damage to the patient

5. A paramedic who forcibly restrains and transports an alert competent patient against his or her will may be guilty of:
   a. Assault
   b. Battery
   c. False imprisonment
   d. All of the above

6. All of the following are reportable patient situations by prehospital personnel, *except:*
   a. Animal bites
   b. Gunshot wounds
   c. Home births
   d. Rape

7. Which of the following statements is true regarding refusal of care if the patient is mentally competent?
   a. It must be written and signed by the patient.
   b. Care may not be refused if a threat to life exists.
   c. Patient should be given no follow-up instructions.
   d. Witnesses should be present and documented.

8. An assigned frequency or pair of frequencies used to carry voice and/or data communications is a:
   a. Channel
   b. Carrier
   c. Dedicated line
   d. Transceiver

9. Radio communications in the United States are regulated by the:
   a. CDC
   b. DEA
   c. FCC
   d. FDA

10. Which of the following pieces of information should routinely be transmitted in a patient radio report?
    a. Patient's name
    b. All past medical history
    c. Complete secondary survey
    d. Chief complaint

11. A portable fire extinguisher that is effective in putting out a fire caused by energized electrical equipment is a class _____ .
    a. A
    b. B
    c. C
    d. E

12. The best time for EMS personnel to approach a patient who is in contact with an electrical current is:
    a. When power is disconnected
    b. When wearing rubberized shoes
    c. When rubber gloves are available
    d. When the patient stops convulsing

13. The area designated for arriving equipment at a mass casualty incident is known as the _____ area.
    a. Command   c. Staging
    b. Mutual aid   d. Transportation

14. A major incident should be declared by:
    a. The highest seniority individual on duty that day
    b. The law enforcement officer with highest rank
    c. The chairperson of the incident command committee
    d. The first crew arriving on the scene of the incident

15. Command has all of the following responsibilities during a mass casualty situation *except:*
    a. Triaging patients   c. Evaluating effectiveness
    b. Assigning sectors   d. Requesting additional resources

16. With regard to helicopter landing site preparation during an emergency, which of the following is *false?*
    a. Flares should be used to light the landing zone at night.
    b. Daytime landing zones should be at least 60 feet by 60 feet.
    c. The area should be flat and free of high grass.
    d. Spotlights should be directed away from the aircraft.

17. *A rescue crew is sent to the scene of a tanker accident at which a large amount of liquid chemical has spilled on the roadway. There is no imminent fire hazard.* What would be the most appropriate gear for rescuers to wear to remove the trucker who has been thrown from the vehicle?
    a. Chemical protective clothing
    b. High-temperature protective clothing
    c. Proximity suits
    d. Structural firefighting clothing

18. Chemical asphyxiants interrupt transport or use of oxygen by the cells and include all of the following, *except:*
    a. Carbon monoxide   c. Hydrogen sulfide
    b. Hydrogen cyanide   d. Mercury

19. Hepatotoxins are substances that cause damage to the:
    a. Brain   c. Liver
    b. Kidneys   d. Lungs

20. The proper emergency management of external contamination by an unknown caustic agent would be to:
    a. Neutralize the substance immediately to reduce pain.
    b. Brush the substance off and flush with large amounts of water.
    c. Brush the substance off and wait for positive identification.
    d. Apply a moist dressing to prevent exposure to the air.

21. The area of a hazardous materials incident that contains the command post and is usually considered "safe," requiring only minimal protective clothing, is the _____ zone:
    a. Hot   c. Cold
    b. Warm   d. Frozen

22. Which physical manifestation occurs because of the "fight-or-flight" response to an alarm reaction?
    a. Decreased pulse   c. Increased digestive rate
    b. Increased blood pressure d. Pupil constriction

23. *Family members are anxiously pacing and crying as you care for a critically ill older patient.* You can best help these people by:
    a. Calmly explaining patient care and giving directions
    b. Allowing them to choose from 10 hospital destinations
    c. Actively involving them in complex patient care efforts
    d. Forcibly removing them from the scene immediately
24. All of the following are stages of death and dying as described by Dr. Elizabeth Kübler-Ross, *except:*
    a. Anger   c. Denial
    b. Acceptance   d. Grief

DIVISION TWO
PREPARATORY

CHAPTER 9
MEDICAL TERMINOLOGY AND THE METRIC SYSTEM

● **READING ASSIGNMENT**

Chapter 9, pp. 100-107, in *Mosby's Paramedic Textbook*

● **OBJECTIVES**

As a paramedic, you should be able to:
1. Describe the purpose of medical terminology.
2. Identify the function of prefixes, suffixes, and root words as they pertain to medical terminology.
3. Apply and interpret medical terminology based on an understanding of a given list of prefixes, suffixes, and root words.
4. Appropriately document information using accepted medical abbreviations.
5. Document with the metric system, using the current notation and units for a given measurement.

● **REVIEW QUESTIONS**

Match the medical terms in Column 2 with the appropriate description in Column 1. Use each term only once.

Column 1	Column 2
_____ 1. Drainage from the ear	a. Adenomegaly
	b. Arthralgia
_____ 2. Pain in the joints	c. Gastroenteritis
	d. Otorrhea
_____ 3. Inflammation of the stomach and intestines	e. Osteomyopathy
_____ 4. Enlargement of a gland	f. Nephrostomy
	g. Neuroma
_____ 5. Tumor of a nerve	h. Hepatitis
_____ 6. Inflammation of the liver	
_____ 7. Opening into the kidney	
_____ 8. Disease of the muscle and bone	

9. Give the root syllable for each of the words in Column 2 of Questions 1 to 8.
   a.
   b.
   c.
   d.
   e.

f.

g.

h.

10. Medical terminology is only useful when communicating with physicians. True/false. If this is false, why is it false?

_____

11. Prefixes in medical terminology often describe location and intensity. True/false. If this is false, why is it false?

_____

12. Rewrite the following paragraph using the appropriate medical terminology for the boldface words or phrases: You are called to evaluate a patient who is **not breathing** and has a **slow heart rate.** You note a **bluish discoloration** of his skin. His family states he had **difficulty breathing,** complained of **loss of sensation** of his right arm, became **unable to speak,** and then **fainted.** His past medical history includes **stroke, heart enlargement,** and **hardening of the arteries.** Home medicines include **drugs to decrease high blood pressure, prevent bad heart rhythms,** and **thin the blood.** Physical examination reveals **paralysis of the right side of the body, high blood pressure,** and **one-sided** facial droop. There is no evidence of **fluid flowing from the ears** or **fluid flowing from the nose.**

_____

_____

_____

_____

_____

_____

_____

_____

_____

_____

_____

_____

13. Rewrite the following paragraph using as many accepted medical abbreviations as possible: *The 78-year-old patient was admitted immediately to intensive care to rule out myocardial infarction. Her chief complaint was shortness of breath. Vital signs were within normal limits except for a blood pressure of 200/100. In the emergency department, she was given nitroglycerin 0.4 milligrams sublingually and*

morphine sulfate two milligrams intravenously. Her past medical history included lung cancer, coronary artery disease, stroke, congestive heart failure, and alcohol abuse.

_____

_____

_____

_____

● STUDENT SELF-EVALUATION

14. The syllable in a medical term that follows the root word and describes the patient's condition or diagnosis is the:
   a. Body   **c.** Suffix
   b. Prefix   **d.** Term

15. The root word *cyto-* means:
   a. Bladder   **c.** Chest
   b. Cell   **d.** Eye

16. Basic units of measurement for the metric system include all of the following, *except:*
   a. Cube   **c.** Liter
   b. Gram   **d.** Meter

17. Pupil size should be documented in:
   a. Millicubics   **c.** Milliliters
   b. Milligrams   **d.** Millimeters

18. Which of the following represents the proper format for metric notation?
   a. 0.75 mg   **c.** .75mg
   b. .75 mg   **d.** 0.75 Mg

19. 10 millimeters equals _____ centimeter(s).
   a. 0.01   **c.** 1
   b. 0.1   **d.** 10

OVERVIEW OF HUMAN SYSTEMS

● **READING ASSIGNMENT**

Chapter 10, pp. 108-179, in *Mosby's Paramedic Textbook*

● **OBJECTIVES**

As a paramedic, you should be able to:

1. Discuss the importance of human anatomy as it relates to the paramedic profession.
2. Describe the anatomical position.
3. Properly interpret anatomical directional terms and body planes.
4. List the structures that compose the axial and appendicular regions of the body.
5. Define the divisions of the abdominal region.
6. List the three major body cavities.
7. Describe the contents of the three major body cavities.
8. Discuss the functions of the cytoplasmic membrane, cytoplasm (and its organelles), and nucleus.
9. Describe the process by which human cells reproduce.
10. Differentiate and describe epithelial, connective, muscle, and nervous tissues.
11. For each of the 11 major organ systems in the human body, label a diagram of anatomical structures, list the functions of the major anatomic structures, and explain how the organs of the system interrelate to perform the specified functions of the system.
12. For the special senses, label a diagram of the anatomical structures of the special senses, list the functions of the anatomical structures of each sense, and explain how the structures of the sense interrelate to perform its specified functions.

● **REVIEW QUESTIONS**

Match the cellular structure from Column 2 with its definition in Column 1. Use each answer only once.

Column 1	Column 2
_____ 1. Cytoplasmic "canals" that transport proteins and other substances	a. Centrioles
_____ 2. Phospholipid layer that forms the outer boundary of the cell	b. Cytoplasm
_____ 3. Organelles that contain enzymes capable of digesting proteins and lipids	c. Cytoplasmic membrane
_____ 4. Mass of cell that lies between the cytoplasmic membrane and nucleus	d. Endoplasmic reticulum
_____ 5. Sacs that package materials for secretion from the cell	e. Golgi apparatus
_____ 6. Control center of the cell that contains genetic material	f. Lysosomes
_____ 7. Structures that are composed of ribonucleic acid and protein and that manufacture enzymes	g. Mitochondria
	h. Nucleus
	i. Ribosomes

_____ **8.** Powerhouse of the cell, responsible for
production of adenosine triphosphate

9. All human cells divide by the process of mitosis throughout the life of a human organism. True/False. If this is false, explain why it is false.

10. The only bone in the human body that does not connect to another bone is the hyoid bone. True/False. If this is false, explain why it is false.

11. Describe the anatomical position.

12. Circle the appropriate directional terms in boldface in the following sentences.
   a. The wrist lies **distal/proximal** to the elbow.
   b. The right nipple is located **medial/lateral** to the sternum.
   c. The cervical spine is **superior/inferior** to the lumbar spine.
   d. The umbilicus is located on the **dorsal/ventral** surface of the body.

13. List the structures that compose:
   a. The appendicular region of the body:

   b. The axial region of the body:

14. Name the anatomical landmarks that divide the abdomen into four quadrants.

15. For each of the following subgroups of tissues, list the tissue type to which it belongs (epithelial, connective, muscle, or nervous), one area of the body where it is found, and at least one specialized function it performs.

Subgroup	Type	Body Area	Function
a. Striated voluntary			
b. Bone			
c. Epithelium			
d. Adipose			
e. Hemopoietic			
f. Striated involuntary			
g. Neurons			
h. Cartilage			
i. Areolar			
j. Nonstriated involuntary			
k. Neuroglia			

16. List the 11 major body systems:

    a.

    b.

    c.

    d.

    e.

    f.

    g.

    h.

    i.

    j.

    k.

17. Label structures of the skin in Fig. 10-1 and list two functions of each.

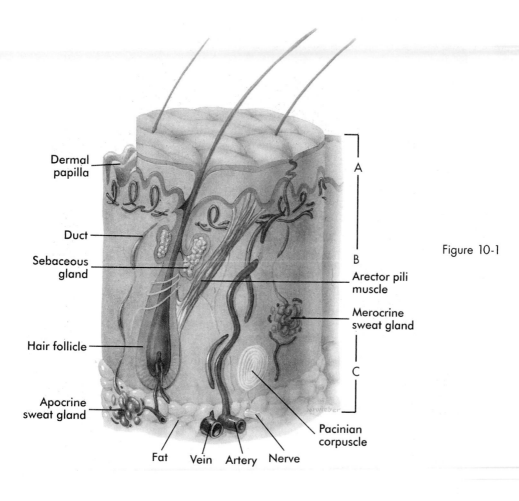

Figure 10-1

	Structure	Functions
a.		
b.		
c.		

18. List three functions of the glands located in the skin.

a.

b.

c.

19. Describe what effect a large third-degree burn that destroys all of the layers of the dermis will have on the skin's function.

20. Label the bones of the human skull in Fig. 10-2.

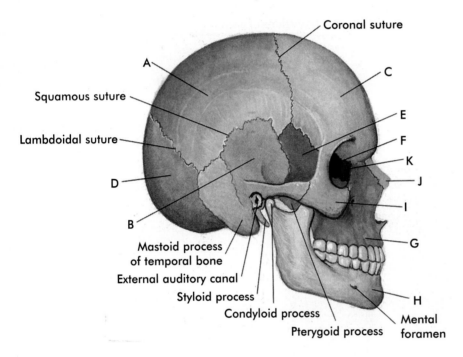

Figure 10-2

a.

b.

c.

d.

e.

f.

g.

h.

i.

j.

k.

21. Label the bony regions of the vertebral column shown in Fig. 10-3 and indicate the number of vertebrae in each region.

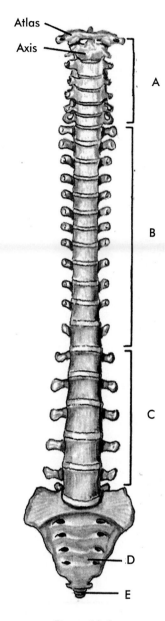

Atlas

Axis

A

B

C

D

E

Figure 10-3

Region	Number
a.	
b.	
c.	
d.	
e.	

22. List two functions of the thoracic cage.
a.
b.

23. Label the structures of the thoracic cage shown in Fig. 10-4.

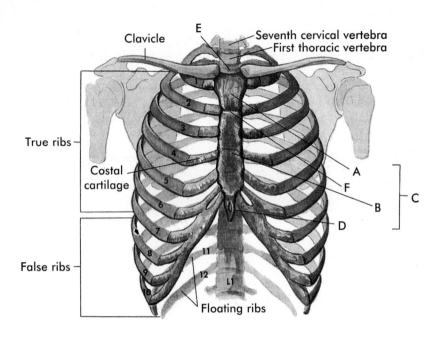

Figure 10-4

a.

b.

c.

d.

e.

f.

24. What problems can occur when a patient sustains a traumatic injury that results in a fractured sternum and multiple fractured ribs?

_____

25. Complete the following sentences that relate to the skeletal system: The pectoral girdle is composed of the (a) _____ and (b)

_____. Its function is to (c)_____

_____.

The point of attachment of the appendicular and axial skeleton occurs at

the (d) _____ joint.

26. Label the diagram of the upper extremity shown in Fig. 10-5.

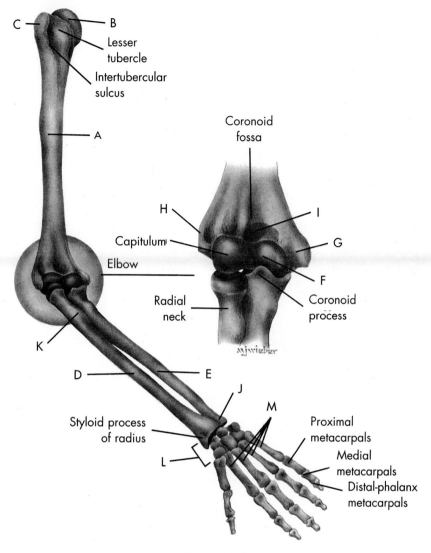

Lesser tubercle

Intertubercular sulcus

Coronoid fossa

Capitulum

Elbow

Radial neck

Coronoid process

Styloid process of radius

Proximal metacarpals

Medial metacarpals

Distal-phalanx metacarpals

Figure 10-5

a.

b.

c.

d.

e.

f.

g.

h.

i.

j.

k.

l.

m.

27. Label Fig. 10-6 of the pelvic girdle.

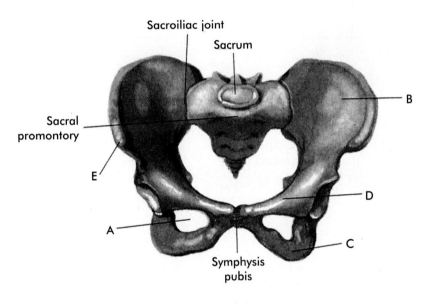

Figure 10-6

a.

b.

c.

d.

e.

28. What are the functions of the pelvic girdle?

29. Label the bones of the lower extremity shown in Fig. 10-7.

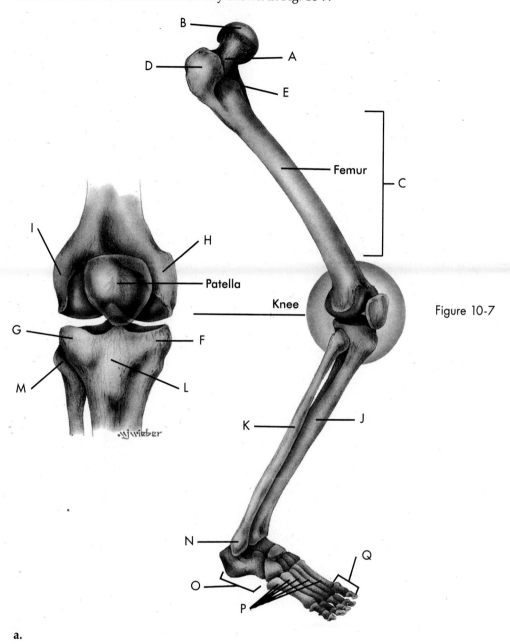

B

A

D

E

Femur

C

I

H

Patella

Knee

Figure 10-7

G

F

M

L

K

J

N

Q

O

P

a.
b.
c.
d.
e.
f.
g.
h.
i.
j.
k.
l.
m.
n.
o.
p.
q.

30. Complete the blanks in the following statements regarding joints: The three major classifications of joints are (a) _____,

_____, and _____. Fibrous

joints have (b) _____ movement. Fibrous joints can

be further divided into sutures found in the (c) _____,

syndesmoses found between the (d) _____ and

_____, and a gomphoses joint, which consists of a

peg in a socket such as the joints between (e) _____

and _____. A synchondroses is a cartilaginous joint
that allows only slight movement and can be found in the chest between the

ribs and the (f) _____. Symphysis joints are another
example of cartilaginous joints and can be found in the chest at the (g)

_____ _____, in the pelvis at

the (h) _____ _____, and in the

spine at the (i) _____ _____.
Synovial joints are classified into six divisions, all of which contain (j)

_____ _____. Joints consisting
of two opposed, flat surfaces, such as the articular processes between

vertebrae, are (k) _____ joints. Joints that consist of
two saddle-shaped, articulating surfaces that allow movement in two
planes and include the carpometacarpal joint in the thumb are (l)

_____ _____. Joints that con-
sist of a convex cylinder of bone that fits into a corresponding concavity in
another bone and permit movement in one plane, such as the elbow and

knee, are known as (m) _____ joints. A cylindrical
bony process that rotates within a ring composed of bone and ligament, such
as the head of the radius where it articulates with the ulna, is a(n)

(n) _____ joint. A wide range of motion is permitted
by shoulder and hip joints, where the head of one bone fits into the socket

of an adjacent bone. These are known as (o) _____

_____ _____ joints. The atlanto-
occipital joint is an example of a modified ball-and-socket joint known as

a(n) (p) _____ joint.

31. Replace the boldface words in the following sentences with the correct terms from the following list. Use each term only once.

Abduction	Excursion	Opposition
Adduction	Extension	Pronation
Depression	Flexion	Rotation
Eversion	Inversion	Supination

  a. The patient has sustained an injury to his elbow and is unable to **rotate his forearm so that the anterior surface is up** or **rotate his forearm so that the anterior surface is down.**_____

  b. To determine whether the patient had an intact neurological function, the paramedic had her **move her thumb and little finger toward each other.**

  c. After he injured his knee, the soccer player had pain when he **bent** and **stretched out** his lower leg._____

  d. An older woman with a hip fracture has a leg that looks shortened and shows external **movement about its axis.** _____

  e. A person with a shoulder separation has a limited ability to **move the arm away from the midline.** _____

  f. The patient with a posterior hip dislocation has the following physical findings: the leg is shortened, internally rotated, and slightly **moved toward the midline.**_____

  g. Ankle sprains are frequently produced by **turning the ankle inward or turning the ankle outward.** _____

  h. Newer splints for the foot can sometimes make casting unnecessary when the desired effect is to prevent **movement from side to side.** _____

  _____

  i. The blow to the head with a baseball bat produced **movement of the temporal bone in an inferior direction.** _____

32. List the three primary functions of the muscular system.

  a.

  b.

  c.

33. Complete the following sentences pertaining to the muscular system: The specialized contractile cells of the muscles are called (a)

_____ _____ . Each muscle fiber is filled with thick and thin threadlike structures known as (b)

_____ . These are composed of the proteins

(c) _____ and _____ . The con-

tractile unit of skeletal muscle fibers is the (d) _____ . During muscle contraction, the two myofilaments slide toward each other and shorten the sarcomere fueled with energy from (e)

_____ .

34. Define the following terms:
  a. Isometric muscle contraction:

_____

  b. Isotonic muscle contraction:

_____

  c. Muscle tone:

_____

35. Describe the role that the muscular system plays in maintaining body temperature.

_____

_____

36. Briefly describe the function of the nervous system.

_____

37. List the primary components of:
   a. The central nervous system:

_____

   b. The peripheral nervous system:

_____

38. List the two subdivisions of the efferent division of the nervous system and briefly describe the function of each.
   a.

_____

   b.

_____

39. Label Fig. 10-8 of the brain.

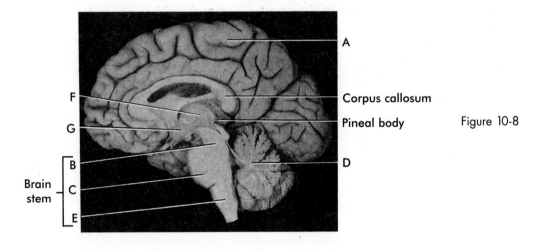

Corpus callosum

Pineal body   Figure 10-8

Brain stem

Figure 10-8

   a.
   b.
   c.
   d.
   e.
   f.
   g.

40. Briefly describe the functions of each of the following components of the brain stem:
   a. Medulla:

_____

   b. Pons:

_____

c. Midbrain:

d. Reticular formation:

e. Hypothalamus:

f. Thalamus:

41. Label Fig. 10-9 of the cerebrum and list one important function of each area.

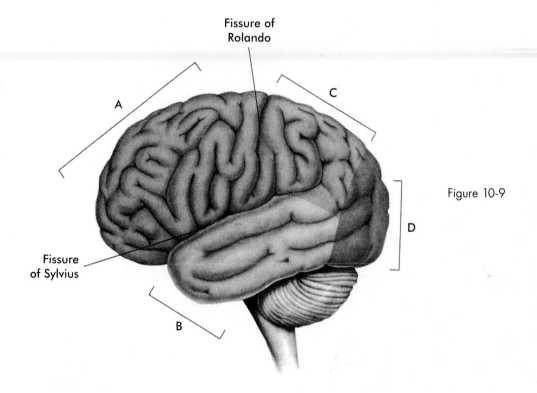

Fissure of Rolando

A

C

Figure 10-9

D

Fissure of Sylvius

B

Area	Function
a.	
b.	
c.	
d.	

42. Briefly describe the major functions of the cerebellum.

43. List two functions of the spinal cord.

a.

b.

44. Complete the following sentences about the meninges: Cerebrospinal

fluid bathes and cushions the (a) _____ and

_____. It is formed in a network of brain capillaries

known as the (b) _____ _____.

45. List the three functional categories of the 12 cranial nerves.

a.

b.

c.

46. For each of the following organs or body systems describe the effects of stimulation by each division of the autonomic nervous system.

Affected Organ	Sympathetic	Parasympathetic
Heart		
Lungs		
Pupils		
Intestine		
Blood vessels		

47. Describe the function of the endocrine system.

_____

_____

48. For each of the following hormones, list the primary target tissue and one action the hormone may have on that tissue.

Hormone	Target	Action
a. Epinephrine		
b. Aldosterone		
c. Antidiuretic		
d. Parathyroid		
e. Calcitonin		
f. Insulin		
g. Glucagon		
h. Testosterone		
i. Thymosin		
j. Oxytocin		
k. Thyroid		

49. Describe how hormones reach their target tissues.

_____

_____

50. List five functions of the circulatory system.

a.

b.

c.

d.

e.

51. Complete the following sentences regarding the components of blood: About 95% of the formed elements in blood are red blood cells, also known

as (a) _____. The primary component of red blood

cells is (b) _____. This gives blood its red color and

allows it to transport (c) _____ from the lungs to the

tissues and to transport (d)_____ _____
from the tissues to the lungs. The remaining 5% of the formed elements in

blood consists of white blood cells called (e) (_____)

and platelets known as (f) (_____). The primary func-

tion of white blood cells is (g) _____. Platelets help

prevent blood loss by activating the formation of (h) _____
to seal off wounds in the blood vessels. The pale yellow fluid that surrounds

these formed elements is (i) _____.

52. Label the structures indicated on Fig. 10-10 of the heart and draw arrows to show the path taken by the blood from the point that it enters the heart from the body until it returns to the body from the heart.

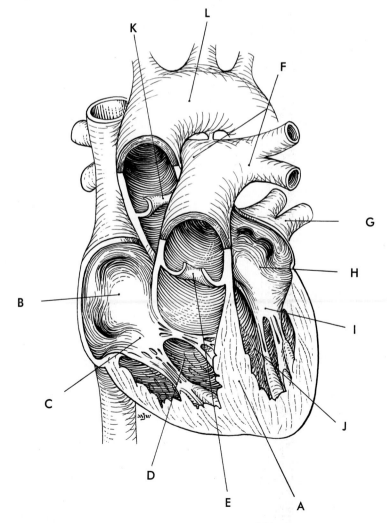

Figure 10-10

a.

b.

c.

d.

e.

f.

g.

h.

i.

j.

k.

l.

53. Name the branches of the circulatory system from the aorta to the cellular level and back to the vena cava.

_____

_____

54. Briefly describe the characteristics of blood vessels that permit vasodilation and vasoconstriction.

_____

_____

55. What structural feature of some veins inhibits the backflow of blood?

_____

56. What is the purpose of an arteriovenous anastomosis (arteriovenous shunt)?

_____

_____

57. List the three basic functions of the lymphatic system.
   a.
   b.
   c.

58. Describe the flow of lymph from its beginning in the tissues until it empties in the circulatory system.

_____

_____

_____

59. Label Fig. 10-11 of the upper airway and list one function of each structure named.

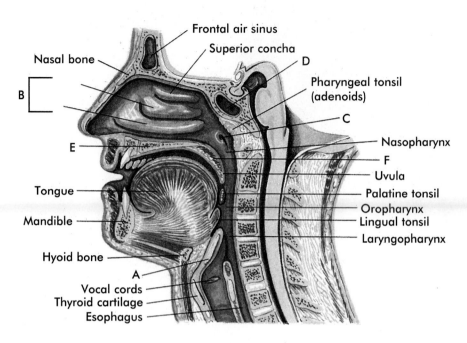

Figure 10-11

	Structure	**Function**
a.		
b.		
c.		
d.		
e.		
f.		

60. Label Fig. 10-12 of the larynx.

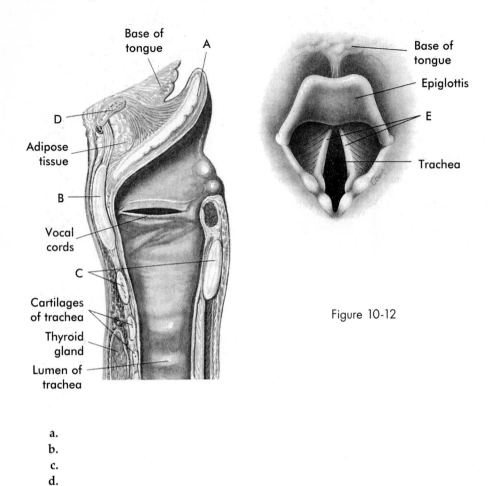

Figure 10-12

a.

b.

c.

d.

e.

61. Label Fig. 10-13 of the lower airway.

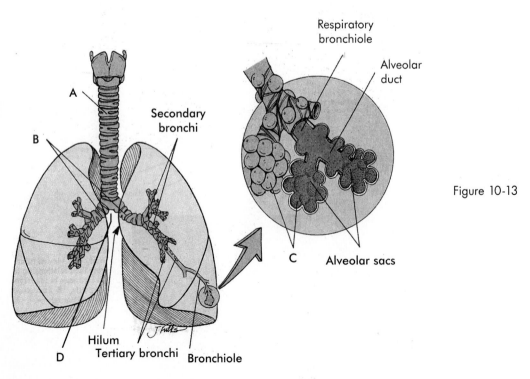

Figure 10-13

a.

b.

c.

d.

62. Describe how the structure of the trachea protects the airway.

_____

_____

63. Describe what happens to the bronchioles that causes wheezing during an asthma attack.

_____

_____

64. Describe the anatomical feature of the alveoli that:
   a. Permits the movement of oxygen to the blood and CO_2 from the blood:

_____

   b. Prevents collapse of the alveoli:

_____

65. Describe the location of the lungs in the chest cavity.

_____

66. List the divisions of:
   a. The right lung:

_____

   b. The left lung:

_____

67. Describe the functions of:
   a. The pleural space:

_____

   b. The pleural fluid:

_____

68. List the functions of the digestive system.

_____

69. As a cheeseburger passes through the digestive tract, many digestive juices act on it to convert the food into a useable form for the body. For each area of the digestive tract listed, name a digestive juice excreted and briefly describe its function.

Area	Digestive Juice	Function
a. Mouth		
b. Stomach		
c. Pancreas		
d. Liver		
e. Large intestine		

70. List the functions of the urinary system.

_____

71. List two specific functions of the kidneys in addition to urine production.

   a.

   b.

72. The basic functional unit of the kidney is the (a) _____.

   It produces urine by a three-step process: (b) _____,

   (c) _____ and (d) _____.

73. For each of the following, state whether it increases or decreases urine production.

   a. Aldosterone:

   b. Atrial natriuretic factor:

   c. Large increase in blood pressure:

   d. Shock:

74. Label Fig. 10-14 of the male reproductive system.

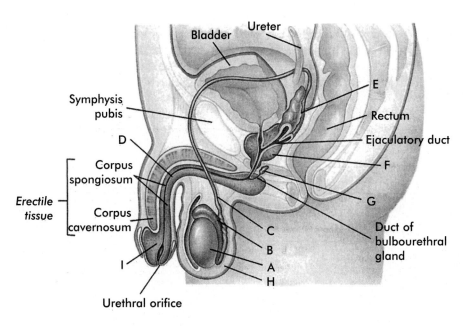

Figure 10-14

   a.

   b.

   c.

   d.

   e.

   f.

   g.

   h.

   i.

75. Label Fig. 10-15 of the female reproductive system.

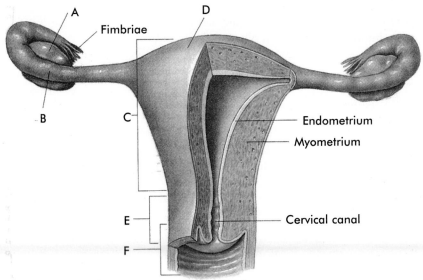

A

Fimbriae

D

B

C

Endometrium

Myometrium

E

Cervical canal

F

Figure 10-15

a.

b.

c.

d.

e.

f.

76. Label Fig. 10-16 of the female perineum.

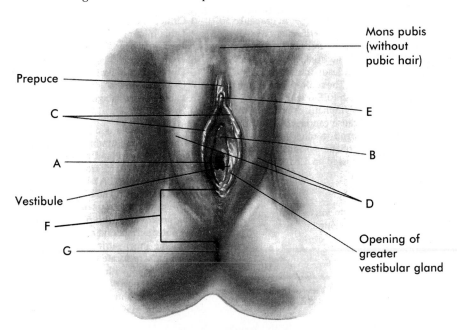

Mons pubis (without pubic hair)

Prepuce

C

A

Vestibule

F

G

E

B

D

Opening of greater vestibular gland

Figure 10-16

a.

b.

c.

d.

e.

f.

g.

77. Complete the following sentences pertaining to the olfactory sense: Receptors for the olfactory nerves lie in the upper part of the (a)

_____ cavity. When olfactory cells are stimulated by airborne molecules, the nerve impulses travel in the olfactory bulb and

(b) _____ _____. The brain

interprets the impulses as specific odors in the (c) _____

and (d) _____ centers.

78. Complete the following sentences pertaining to the sense of taste: Sensory structures that detect taste stimuli in the mouth are (a)

_____ _____. Taste buds are

most commonly found in the mouth on the (b) _____.

However, they are also found on the (c) _____,

_____, _____, and

_____. The four basic tastes that are detected

are: (d) _____, _____,

_____ and _____.

79. Complete the following sentences pertaining to the sense of vision: The sensation of vision is transmitted from the eye to the brain by way of

the (a) _____ nerve. Impulses that travel from the brain to control the movements of the eye are relayed by the (b)

_____ nerve. The avascular, transparent structure that bends and refracts light as it enters the eye is the (c)

_____. The size of the pupil and therefore the amount of light that enters the eye through it is controlled by the (d) _____. The inner sensory layer of the retina contains two types of photoreceptor cells. The receptors that are responsible for

night vision are the (e) _____, and the receptors that

permit daytime and color vision are the (f) _____.
The eye has two compartments. The anterior chamber is filled with (g)

_____ humor, and the posterior chamber contains

(h) _____ humor. The humor in both chambers helps

maintain (i) _____ _____.

80. List the function of each of the following accessory structures of the eye.
   a. Eyebrows:

b. Eyelids:

_____

c. Lacrimal glands:

_____

81. Complete the following sentences pertaining to the tissues associated with hearing and balance: The external and middle ear are involved in (a)

_____, and the inner ear plays a role in (b)

_____ and _____. The senses

of hearing and balance are transmitted by the (c) _____
nerve. Sound is picked up by the external ear prominence known as the

(d) _____ and transmitted through the external auditory

meatus into the (e) _____ canal. At the end of this

canal, vibration of the (f) _____ _____
is produced. These vibrations are picked up and transmitted to the oval
window by the auditory ossicles of the middle ear. These three bones are

the (g) _____, _____, and

_____. Finally, in the inner ear inside the cochlea

lies the hearing sense organ called the (h) _____

_____ _____. The two other
structures within the inner ear involved in balance are the (i)

_____ and (j) _____.

● STUDENT SELF-EVALUATION

82. You find your patient lying face-up on his back. This is the _____ position.
    a. Anatomical   c. Prone
    b. Lateral recumbent d. Supine
83. A teenage football player has collapsed following a sharp blow to the left upper quadrant of the abdomen. You suspect injury to the _____:
    a. Appendix   c. Liver
    b. Gallbladder   d. Spleen
84. Structures in the mediastinum include all of the following, *except:*
    a. Esophagus   c. Thyroid
    b. Heart   d. Trachea
85. Cardiac muscle cells are:
    a. Striated voluntary   c. Nonstriated voluntary
    b. Striated involuntary   d. Nonstriated involuntary
86. The actual conducting cells of the nervous system are the:
    a. Dendrites   c. Neurons
    b. Neuroglia   d. Synapses
87. Functions of the integumentary system include all of the following, *except:*
    a. Infection barrier   c. Movement
    b. Injury protection   d. Temperature regulation

88. The scapula and clavicle comprise the:
    a. Pectoral girdle   c. Thorax
    b. Pelvic girdle   d. Vertebral disks
89. An indoor soccer player has sustained an injury resulting in marked swelling and pain at the inner aspect of the ankle. You would describe this to an on-line physician as pain and swelling at the area of the:
    a. Lateral malleolus   c. Olecranon
    b. Medial malleolus   d. Patella
90. Muscle fiber contractions are initiated when stimulated by:
    a. Actin and myosin   c. Myofilaments
    b. Motor neurons   d. Sarcomeres
91. The primary action of the frontal lobe of the cerebral cortex is to:
    a. Receive and integrate visual input
    b. Evaluate olfactory and auditory input
    c. Receive and interpret sensory information
    d. Initiate voluntary motor function
92. The spinal cord ends at the _____ vertebrae.
    a. Twelfth thoracic   c. Sacral
    b. Second lumbar   d. Coccygeal
93. The innermost meningeal layer, which adheres to the brain and spinal cord is the _____ mater.
    a. Arachnoid   c. Dura
    b. Choroid   d. Pia
94. The component of the endocrine system that transmits information from the gland to its target body part is the:
    a. Enzyme   c. Neurotransmitter
    b. Hormone   d. Synapse
95. The formed element in blood that contains hemoglobin and carries oxygen is the:
    a. Erythrocyte   c. Leukocyte
    b. Immunoglobulin   d. Platelet
96. Which blood vessel(s) carries(y) blood from the heart to the systemic circulation?
    a. Aorta   c. Pulmonary veins
    b. Pulmonary arteries   d. Vena cava
97. Cardiac electrical impulse conduction is normally initiated in the:
    a. Atrioventricular node c. Purkinje fibers
    b. Bundle of His   d. Sinoatrial node
98. Lymph nodes filter foreign substances and are located in all of the following body regions, *except:*
    a. Axillary   c. Inguinal
    b. Cervical   d. Temporal
99. The airway division that is involved in the production of speech and that serves as a protective sphincter to prevent liquids and solids from entering the lungs is the:
    a. Larynx   c. Pharynx
    b. Propharynx   d. Trachea
100. The functional unit of the respiratory system where gas exchange occurs between the lungs and the blood is the:
    a. Alveolus   c. Capillary
    b. Bronchus   d. Trachea
101. The major site of nutrient absorption in the intestines is the:
    a. Colon   c. Ileum
    b. Duodenum   d. Jejunum
102. Liver function includes all of the following actions, *except:*
    a. Bile production   c. Hormone secretion
    b. Drug detoxification   d. Plasma protein synthesis

103. Which of the following statements is *true* with regard to renal function?
   a. All fluid filtered from the glomerulus becomes urine.
   b. Healthy people produce 180 L of urine per day.
   c. Water and other nutrients are reabsorbed in the tubules.
   d. Potassium and ammonia are secreted into the blood.
104. Which of the following hormones influences urine production?
   a. Aldosterone   c. Oxytocin
   b. Glucagon   d. Testosterone
105. Sperm production occurs in the:
   a. Epididymis   c. Seminal vesicle
   b. Prostate   d. Testes
106. When the nasal receptors of the olfactory neurons are stimulated, messages are sent for interpretation to the olfactory and _____ centers of the brain.
   a. Frontal   c. Pontine
   b. Medullary   d. Thalamic
107. The hearing sense organ is the:
   a. Cochlea   c. Semicircular canal
   b. Organ of Corti   d. Vestibule

CHAPTER 11
GENERAL PATIENT ASSESSMENT

● **READING ASSIGNMENT**

Chapter 11, pp. 180-217, in *Mosby's Paramedic Textbook*

● **OBJECTIVES**

As a paramedic, you should be able to:
 1. Establish priorities of care based on life-threatening conditions.
 2. Distinguish between patient assessment and patient management.
 3. Explain the purpose of the primary and secondary surveys.
 4. Detail in the correct order the assessment of each component of the primary survey.
 5. Identify potentially life-threatening conditions that can be discovered in the primary survey.
 6. Discuss patient management techniques that may be used if abnormalities are found in the primary survey.
 7. Differentiate between resuscitation procedures for medical patients and trauma patients.
 8. Describe the examination techniques for inspection, palpation, and auscultation.
 9. Explain in detail the physical examination for each component of the secondary survey.
10. Apply effective patient interviewing techniques to given scenarios.
11. Describe the essential elements of the patient history.
12. Describe the process of patient reevaluation.
13. Describe special considerations in assessing pediatric, geriatric, disabled, and non-English-speaking patients.

● **REVIEW QUESTIONS**

Match the sign in Column 2 with its definition in Column 1. Use each term only once.

Column 1	Column 2
_____ **1.** Persistent respiratory rate less than 12 breaths/min	**a.** Biot's
_____ **2.** Normal breath sounds heard over most lung fields	**b.** Bradypnea
_____ **3.** Low-pitched, rumbling expiratory sounds	**c.** Cheyne-Stokes
_____ **4.** Crowing sound associated with upper airway narrowing	**d.** Crackles
_____ **5.** Crescendo-decrescendo sequence of respirations followed by apnea	**e.** Rhonchi
_____ **6.** Irregular respirations interrupted by apneic periods	**f.** Stridor
_____ **7.** End inspiratory sounds associated with fluid in the small airways	**g.** Vesicular
_____ **8.** High-pitched airway noise resulting from lower airway narrowing	**h.** Wheezes

9. The purpose of the secondary survey is to find and treat all injuries. True/False. If this is false, why is it false?

_____

_____

10. Packaging may include airway control, intravenous fluid administration, fracture stabilization, bandaging, and extrication. True/False. If this is false, why is it false?

_____

_____

11. *You are called to the scene of a neighborhood disturbance in an area well known for its gang violence. On arrival, you are told that several people have been shot. A heated exchange is occurring among the large crowd gathered outside. The victims are still inside, and there is a report of smoke sighted in the rear of the apartment complex where they are located.* What potential hazards must be considered by EMS personnel on this scene?

_____

_____

12. What measures may be taken in the situation in Question 11 to minimize risk of injury to the paramedic crew?

_____

_____

13. List the six critical elements of patient assessment.
   a.
   b.
   c.
   d.
   e.
   f.

14. List the five components of the primary survey (using the mnemonic *ABCDE*) and describe what techniques you will perform during your patient assessment in each of the five areas.

	Component	**Techniques**
a.		

_____

| b. | | |

_____

| c. | | |

_____

d.

_____

e.

_____

15. List one life-threatening condition that you may discover in your assessment in each of the first three areas of the primary survey and describe a patient management technique for each.

	Life Threat	**Management**
a.		
b.		
c.		

16. *You are called to the scene of an accident in which a person was struck by an automobile. On arrival, you note a middle-aged victim whose forearm is nearly amputated. The wound is spurting bright red blood. The patient has noisy agonal respirations at approximately 8/min. His skin is pale, cyanotic, and diaphoretic. His pulse is thready and very rapid. Multiple loose teeth and blood fill the oral cavity. Establish your priorities of care and describe the sequence in which you will manage this patient.*

_____

_____

17. For the scenario described in Question 16, what other assessment parameters do you need to make as quickly as possible?

_____

18. List four general resuscitation measures commonly used for:
    a. A medical patient:

    _____

    b. A trauma patient:

    _____

19. Describe the correct method of performing each of the following patient assessment techniques:
    a. Inspection:

    _____

b. Palpation:

_____

c. Auscultation:

_____

20. List the steps of the secondary survey.

_____

_____

21. For each of the following deviations from normal pupil response, list a cause:

Abnormality	Cause
a. Dilated/unresponsive	
b. Constricted/unresponsive	
c. Unequal/one dilated and unresponsive	
d. Dull/lackluster	

22. _Your patient is a teenage assault victim who was struck repeatedly on the head with a baseball bat._ Outline your secondary survey of this patient's head and neck, detailing specific examination techniques and the types of normal or abnormal findings for which you would look.

_____

_____

_____

_____

23. _You are called to evaluate a patient whose chief complaint is difficulty breathing._ Describe your history-taking process with this patient, including any helpful mnemonic you may use.

_____

_____

24. For the patient in Question 23, explain your assessment of the thorax.

_____

_____

25. _Your 56-year-old patient has a history of right-upper-quadrant abdominal pain, malaise, nausea, and vomiting. He is jaundiced and complains of itching. Past history reveals heavy alcohol use. You suspect hepatitis._ Describe your physical examination of this patient's abdomen.

_____

_____

26. _You are examining a patient involved in a motor vehicle collision whose automobile was struck on his side. The patient complains of considerable pain in the pelvic area. The primary survey has been completed. The patient's pulse is elevated, but blood pressure is within normal limits._ Describe your secondary survey of this patient's pelvic area.

27. *Your crew arrives at the home of an older patient whose family states that she complained of weakness on one side, stumbled, and fell down five steps. No life-threatening conditions are found in the primary survey, and vital signs assessment reveals a moderately elevated blood pressure and pulse. The patient is slightly confused but cooperative. You suspect a cerebrovascular accident.* Describe your assessment of this patient's extremities.

28. *A painter has fallen approximately 20 feet, striking a scaffold rail with his lower back. Primary survey and vital signs are normal.* Outline your secondary survey of this patient's back.

29. Explain how a paramedic should approach a patient to best yield an effective patient examination and interview.

30. Rewrite the following patient interview questions to make them more effective in eliciting appropriate information:
   a. Is the pain right here in this spot?
   b. Are you depressed?
   c. Does your indigestion get worse after meals?
   d. So you called us because your chest hurts?
   e. Is the pain sharp?

31. For each of the following categories, give one example of social information that may be significant in a patient's past medical history.
   a. Habits:

   b. Home conditions:

   c. Occupation:

   d. Environment:

   e. Military record:

   f. Religious preference:

32. List four general guidelines that are helpful when approaching a pediatric patient.

a.

b.

c.

d.

33. Describe two specific developmental differences of the children in each of the following age groups that influence patient assessment.

a. Birth to 6 months:

_____

b. 7 months to 3 years:

_____

c. 4 to 10 years:

_____

d. Adolescence:

_____

34. Describe two special considerations and techniques that may be useful when caring for each of the following patient groups:

a. Older patient:

_____

b. Deaf patient:

_____

c. Blind patient:

_____

d. Brain injured or developmentally disabled patient:

_____

e. Non-English-speaking patient:

_____

● **STUDENT SELF-EVALUATION**

35. Recognition and management of life-threatening conditions should be the priority of the:

a. Primary survey
c. Definitive field management
b. Secondary survey
d. Re-evaluation

36. Which of the following can cause airway obstruction?

a. Emphysema
c. Hyperventilation
b. Flail chest
d. Vomitus

37. Signs and symptoms of inadequate circulation include all of the following, *except:*

a. Capillary refill less than 2 seconds
b. Decreased level of consciousness
c. Pale, cool, diaphoretic skin
d. Patient complains of thirst

38. Which of the following is the clearest way to report an altered level of consciousness?

a. Obtunded   c. Stuporous
b. Semiconscious   d. Unresponsive to pain

39. Prehospital resuscitation procedures for trauma patients will *most frequently* include:
    a. Blood samples for analysis   c. Electrical therapy
    b. Cervical spine immobilization   d. Medication administration

40. Using an adult blood pressure cuff to evaluate a child's blood pressure can result in:
    a. False-low reading   c. Normal reading
    b. False-high reading   d. Lack of audible sounds

41. To verify that vision is present the paramedic should:
    a. Assess bilateral pupil response to light.
    b. Ask the patient to count fingers.
    c. Lightly touch the cornea with a cotton swab.
    d. Palpate the globe for firmness.

42. A bubbling, crackling sensation that is due to air in the tissues and that is present on palpation of the neck may indicate:
    a. Air embolus   c. Pulsus paradoxis
    b. Pneumomediastinum   d. Subcutaneous emphysema

43. Bronchial breath sounds should normally be:
    a. Auscultated over the trachea
    b. Low pitched and soft
    c. Auscultated over the bronchi
    d. Not heard with a normal stethoscope

44. Simultaneous palpation of the apical and carotid pulses whereby each apical beat is not transmitted is known as:
    a. Mean arterial pressure   c. Pulsus paradoxis
    b. Pulse deficit   d. Pulse pressure

45. All of the following may cause muffled heart sounds, *except:*
    a. Cardiac tamponade   c. Obstructive lung disease
    b. Obesity   d. Tension pneumothorax

46. In a patient who has fractured the neck of the femur, the affected extremity will frequently be:
    a. Shortened and externally rotated
    b. Lengthened and externally rotated
    c. Shortened and internally rotated
    d. Lengthened and internally rotated

47. Which of the following statements is *true* regarding cervical spine assessment?
    a. All seven cervical vertebrae should be palpable on adults.
    b. Fractures can easily be assessed by palpation.
    c. Range of motion should be assessed in patients with neck pain.
    d. Trauma patients with a decreased level of consciousness should have cervical spine immobilization.

48. A young child has an obvious fractured lower leg. Which of the following statements is *false* regarding care of this patient?
    a. Remain calm and confident.
    b. Separate the parents from the child.
    c. Establish rapport with the parents.
    d. Be honest with child and parents.

49. Which of the following statements is *true* regarding the physical examination of a 2-year-old child?
    a. Abdominal breathing is normal in this age group.
    b. Patient modesty should be a primary concern.
    c. Explanations should be given for each activity.
    d. Separation anxiety will not be a problem.

50. When examining the older patient, the paramedic should:
   a. Always speak loudly because most of these patients are deaf.
   b. Assume that memory impairment is present.
   c. Anticipate multiple health problems and medicines.
   d. Address the patient as *honey* or *dear* to appear friendly.

51. *A blind patient has fallen down a flight of steps and has many bruises and an obvious fracture to the wrist.* When caring for this patient the paramedic should:
   a. Speak loudly because blind persons are often deaf too.
   b. Assume a mental handicap and treat the patient as a child.
   c. Explain each procedure simply but thoroughly.
   d. Make no adjustment in patient approach and examination.

AIRWAY AND VENTILATION

● READING ASSIGNMENT

Chapter 12, pp. 218-281, in *Mosby's Paramedic Textbook*

● OBJECTIVES

As a paramedic, you should be able to:
 1. Describe the function and location of the anatomical structures of the upper and lower airways.
 2. Explain the mechanics of respiration.
 3. Relate the partial pressures of gases in the blood and lungs to atmospheric gas pressures.
 4. Describe pulmonary circulation.
 5. Explain the process of exchange and transport of gases in the body.
 6. Describe voluntary, chemical, and nervous regulation of respiration.
 7. Discuss the assessment and management of medical or traumatic obstruction of the airway.
 8. Describe preventative measures, assessment, and management for aspiration by inhalation.
 9. Describe the use of manual airway maneuvers based on knowledge of their indications, contraindications, potential complications, and techniques.
10. Describe the use of mechanical airway adjuncts in airway management based on knowledge of their indications, contraindications, potential complications, and insertion techniques.
11. Describe assessment techniques and devices used to ensure adequate oxygenation and elimination of carbon dioxide.
12. Discuss methods for patient ventilation based on knowledge of their indications, contraindications, potential complications, and use.
13. Explain variations in assessment and management of airway problems in pediatric and older patients.
14. Describe the use of oxygen regulators.
15. Given a patient scenario, select the correct oxygen delivery device based on knowledge of proper indications and contraindications.

● REVIEW QUESTIONS

Match the lung volume in Column 2 with its description in Column 1. Use each term only once.

Column 1	Column 2
_____ 1. The air inhaled and exhaled during a normal respiratory cycle (500 to 600 ml)	a. Expiratory reserve volume
_____ 2. Quantity of air moved on deepest inspiration and expiration	b. Inspiratory reserve volume
_____ 3. Tidal volume multiplied by respiratory rate	c. Minute volume
_____ 4. Air remaining in respiratory passages after a forceful exhalation	d. Residual volume
_____ 5. Amount of air that can be forcefully exhaled after a normal breath is exhaled	e. Tidal volume
	f. Vital capacity

6. Internal respiration is the transfer of oxygen and carbon dioxide between the blood capillaries and alveoli. True/false. If this is false, why is it false?

_____

7. pH is a measurement that reflects hydrogen ion concentration. True/false. If this is false, why is it false?

_____

8. The pressure regulator attached to an oxygen cylinder permits administration of a specific amount of oxygen. True/false. If this is false, why is it false?

_____

9. Describe the *mechanical* process by which air is moved into and out of the lungs.

_____

_____

_____

10. Complete the sentences in the following paragraph: At sea level, atmospheric pressure is (a) _____. The pressure in the alveoli is known as the (b) _____ pressure. Changes in this pressure are due to changes in the (c) _____ size. During inspiration, the pressure in the alveoli will (d) _____ approximately 1 mm Hg relative to atmospheric pressure, whereas during exhalation the pressure will (e) _____ by 1 mm Hg. The ability of the lungs to expand during changes in pressure is known as (f) _____. This ability can be impaired by diseases such as (g) _____, _____, and _____.

11. The major blood vessels that carry deoxygenated blood to the lungs are the

    (a) _____ _____. Oxygenated blood is carried away from the lungs by the (b) _____

    _____.

12. *Your patient is a 70-year-old man with chronic bronchitis and emphysema who experienced an acute onset of shortness of breath while at the grocery store.* Describe your secondary assessment of this patient's head, neck, chest, and abdomen. (Be specific when describing the muscle groups that you will inspect to help determine his degree of distress.)

_____

_____

13. The partial pressure of nitrogen (P_{N_2}) = (a) _____ percent × atmospheric pressure (b) _____ mm Hg = (c) _____ mm Hg. The partial pressure of oxygen (P_{O_2}) = (d) _____ percent × atmospheric pressure (e) _____ mm Hg = (f) _____ mm Hg.

14. List three physiological factors that can increase the work of breathing.

   a.

   b.

   c.

15. Describe the *structural* aspects of the lung that explain the following:

   a. Normal lung expansion:

   _____

   _____

   b. Alveolar collapse that occurs secondary to decreased surfactant in a premature infant:

   _____

   _____

   c. Poor ventilation during an asthma attack:

   _____

   _____

16. Each of the diagrams in Fig. 12-1 represents solutions separated by a semipermeable membrane. In each illustration, indicate whether the process of diffusion will cause a net movement of solute particles to the *left* or *right* or *not at all.*

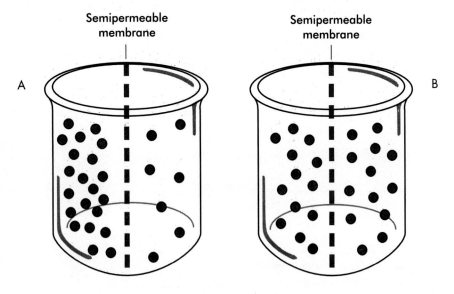

Figure 12-1

a. _____   **b.** _____

17. Outline the mechanism by which gases are exchanged between the alveoli and the blood. Be specific with regard to the partial pressures of the gases at each state of this process.

_____

_____

18. Indicate whether each of the following substances is *acidic, basic,* or *neutral:*
    a. Human blood—pH 7.40:
    b. Urine—pH 6.0:
    c. Gastric juice—pH 0.8:
    d. Oven cleaner—pH 13.8:
    e. Distilled water—pH 7.0:
    f. Milk of Magnesia—pH 10.5:
19. Complete the following sentences:
    a. The primary way that oxygen is transported in the blood is by a

       chemical bond to _____.
    b. P_{O_2} describes the oxygen level dissolved in blood

       _____.

    c. The amount of carbon dioxide present in the venous blood is influenced

       by the rate and type of _____.
    d. Carbon dioxide is transported in the blood in three forms:

       _____, _____

       _____, and _____.
20. In one sentence describe the physiological basis for poor blood oxygenation in the following patients:
    a. *A 23-year-old woman who is completely paralyzed from Guillain-Barré syndrome:*

_____

    b. *A 52-year-old patient with pneumonia:*

_____

    c. *An 8-year-old with an acute asthma attack:*

_____

    d. *A 42-year-old with massive head trauma caused by a motor vehicle crash:*

_____

21. Briefly explain the action of each of the following mechanisms that control respiration:
    a. Inspiratory centers:

_____

    b. Expiratory centers:

_____

    c. Hering-Breuer reflex:

_____

    d. Pneumotaxic center:

_____

e. Apneustic center:

22. For each of the following scenarios, briefly explain why the patient's respirations will increase or decrease or be unchanged.
    a. *A 3-year-old who loses consciousness from breath-holding secondary to a temper tantrum:*

    b. *A 34-year-old with a morphine overdose:*

    c. *A 17-year-old football player with a dislocated shoulder:*

    d. *A hostage with no apparent injuries who has just been freed:*

    e. *A student who is sleeping in class:*

    f. *An individual who suffers from chronic obstructive pulmonary disease who has fallen and for whom an oxygen level of 10 L/min is being administered by non-rebreather mask:*

    g. *A lost snow skier who has a core temperature of 84° F (28.9° C):*

23. Briefly describe the benefit of the following modified forms of respiration:
    a. Cough:

    b. Sneeze:

    c. Hiccough:

    d. Sigh:

24. For each of the following scenarios identify the pathological condition or injury you would suspect and list the signs and symptoms that the patient may develop:
    a. *A 50-year-old man unable to speak after choking on a piece of steak:*

    b. *A nursing home patient with shortness of breath after "inhaling" some food:*

    c. *A 17-year-old hockey player who has difficulty speaking after being struck across the neck by a stick:*

38. Which of the following patients is most likely to have a decreased minute volume?
   a. A 17-year-old with deep respirations and signs of hyperventilation
   b. A 20-year-old patient with a head injury with shallow, slow respirations
   c. A 45-year-old with a possible myocardial infarction and whose respirations are 16 breaths/min and normal
   d. A 30-year-old in early shock with an increased respiratory rate

39. Your patient is on a pulse oximeter and the reading is 100% saturation. This means that:
   a. The patient is on 100% oxygen by mask.
   b. The partial pressure of oxygen is 100.
   c. All hemoglobin has converted to oxyhemoglobin.
   d. The blood will not carry any more oxygen.

40. An example of decreased oxygenation secondary to increased resistance in the airways is a person suffering from:
   a. Asbestosis   c. Poliomyelitis
   b. Asthma   d. Tuberculosis

41. The tissues of a patient with anemia may not be well oxygenated because:
   a. The blood will not reach all tissue to off-load oxygen.
   b. The respiratory drive in the brain will be depressed.
   c. There will be insufficient red blood cells to carry oxygen.
   d. The pulmonary vessels will not be well perfused with blood.

42. Respiratory chemoreceptors in the medulla, aortic bodies, and carotid bodies are stimulated by changes in all of the following, *except:*
   a. Blood pressure   c. Oxygen
   b. Carbon dioxide   d. pH

43. If a person appears to be choking but can still speak and cough, the rescuer should:
   a. Deliver five back blows.
   b. Perform the Heimlich maneuver.
   c. Administer five chest thrusts.
   d. Not intervene but just observe.

44. The most frequent cause of any airway obstruction in the unconscious adult is:
   a. Hot dogs   c. Tongue
   b. Steak   d. Vomitus

45. You arrive at a private residence, where you find an unconscious 52-year-old man. You open his airway and determine that he is not breathing. You attempt to ventilate his lungs, but the airflow is blocked. What is your next step?
   a. Assess the pulse.
   b. Reposition the head.
   c. Administer 5 abdominal thrusts.
   d. Perform a cricothyrotomy.

46. Your patient attempted suicide by hanging. She is hoarse and has hemoptysis and stridor. You suspect:
   a. Laryngeal fracture   c. Foreign body obstruction
   b. Laryngeal spasm   d. Tracheal injury

47. All of the following are potential complications of nasopharyngeal airway insertion, *except:*
   a. It is poorly tolerated by sedated patients with gag reflexes.
   b. It may enter the esophagus if it is of excessive length.
   c. It may cause injury and bleeding to the nasal mucosa.
   d. It may become obstructed with blood or mucus.

48. To ensure adequate ventilation when an esophageal obturator airway is used, the paramedic must be certain that:
  a. The tube passes into the trachea.
  b. There is a tight mask seal.
  c. The patient is less than 5 feet tall.
  d. Breath sounds are audible over the gastric area.

49. The pharyngeal tracheal lumen airway may be used successfully if the tube is placed in:
  a. The esophagus   **c.** The right mainstem bronchus
  b. The trachea   **d.** The esophagus or trachea

50. If 30 seconds have elapsed from the last ventilation and tracheal intubation has not been accomplished, the paramedic should:
  a. Remove the tube, hyperventilate, and try again.
  b. Continue if intubation can be done in a few more seconds.
  c. Insert an esophageal obturator airway.
  d. Have another paramedic attempt the skill.

51. Which of the following statements is true regarding percutaneous transtracheal ventilation?
  a. Demand valves may be used to provide adequate ventilations.
  b. It is a good long-term airway-management device.
  c. It minimizes the risk of aspiration.
  d. The high pressures generated may cause pneumothorax.

52. Which of the following is *not* an advantage of the bag-valve-mask device?
  a. It allows delivery of high oxygen concentrations.
  b. It can give the rescuer a sense of the patient's lung compliance.
  c. It is easily used by one rescuer to deliver ventilations.
  d. It can provide a wide range of inspiratory pressures.

53. The demand valve set in the demand mode should ideally be used to assist ventilations in a:
  a. Patient with chronic obstructive pulmonary disease
  b. Breathing patient with dyspnea
  c. Pediatric patient
  d. Patient with apnea

54. Which of the following statements is true regarding patient suctioning?
  a. Hyperventilation for 2 minutes should precede suctioning.
  b. Suction should be applied for a maximum of 30 seconds.
  c. Coughing may cause decreased intracranial pressure.
  d. Suction should be set between 200 and 300 mm Hg.

55. The patient who is on a nasal cannula at 5 L/min will be receiving approximately _____ oxygen.
  a. 36%   **c.** 44%
  b. 40%   **d.** 50%

56. Your patient has been removed from a smoky building and is confused and tachycardic. What is the appropriate oxygen-delivery device for this person?
  a. Nasal cannula   **c.** Simple face mask
  b. Nonrebreather mask   **d.** Venturi mask

CHAPTER 13
SHOCK

● **READING ASSIGNMENT**

Chapter 13, pp. 282-333, in *Mosby's Paramedic Textbook*

● **OBJECTIVES**

As a paramedic, you should be able to:
1. Differentiate aerobic from anaerobic metabolism.
2. Describe the role of the heart, vasculature, and lungs in tissue perfusion.
3. Describe the constituents of blood and their functions.
4. Distinguish among the fluid compartments of the body.
5. Explain the various mechanisms for moving fluid and electrolytes among the body fluid compartments.
6. Describe the assessment and management of a patient with an imbalance of fluids, electrolytes, or both.
7. Discuss prehospital interventions for acid-base imbalances not corrected by the body's compensatory mechanisms.
8. Describe the role of negative feedback mechanisms in maintaining normal tissue perfusion.
9. Discuss the factors that influence microcirculation.
10. Recognize the stages in the progression of shock from vasoconstriction to death.
11. Differentiate the etiologies, signs, symptoms, and management of each classification of shock.
12. Describe the body's response to shock during the compensated, uncompensated, and irreversible stages of the syndrome.
13. Discuss factors that influence an individual's physiological response to shock.
14. Outline the physical examination of a patient in shock.
15. Discuss the indications, contraindications, complications, and techniques of intervention for shock.

● **REVIEW QUESTIONS**

Match the blood component in Column 2 with its definition in Column 1. Use each term only once.

Column 1	Column 2
_____ 1. Provides oxygen to and removes carbon dioxide from cells	a. Albumen
_____ 2. Forms sticky plugs and initiates clotting	b. Erythrocytes
_____ 3. Destroys red blood cells and bacteria	c. Fibrinogen
_____ 4. Large protein that moves water from tissues into the blood	d. Gamma globulin
_____ 5. Important in human immune response	e. Leukocyte
_____ 6. Blood's solvent through which salts, minerals, and fats travel	f. Plasma
	g. Platelet

7. *Shock* can best be defined as the clinical situation in which the systolic blood pressure is less than 90 mm Hg and the pulse exceeds 120 beats/min. True/false. If this is false, why is it false?

_____

8. A milliequivalent represents the number of milligrams of an anion that will combine with an equal number of cations. True/false. If this is false, why is it false?

_____

9. *You are called to evaluate a 20-year-old butcher who sustained a stab wound to the femoral artery. Evaluation of the patient reveals a large amount of blood loss from an inguinal wound that is spurting bright red blood. The patient is very anxious and confused. Vital signs are blood pressure, 86/70 mm Hg; pulse, 136; respirations, 28; and lungs, clear. The patient's lips and nail beds are pale and cyanotic, and capillary refill is greater than 2 seconds.* List each of the three physiological components necessary for normal cellular oxygenation as measured by the Fick principle and determine whether each has been met.

a.

_____

_____

b.

_____

_____

c.

_____

_____

10. For each of the following situations, describe why the cardiac output will increase or decrease in an otherwise healthy individual.
  a. *Patient has had a myocardial infarction with necrosis of 50% of the heart muscle.*

_____

  b. *Dehydrated patient is given 500 ml of normal saline intravenously.*

_____

  c. *The patient's normal heart rate is 80 and suddenly drops to 40.*

_____

  d. *A paramedic student enters a testing station.*

_____

11. Describe the structural elements of the vascular system that enable it to adjust its size and adapt to pressure changes.

_____

_____

signs are blood pressure, 80 mm Hg by palpation; pulse, 140; and respirations, 40 and labored.

    Classification:

    Interventions:

---

e. *A 72-year-old resident of a nursing home has a fever and is restless and agitated. The urine in the indwelling catheter collection bag is milky and green in color. Vital signs are blood pressure, 94/60 mm Hg; pulse; 132; and respirations, 30.*

    Classification:

    Interventions:

---

f. *A 55-year-old office worker has complained of a pounding sensation in his chest and has fallen from his chair, striking his head on the desk. You note a 5-cm laceration on the frontal area that is freely oozing dark red blood (approximately 20 ml on the floor). The patient is unconscious, and vital signs are blood pressure, 60 mm Hg by palpation; pulse, 180; and respirations, 28.*

    Classification:

    Interventions:

---

31. For each of the situations below, identify whether the patient is in compensated or uncompensated shock and explain why.

    a. *A 48-year-old has sustained second- and third-degree burns to 70% of his body. He is pale, cool, and diaphoretic. His nailbeds are cyanotic, and his vital signs are blood pressure, 84/76 mm Hg; pulse, 136; and respirations, 32.*

---

    b. *A 22-year-old passenger in a high-speed motor vehicle crash was restrained with a lap belt. She complains of severe abdominal pain. Her skin is cool and pale. Vital signs are blood pressure, 110/86 mm Hg; pulse, 128; and respirations, 28.*

---

32. Describe the characteristics of irreversible shock.

---

33. List three conditions, situations, or characteristics that decrease a patient's ability to compensate in shock.

    a.

    b.

    c.

34. For each of the following scenarios, select the appropriate intervention(s) indicated from the following list. Briefly justify your answer.

Pneumatic antishock garments   Drug therapy

Rapid fluid replacement   Blood transfusions

Intraosseous infusion

a. A 72-year-old after a myocardial infarction with pulmonary edema and vital signs of blood pressure, 86/60 mm Hg; pulse, 124; and respirations, 28.

_____

b. A 2-year-old who was struck by an automobile and who has suspected multiple pelvic and abdominal injuries. Vital signs: blood pressure, unobtainable; pulse, 170 carotid and very weak; and respirations, 40 and shallow.

_____

c. A 44-year-old with a sudden onset of dizziness followed by syncope. Vital signs: blood pressure, 86/68 mm Hg; pulse, 44; and respirations, 20.

_____

d. An 18-year-old stung by a bee at a park has generalized redness and hives and is acutely short of breath. Vital signs: blood pressure, 70 mm Hg by palpation; pulse, 132; and respirations, 36.

_____

e. A 53-year-old woman with heavy abdominal bleeding for 1 week and who becomes lethargic and confused. Vital signs: blood pressure, 66 mm Hg by palpation; pulse, 136; and respirations, 32.

_____

f. A 19-year-old who sustains a gunshot wound to the chest. Vital signs: blood pressure, 106/88 mm Hg; pulse, 128; and respirations, 24.

_____

35. Briefly explain the steps in the insertion of a peripheral intravenous line, as illustrated in Fig. 13-1.

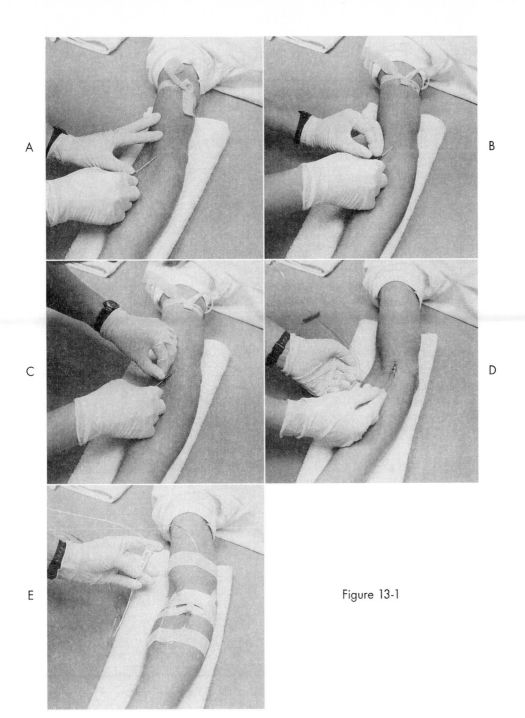

Figure 13-1

   a.

   b.

   c.

   d.

   e.

36. List three complications of intravenous line placement for each of the following approaches:

  a. Peripheral site:

  b. Internal jugular and subclavian sites:

c. Femoral site:

---

37. In each of the following situations, calculate the drops/min at which you will regulate your intravenous fluid to deliver the appropriate volume of fluid.
    a. *The physician orders an intravenous fluid to run at 30 cc/hour (drop factor, 60 drops/ml).* Drops/minute = _____.
    b. *You want to give a fluid challenge of 200 ml over 20 minutes (drop factor, 10 drops/ml).* Drops/minute = _____.
    c. *You need to infuse a drug mixed in 50 ml of fluid over 15 minutes (drop factor, 15 drops/ml).* Drops/minute = _____.
    d. *The physician orders 150 ml of lactated Ringer's solution to infuse in 2 hours (drop factor, 15 drops/ml).* Drops/minute = _____.
    e. *You are told to give 275 ml over 2 hours (drop factor, 10 drops/ml).* Drops/minute = _____.
    f. *The intravenous drug must run in at 0.5 ml/min (drop factor, 60 drops/ml).* Drops/minute = _____.
    g. *You want to push 500 ml in over an hour (drop factor, 10 drops/ml).* Drops/minute = _____.

● STUDENT SELF-EVALUATION

38. *Shock* is best defined as:
    a. Systolic blood pressure less than 90 mm Hg
    b. Greater than 25% loss of circulating blood
    c. Inadequate perfusion of the capillaries
    d. Blood flow deficit to the myocardium
39. Cardiac output is equal to:
    a. Heart rate × stroke volume
    b. Heart rate × peripheral vascular resistance
    c. Preload × myocardial contractility
    d. Preload × stroke volume
40. According to the Fick principle:
    a. Glucose must be available for cellular oxygenation.
    b. Precapillary and postcapillary sphincters must be open for adequate flow.
    c. Red blood cells must be able to load and unload oxygen.
    d. The pH should be at least 6.5 for adequate perfusion to occur.
41. The greatest determinant of afterload (peripheral vascular resistance) is the blood:
    a. Vessel diameter   c. Viscosity
    b. Vessel length   d. Volume
42. A decrease in peripheral vascular resistance will cause the container size of the body to _____ and the blood pressure to _____.
    a. Decrease, decrease   c. Increase, increase
    b. Decrease, increase   d. Increase, decrease
43. The blood cells responsible for transporting approximately 99% of the oxygen carried to body tissues are the:
    a. Erythrocytes   c. Plasma proteins
    b. Leukocytes   d. Platelets
44. Which of the following is an important anion found in body fluids?
    a. Calcium   c. Magnesium
    b. Hydrogen   d. Phosphate

45. Which of the following electrolytes is found predominantly in the *intracellular* fluid?
a. Bicarbonate   c. Potassium
b. Chloride   d. Sodium

46. One thousandth the molecular weight divided by the charges on an ion is expressed as:
a. mEq   c. ml
b. mg   d. moles

47. The flow of fluid across a semipermeable membrane from a lower concentration to a higher concentration is:
a. Active transport   c. Facilitated diffusion
b. Diffusion   d. Osmosis

48. A solution that has a concentration of solute particles equal to that inside the cells is a(n) _____ solution.
a. Atonic   c. Hypotonic
b. Hypertonic   d. Isotonic

49. When it is desirable to administer a fluid that will rapidly move out of the intravascular space, you would select:
a. D50W   c. 0.45% normal saline
b. Lactated Ringer's solution   d. 0.9% normal saline

50. *Your patient is a 65-year-old woman who has had vomiting and diarrhea for 3 days. Skin turgor is poor, and the patient states that she has lost 10 pounds and has not urinated in 12 hours.* The fluid of choice for this patient is:
a. D5W   c. 0.45% normal saline
b. 0.9% normal saline   d. D50W

51. *You are called to transport a 56-year-old patient with a history of renal failure who missed his last dialysis session. He is complaining of nausea, abdominal distention, weakness, and irritability.* You suspect:
a. Hypercalcemia   c. Hypernatremia
b. Hyperkalemia   d. Hyperuria

52. Which of the following is true regarding hypomagnesemia?
a. It is often accompanied by hypercalcemia.
b. It results from antacid abuse.
c. It causes hypoactive reflexes.
d. It causes cardiac dysrhythmias.

53. Prolonged diarrhea may result in all of the following, *except:*
a. Hypocalcemia   c. Hypomagnesemia
b. Hypokalemia   d. Hyponatremia

54. Which acid-base disturbance would you anticipate in a patient with severe flail chest?
a. Metabolic acidosis   c. Respiratory acidosis
b. Metabolic alkalosis   d. Respiratory alkalosis

55. Lactic acidosis is harmful to the body because it:
a. Increases the basal metabolic rate
b. Decreases the force of cardiac contraction
c. Increases the response to catecholamines
d. Can cause severe hypertension

56. The patient with metabolic acidosis and adequate spontaneous ventilations will typically have:
a. Decreased pH and decreased pCO_2
b. Decreased pH and increased pCO_2
c. Increased pH and decreased pCO_2
d. Increased pH and increased pCO_2

57. Exchange of nutrients and metabolic products takes place in the:
a. Arterioles   c. Metarterioles
b. Capillaries   d. Thoroughfare channels

58. Dilation of the precapillary sphincter while the postcapillary sphincter remains constricted during lactic acidosis will result in:
   a. No net movement of fluid between the fluid compartments
   b. Loss of vascular fluid into the interstitial spaces
   c. Movement of fluid from interstitial to the intravascular spaces
   d. Fluid shunting around the capillaries through the venules
59. Carotid baroreceptor stimulation when a person is hypertensive will cause:
   a. Decreased urine output
   b. Peripheral vasoconstriction
   c. Decreased heart rate
   d. Increased myocardial contractility
60. Sympathetic vasoconstriction during shock will result in:
   a. Tachycardia
   b. Pupil dilation
   c. Increased container size
   d. Pale, cool skin
61. The central nervous system ischemic response is initiated when:
   a. Blood pressure falls below 90 mm Hg.
   b. Aortic and carotid chemoreceptors are stimulated.
   c. Bradycardia and vasodilation are present.
   d. Blood flow decreases in the vasomotor center.
62. Which of the following hormonal mechanisms will increase urine production?
   a. Adrenal medullary mechanism
   b. Atrial natriuretic mechanism
   c. Renin-angiotension-aldosterone mechanism
   d. Vasopressin mechanism
63. In stage two of the progression of shock, fluid:
   a. Is pulled into the intravascular space because of vasoconstriction
   b. Leaks out of the intravascular space because of vasoconstriction
   c. Is pulled into the intravascular space because of increased hydrostatic pressure
   d. Leaks out of the intravascular space because of increased hydrostatic pressure
64. Which of the following shock states will *not* present with vasodilation?
   a. Anaphylactic
   b. Cardiogenic
   c. Neurogenic
   d. Septic
65. *Your patient was stabbed in the abdomen 20 minutes ago. Vital signs are blood pressure, 80/50 mm Hg; pulse, 136; and respirations, 26. He is anxious and very pale. He is probably in which stage of shock?*
   a. Compensated
   b. Irreversible
   c. Transitional
   d. Uncompensated
66. Increases in peripheral vascular resistance can be indirectly measured by noting the patient's:
   a. Diastolic blood pressure
   b. Jugular distention
   c. Pulse rate
   d. Systolic blood pressure
67. In which of the following is the pneumatic antishock garment considered helpful?
   a. Cardiogenic shock
   b. Pelvic fractures
   c. Penetrating chest injuries
   d. Pulmonary edema
68. Which of the following fluids is a colloid solution?
   a. Dextran
   b. 0.45% sodium chloride
   c. Lactated Ringer's solution
   d. Normal saline
69. Which of the following blood recipients could safely be given type AB blood:
   a. Type A
   b. Type B
   c. Type AB
   d. Type O
70. *You arrive at the emergency department with a patient who has been vomiting bright red blood and who is exhibiting signs and symptoms of shock. Which fluid would be most beneficial to him at this time?*

a. Blood plasma   **c.** Packed red blood cells
b. Dextran   **d.** Plasmanate

71. *Your patient has fallen 30 feet from scaffolding and is anxious and confused and in obvious shock.* Which of the following indicates your priorities of care, in the proper order.
    a. Rapid transport, oxygen, intravenous therapy
    b. Oxygen, intravenous therapy, rapid transport
    c. Intravenous therapy, rapid transport, oxygen
    d. Oxygen, rapid transport, intravenous therapy

72. In the absence of spinal or head injury, the hypovolemic patient in shock should be placed in the _____ position.
    a. Lateral recumbent   **c.** Supine hypotension
    b. Modified Trendelenberg   **d.** Trendelenberg

73. Appropriate initial prehospital management techniques for the patient in hypovolemic shock would include all of the following, *except:*
    a. Crystalloid fluid replacement   **c.** Pneumatic antishock garment
    b. External hemorrhage control   **d.** Vasoactive drug therapy

74. Fluid therapy in cardiogenic shock should be slowed to the to-keep-open rate if:
    a. Lung crackles (rales) increase.
    b. Jugular vein distention decreases.
    c. Heart rate decreases.
    d. Peripheral edema increases.

75. The treatment of choice for the patient in severe anaphylactic shock is:
    a. Antihistamines   **c.** Fluid challenge
    b. Epinephrine   **d.** Pneumatic antishock garments

76. *You suspect that your patient has a ruptured ectopic pregnancy. She is in profound shock.* Which intravenous catheter will you select?
    a. 14 gauge, 1½ inch   **c.** 18 gauge, 1½ inch
    b. 14 gauge, 3 inch   **d.** 18 gauge, 3 inch

77. *You are transferring a patient with a jugular central line. Suddenly, the patient becomes unconscious, cyanotic, and tachycardic. You note that the intravenous tubing has been disconnected from the central line catheter.* The patient should immediately be positioned on his:
    a. Left side with his head down
    b. Left side with his head up
    c. Right side with his head down
    d. Right side with his head up

78. You wish to administer an intravenous fluid at 30 ml/hr. The infusion set delivers 60 drops/ml. How fast will you run it?
    a. 15 drops/min   **c.** 60 drops/min
    b. 30 drops/min   **d.** 120 drops/min

79. A 200-ml fluid challenge is to be infused over 20 minutes. The drop factor is 10 drops/ml. How fast will you run it?
    a. 1 drop/min   **c.** 100 drops/min
    b. 33 drops/min   **d.** 400 drops/min

CHAPTER 14
EMERGENCY PHARMACOLOGY

● READING ASSIGNMENT
Chapter 14, pp. 334-395, in *Mosby's Paramedic Textbook*

● OBJECTIVES
As a paramedic, you should be able to:
1. List five sources of drugs.
2. Identify the four different types of drug names.
3. Outline drug standards and legislation pertinent to the paramedic.
4. Describe the role of drug-control agencies.
5. Distinguish among drug forms.
6. Explain the meaning of drug terms necessary to safely interpret information in drug-reference sources.
7. Discuss factors that influence drug absorption, distribution, and elimination.
8. Describe how drugs react with receptors to produce their desired effects.
9. Outline assessment techniques performed and documented to evaluate the effectiveness of drug therapy.
10. Calculate and correctly measure or infuse the correct volume of drug to be administered for a given situation.
11. Describe steps for ensuring safe administration of drugs.
12. Explain techniques of drug administration by enteral and parenteral routes.
13. Identify special considerations for administering pharmacological agents to pediatric and older patients.
14. List the class, actions, onset, duration, indications, contraindications, adverse reactions, drug interactions, dosage, routes of administration, and special considerations for the drugs listed in the Emergency Drug Index.
15. Outline drug actions and considerations for care of the patient who is given drugs that affect the nervous, cardiovascular, respiratory, endocrine, and gastrointestinal systems.

● REVIEW QUESTIONS
Match the appropriate drug form in Column 2 with its description in Column 1. Use each drug form only once.

Column 1	Column 2
_____ 1. Semisolid medicine in a greasy base externally applied to the skin	a. Capsule
_____ 2. A sweetened alcohol and water solution	b. Elixir
_____ 3. Drug ground into loose granules	c. Emulsion
_____ 4. Drug compressed into small disk	d. Extract
_____ 5. Drug dissolved in sugar and water	e. Liniment
	f. Lotion
	g. Aqueous suspension (magma)
_____ 6. Flat or round medicine held in mouth until dissolved	h. Ointment
_____ 7. Gelatin-covered, dry drug preparation	i. Tablets
_____ 8. Suspension of fat or oil in water with an agent that decreases surface tension	j. Powder
	k. Aqueous solution
	l. Troche

_____ **9.** Suspension of insoluble particles
in water

10. Pharmacodynamic interactions describe the effects of the drug on the body.
True/false. If this is false, why is it false?

_____

_____

11. If a drug binds to a receptor site and does not cause or prevents a physiological response, it is called an *antagonist.* True/false. If this is false, why is
it false?

_____

_____

12. List five sources of drugs.
   a.
   b.
   c.
   d.
   e.

13. Complete the following sentences by listing the appropriate drug name: The
precise composition and molecular structure of a drug is described in its

(a) _____ name. The name that is not protected by
law and denotes pharmacologically similar drugs is known as the (b)

_____ name. The copyrighted name of the drug
designated by the company that manufactures it is the (c)

_____ name. The initials *USP* or *NF* follow the (d)

_____ name.

14. In one sentence, describe how the following drug standards or legislation influences medication administration and distribution in the United States.
   a. Pure Food and Drug Act (1906):

_____

   b. Federal Drug and Cosmetic Act (1938):

_____

   c. Harrison Narcotic Act (1914):

_____

15. List the agency responsible for each of the following aspects of drug control:
   a. It has the power to suppress false or misleading advertising regarding
       drugs to the general public.

_____

   b. It is responsible for enforcing the federal Food, Drug, and Cosmetic Act.

_____

   c. It monitors the distribution of controlled substances.

_____

d. It regulates biological products like antitoxins.

___

16. Refer to the *Physician's Desk Reference (PDR)*, a common drug reference source, to find the answers to the following questions:
   a. What is the indication for the drug beclomethasone?

___

   b. List the contraindications and side effects of this drug.

___

17. Select the appropriate drug term from the following list to complete the sentences:

Antagonism	Potentiation
Contraindications	Side effect
Cumulative action	Stimulant
Depressant	Summation
Drug allergy	Synergism
Drug dependence	Therapeutic action
Drug interaction	Tolerance
Idiosyncrasy	Untoward effect

   a. An abnormal or peculiar response to a drug that is possibly caused by

   a genetic deficiency is _____.
   b. Caffeine and Ritalin are examples of drugs that exhibit a(n)

   _____ effect.
   c. A drug action caused by an immunological response to a previous

   exposure is a(n) _____ reaction.
   d. Nalaxone's desired effect on narcotics is attributed to _____

   _____.
   e. The enhancement of the effects of one drug caused by the concurrent

   administration of a second drug is _____.
   f. An undesirable effect of a drug that is harmful to the patient is a(n)

   _____.
   g. The combined action of two drugs that is greater than the sum of each

   individual agent acting independently is _____.
   h. The intense physical or emotional disturbance possibly resulting when a narcotic is withheld from a person who frequently uses it is a result of

   _____.
   i. A drug that diminishes a person's central nervous system function is a

   _____.
   j. The ability of atropine to increase the heart rate is known as the desired

   effect, or _____.
   k. The list of factors used to describe situations when medication adminis-

   tration would be harmful is the _____.

l. Concurrent administration of drugs such that one agent modifies the

actions of the other is _____.

m. A decreased response to a drug after repetitive doses, which necessitates higher doses to achieve the desired effect, is _____

_____.

n. When repeat administration of drugs results in absorption that exceeds metabolism and excretion, the increased effect that results is known as

_____.

18. List six factors that influence the rate and extent to which a drug is absorbed in the body.

    a.

    b.

    c.

    d.

    e.

    f.

19. *You need to administer acetaminophen to a child who has been vomiting repeatedly.*

What enteral route will you choose? _____

20. When giving epinephrine to an asthmatic patient, a slow and sustained effect is desirable to minimize side effects and prolong the drug's effects. You

will administer the drug by the _____ route.

21. *Your 76-year-old patient has a heart rate of 34 and a blood pressure of 70 by palpation. You wish to give atropine to increase the heart rate.* What route will you

choose? _____

22. List the four medications that may be administered via an endotracheal tube when intravenous therapy cannot be established in a critically ill patient.

    a.

    b.

    c.

    d.

23. *A 3-month-old is in hemorrhagic shock after sustaining a gunshot wound to the abdomen.* After intravenous attempts are unsuccessful, what route will you

consider for fluid volume resuscitation? _____

24. The rate of drug absorption by the pulmonary route is *faster* or *slower* than

the subcutaneous route? _____

25. List the two physiological barriers to drug distribution within the body.

    a.

    b.

26. *A 70-year-old patient is experiencing chest pain. The monitor reveals ventricular ectopy. In consultation with medical direction, you administer nitroglycerin and lidocaine.* Describe the assessment techniques you will use to determine the effects of the medications you have administered.

_____

_____

● MATH SKILLS

The following questions are a brief review of basic math skills necessary for drug dose calculation. It is intended as a refresher. If these concepts are not understood, references should be consulted or tutoring sought before proceeding to the next section.

Fractions

A fraction is part of a whole number or one number divided by another number. A fraction consists of two parts, the numerator and the denominator:

$$\frac{a}{b} \quad \begin{array}{l} a \text{ is the numerator} \\ \hline b \text{ is the denominator} \end{array}$$

The denominator indicates the number of equal parts into which the whole is separated. The numerator tells how many parts are being considered (Fig. 14-1).

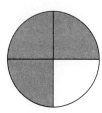

Figure 14-1

Example: $\dfrac{3}{4}$ $\quad\begin{array}{l}\text{Numerator is 3, so 3 parts are being used.}\\ \hline \text{Denominator is 4, so there are four equal parts.}\end{array}$

A fraction that has the same numerator and denominator equals the whole number 1 (Fig. 14-2).

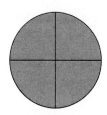

Figure 14-2

Example: $\dfrac{4}{4} = 1$

27. Identify the numerator and denominator of the following fractions:

  a. $\dfrac{7}{8} = $ _____   **b.** $\dfrac{6}{13} = $ _____

When the numerator and denominator of the fraction are multiplied by the same number, the value of the fraction remains unchanged.

Example: $\dfrac{1 \times 2}{2 \times 2} = \dfrac{2}{4} = \dfrac{1}{2}$

A fraction may be reduced to lower terms by dividing the numerator and denominator by the largest whole number that will go evenly into both of them.

Example: $\dfrac{100}{1000} = \dfrac{100 \div 100}{1000 \div 100} = \dfrac{1}{10}$

28. Reduce the following fractions to lowest terms:

a. $7/28$	**d.** $6/36$	**g.** $24/120$	**j.** $10/25$
b. $9/12$	**e.** $25/125$	**h.** $9/25$	**k.** $17/23$
c. $4/8$	**f.** $18/72$	**i.** $1000/10,000$	**l.** $16/24$

An improper fraction has a larger numerator than denominator.

Example: $\frac{8}{4}$

To change an improper fraction to a whole number, divide the numerator by the denominator:

Example: $^8/_4 = 8 \div 4 = 2$ (Whole number)

           $^7/_4 = 7 \div 4 = 1^3/_4$ (This is a mixed number because it has a whole number plus a fraction.)

29. Convert the following to whole numbers or mixed fractions.
     a. $^{75}/_5$ **b.** $^{24}/_{12}$ **c.** $^{12}/_4$ **d.** $^{15}/_6$

To change a mixed number into an improper fraction, multiply the whole number by the denominator of the fraction and add the numerator of the fraction to the result.

Example: $4\frac{1}{2} = \frac{(4 \times 2) + 1}{2} = \frac{9}{2}$

30. Change each of the following mixed numbers to improper fractions:
     a. $5^3/_8$ **b.** $1^3/_4$ **c.** $3^1/_{12}$ **d.** $15^2/_3$

To change a fraction to equivalent fractions in which both terms are larger, multiply the numerator and denominator by the same number.

Example: Enlarge $^2/_5$ to the equivalent fraction in tenths.

$$\frac{2}{5} \times \frac{2}{2} = \frac{4}{10}$$

31. Change the following fractions to the equivalent fraction indicated.
     a. $\frac{6}{8} = \frac{x}{24}$ **b.** $\frac{12}{15} = \frac{x}{60}$ **c.** $\frac{79}{100} = \frac{x}{100,000}$

To compare fractions with different denominators, find the lowest common denominator. The lowest common denominator is the smallest number that is divisible by the denominators.

Example 1:   What is the lowest common denominator of $^1/_2$, $^3/_5$, and $^7/_{10}$? The denominators are 2, 5, and 10. Because 10 is divisible by 2 and 5, it is the lowest common denominator.

Example 2:   What is the lowest common denominator of $^1/_3$ and $^2/_5$? Because 5 is not divisible by 3, multiply the larger denominator by 2, 3, 4 and so on. Each time, determine whether the product is divisible by 3:
$5 \times 2 = 10$ 10 is not divisible by 3.
$5 \times 3 = 15$ 15 is divisible by 3, so 15 is the lowest common denominator.

32. Find the lowest common denominator.
     a. $^1/_9$ and $^1/_5$ **b.** $^2/_3$ and $^1/_{12}$ **c.** $^1/_3$, $^2/_6$ and $^3/_8$
33. Circle the correct response:
     a. $^3/_8$ *is greater than, less than, or equal to* $^9/_{24}$.
     b. $^8/_9$ *is greater than, less than, or equal to* $^5/_8$.
     c. $^2/_5$ *is greater than, less than, or equal to* $^7/_{10}$.

To add or subtract fractions:
   1. **Convert all fractions to equivalent fractions using the lowest common denominator.**
   2. **Add or subtract the numerator and place over the common denominator.**
   3. **Simplify to the lowest terms.**

Example: $\frac{5}{9} + \frac{2}{6} = \frac{5(2)}{9(2)} + \frac{2(3)}{6(3)} = \frac{10}{18} + \frac{6}{18} = \frac{16}{18} \div \frac{2}{2} = \frac{8}{9}$

34. Add the following fractions and mixed numbers:
     a. $^7/_8 + ^2/_5 + ^1/_{10}$ **b.** $1^1/_4 + 2^2/_3$
35. Subtract the following fractions and mixed numbers:
     a. $1^3/_5 - ^6/_{10}$ **b.** $2^3/_4 - ^5/_6$

To multiply fractions:
   1. Change mixed numbers to improper fractions.
   2. Multiply numerators.
   3. Multiply denominators.
   4. Simplify to the lowest terms.

Example: $\dfrac{3}{4} \times \dfrac{4}{5} = \dfrac{12}{20} \div \dfrac{4}{4} = \dfrac{3}{5}$

36. Multiply the following fractions and mixed numbers:
   a. $\frac{5}{6} \times \frac{11}{13}$ c. $6\frac{7}{8} \times 2$
   b. $8\frac{1}{2} \times 3$ d. $\frac{1}{3} \times \frac{7}{8}$

To divide fractions:
   1. Change mixed numbers to improper fractions.
   2. Turn the number after the division sign (÷) upside-down.
   3. Follow the steps for multiplication of fractions.
   4. Simplify to the lowest terms.

Example: $\dfrac{4}{5} \div \dfrac{2}{3} = \dfrac{4}{5} \times \dfrac{3}{2} = \dfrac{12}{10} \div \dfrac{2}{2} = \dfrac{6}{5} = 1\dfrac{1}{5}$

37. Divide the following fractions:
   a. $\frac{3}{8} \div \frac{3}{10}$ b. $2\frac{1}{2} \div \frac{7}{11}$

Decimals

All whole numbers are to the left of the decimal; all decimal fractions are to the right of the decimal (Fig. 14-3).

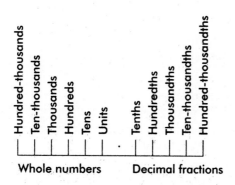

Figure 14-3

38. Write the decimal notation for the following examples:
   a. 3 and 4 tenths
   b. 5 and 35 hundredths
   c. 62 thousandths

To convert a fraction into a decimal:
   1. Divide the numerator by the denominator.
   2. Place the decimal point in the proper position.

Example: $\dfrac{3}{5} = 3 \div 5 = 5\overline{)3.0}^{\,0.6}$

39. Change the following fractions to decimals:
   a. $\frac{1}{4}$ b. $\frac{7}{25}$ c. $\frac{3}{150}$

To convert a decimal to a fraction:
   1. Write the numerator of the fraction as the numbers expressed in the decimal.
   2. Write the denominator of the fraction as the number 1 followed by the number of zeros as there are places to the right of the decimal point.

3. **Simplify the fraction to the lowest terms.**

Example: $0.234 = x$
Numerator = 234
Denominator = 1 + 3 zeros = 1000

Simplify: $\dfrac{234}{1000} = \dfrac{234}{1000} \div \dfrac{2}{2} = \dfrac{117}{500}$

40. Change the following decimals to fractions:
    a. 0.5   **b.** 3.24   **c.** 6.007

To add or subtract decimals:
    1. Line up the decimal points.
    2. Add zeros to make all decimal numbers equal 1 length.
    3. Add or subtract as with whole numbers.
    4. Place the decimal point in the sum.

Example: $0.6 + 4.23 + 1.123 = x$
Line up the decimal points: 0.6
        4.23
        1.123

Add zeros: 0.600
        4.230
        1.123
Add as whole numbers: 5.953
Place decimal point in the sum

41. Add the following decimals:
    a. $0.03 + 0.12 + 0.32$ **b.** $0.26 + 0.01 + 0.75$

42. Subtract the following decimals:
    a. $91.5 - 62.5$ **b.** $17 - 3.42$

To multiply decimals:
    1. Multiply as with whole numbers.
    2. Count the total number of decimal places in the decimals multiplied.
    3. Place the decimal point in the answer to the left of the total decimal places calculated in step 2.
    4. When multiplying a decimal by a power of ten, move the decimal point the same number of places to the right as there are zeros in the multiplier.

Example 1: $1.25 \times 3.3 = x$
        1.25 (two decimal places)
    $\times$ 3.3 (one decimal place)
        4.125 (the decimal point is placed to the left of three decimal places)

Example 2: $3.46 \times 10 = 3.4.6 = 34.6$

43. Multiply the following decimals:
    a. 3.62×0.02 **c.** 7.25×0.03 **e.** 2.9×10
    b. 27×0.04 **d.** 4.256×100 **f.** 7.052×1000

To divide decimals
    1. If the divisor (number you are dividing by) is a whole number, divide as you would with whole numbers. Place the decimal place in the answer in the same place it was in the answer to be divided.
    2. If the divisor (number you are dividing by) is a decimal, make it a whole number by moving the decimal place to the end of the divisor. Move the decimal in the number being divided by the same number of places.
    3. If the divisor is a power of ten, move the decimal point to the left as many places as there are zeros in the divisor.

Example 1: $25.5 \div 5 = 5\overline{)25.5} = 5.1$

Example 2: $25.5 \div 0.5 = 0.5\overline{)25.5} = 5\overline{)255.} = 51$

Example 3: $25.5 \div 10 = 2.55 \ (2.5.5)$

44. Divide the following:
    a. $0.25 \div 5$ **d.** $0.16 \div 0.04$
    b. $5.16 \div 2$ **e.** $14.237 \div 100$
    c. $4 \div 0.5$ **f.** $0.17 \div 10$

Rounding decimal fractions:
Most drug calculations require rounding to the hundredth or greater. This depends on the individual example. To round off, consider the number in the next position to the right. If the number is greater than or equal to 5, increase the number being considered by 1. If it is less than 5, do not increase the number being considered.

Example 1:   Round off 0.74 to the nearest tenths. Because the number in the hundredths column is less than 5, the answer will be 0.7.

Example 2:   Round off 0.24555 to the nearest hundredths. Because the number in the thousandths column is 5, the answer will be 0.25.

45. Round off the following examples to the nearest tenth:
    a. 7.6245   **b.** 0.081   **c.** 0.851
46. Round off the following examples to the nearest hundredth:
    a. 0.10423   **b.** 5.6258   **c.** 892.02975

Ratios
Ratios indicate the relationship of one quantity to another. They indicate division and may be expressed as:

$\frac{a}{b}$, a to b, or a:b

Example: 5 gallons of gas for 6 dollars means the ratio of gas to dollars is:

$\frac{5}{6}$, 5 to 6, or 5:6

47. Write the ratio for the following examples.
    a. The heart ejects approximately 5000 ml of blood every 60 seconds.
    b. Approximately 6000 cc of air is moved in and out of the lungs every 60 seconds.
    c. The intravenous line delivers 100 ml every 30 minutes.
    d. There are 100 mg of the drug in 10 ml of solution.

To simplify a ratio that compares two measures divide the denominator into the numerator to calculate unit rate.

Example: On a routine transfer we traveled 120 miles in 2 hours.

$$\text{The unit rate} = \frac{120 \text{ miles}}{2 \text{ hours}} = 60 \text{ miles per hour.}$$

48. Calculate the unit rate for each of the following (based on the examples in Question 47):
    a. How many milliliters of blood are ejected from the heart each second?
    b. How much air is moved in and out of the lungs each second?
    c. How much fluid is being delivered each minute?
    d. How many milligrams are in each milliliter.

A proportion shows the relationship between two different ratios. To determine whether a proportion is true (equivalent):
1. If the proportion is expressed as a fraction, ($\frac{1}{2} = \frac{2}{4}$), multiply the cross products and then determine whether the proportion is equivalent.

Example: $\frac{1}{2} = \frac{2}{4}$ $\frac{1}{2} \bowtie \frac{2}{4}$ $1 \times 4 = 4$ and $2 \times 2 = 4$; $4 = 4$; therefore the proportion is true.

 2. If the proportion is expressed as a ratio (2:5::4:10), multiply the two inside numbers (5 × 4 = 20) and the two outside numbers (2 × 10 = 20). 20 = 20; therefore the proportion is equivalent.

49. Determine whether each of the following proportions is true:

 a. $\frac{5}{10} = \frac{1}{2}$ **b.** $\frac{4}{6} = \frac{8}{10}$ **c.** $\frac{25}{75} = \frac{1}{3}$

To solve a proportion problem when one of the numbers is unknown (x):

 1. Use either proportion methods demonstrated previously.

 2. Make x stand alone by dividing both sides of the equation by the number on the side of x.

 3. Solve for x.

Example 1: $\frac{17}{20} = \frac{x}{100}$ $20x = 17 \times 100 = \frac{20x}{20} = \frac{17 \times 100}{20}$

      $x = \frac{17 \times 100}{20}$

      $x = 85$

Example 2: $17:20::x:100$ $20x = 17 \times 100$

      $\frac{20x}{20} = \frac{17 \times 100}{20}$

50. Solve for x in the following problems:

 a. $\frac{2}{4} = \frac{x}{6}$ **c.** $\frac{2}{3} = \frac{7}{x}$ **e.** $3:5::x:45$ **g.** $x:35::80:100$

 b. $\frac{1}{4} = \frac{x}{16}$ **d.** $\frac{5}{4} = \frac{x}{12}$ **f.** $4:9::16:x$ **h.** $1.5:3::x:18$

Simplifying a problem by canceling common elements will make problem solving easier.

Example 1: $x = \frac{12 \times 10}{20} = 6$ Zeros cancel. Then 2 divides into 12 six times

Example 2: $x = \frac{1\,mg \times 1\,ml}{1\,mg} = 1\,ml$ *mg* cancels *mg*. 1 ml is left.

51. Simplify the following problems as much as possible and then solve:

 a. $x = \frac{10 \times 150}{50}$

 b. $x = \frac{25 \times 2}{50}$

 c. $x = \frac{2500 \times 500}{20,000}$

 d. $x = \frac{1\,g \times 1\,L}{1\,g}$

 e. $x = \frac{2\,mg \times 1\,cc}{10\,mg}$

 f. $x = \frac{10\,mg \times 10\,ml}{100\,mg}$

Percentages

 Percent (%) is a portion of a whole divided by 100.

 1. To change a percent to a decimal, drop the percent sign and move the decimal two places to the left.

Example: $15.0\% = 0.15$

   2. **To change a decimal to a percent, move the decimal two places to the right and add the percent sign.**

Example: 0.76 = 76%

   3. **To change a fraction to a percent, convert it to a decimal and follow rule 2 above.**

Example: $\frac{2}{5}$ = 0.2   0.2 = 20%

52. Change the following percentages to decimals:
   a. 25%   **b.** 110%   **c.** 0.5%
53. Convert the following decimals to percentages:
   a. 0.34   **b.** 2.29   **c.** 0.07
54. Express the following as percentages:
   a. $\frac{34}{50}$ **b.** $\frac{100}{500}$ **c.** $\frac{3}{7}$
55. Rewrite the following fractions as ratios, decimals, and percentages:

Fraction	Ratio	Decimal	Percentage
a. $\frac{5}{6}$			
b. $\frac{1}{20}$			
c. $\frac{7}{33}$			

56. Solve the following:
   a. 15% of 75   **b.** 0.5% of 250

   This is the end of the refresher. Refer to reference sources listed at the end of the textbook chapter if additional practice is necessary.

● UNITS OF MEASURE AND DRUG DOSE CALCULATIONS

57. In the metric system the primary unit of volume is the (a)

   _____, the primary unit of mass (weight) is the

   (b) _____, and the primary unit of length is the

   (c) _____.
58. List the four metric weight units commonly used in the prehospital environment, beginning with the largest and ending with the smallest.
   a.
   b.
   c.
   d.
59. Each of the units listed in Question 58 differs in value from the next unit

   by _____.
60. To convert from one unit to the next smallest unit in Question 58, one must

   move the decimal point three places to the right or left? _____
61. To convert from one unit to the previous unit (example unit 58d to unit 58c), one must move the decimal point 3 places to the right or left?

   _____
62. Convert the following units of weight to the units indicated.
   a. 2 kg = _____ g   **e.** 400 mcg = _____ mg
   b. 4 mg = _____ mcg   **f.** 350 mg = _____ g
   c. 2 g = _____ mg   **g.** 0.25 mg = _____ mcg
   d. 600 mg = _____ kg   **h.** 12.5 g = _____ mg

63. Convert the following units of volume to the units indicated.
    a. 1 cc = _____ ml   c. 250 ml = _____ L
    b. 10 ml = _____ cc   d. 0.33 L = _____ ml

64. The primary unit of mass in the apothecary system is the _____

   _____.

65. The primary unit of volume in the apothecary system is the _____

   _____.

66. If the physician orders acetaminophen gr X, how many milligrams will

    you give? _____

67. *Your patient has chest pain and medical direction orders nitroglyc-erin gr $^1/150$. How many milligrams will you administer?*

    (a) _____ *When it is time for a second nitroglycerin, the patient's blood pressure is slightly low, so this time the physician orders nitroglycerin gr $^1/200$. How many milligrams will you give?*

    (b) _____.

68. Convert the following measures in the household system to the units indicated:
    a. 1 T = _____ t   d. 1 gl = _____ qt
    b. 1 lb = _____ oz   e. 1 f oz = _____ T
    c. 1 pt = _____ oz   f. 1 c = _____ f oz

69. Convert the following measures in the household system to the appropriate metric units:
    a. 1 tsp = _____ ml   d. 1 qt = _____ ml
    b. 1 T = _____ ml   e. 22 lb = _____ kg
    c. 1 f oz = _____ ml   f. 110 lb = _____ kg

70. Convert the following measures to the appropriate units indicated:
    a. *A patient's family tells you that he lost about a cup of blood from a head wound.* You will relay to medical direction that the estimated blood loss is approximately _____ ml
    b. *A patient vomits roughly a quart of coffee-grounds emesis.* This is equal to ___ ml
    c. *You give the patient 1 ounce or* _____ *ml of syrup of ipecac. This will be followed by 16 oz of warm water.* This is equal to _____ ml of water.
    d. *A parent reads a drug label and instead of administering 2 ml of a drug, accidentally gives 2 oz of a drug.* How many milliliters in excess of the prescribed dose did they give? _____ ml
    e. The human body normally contains about 5 L of blood, or _____ qt.
    f. *A pregnant woman states that her membranes have ruptured and about a pint of amniotic fluid leaked out.* This is equal to _____ ml.
    g. *A premature newborn infant you have just delivered weighs 2 pounds, or* _____ kg (_____ g).

71. Identify the following information from the drug label or package in Fig. 14-4.

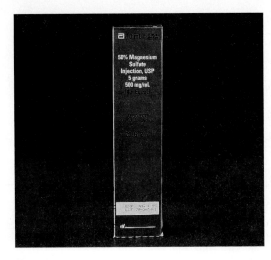

**50% Magnesium
Sulfate
Injection, USP
5 grams
500 mg/mL**

Figure 14-4

a. Drug name:
b. Expiration date:
c. Total volume:
d. Total drug:
e. Concentration of drug:

72. Convert the following drug concentrations into the total number of grams:
a. Calcium chloride 10% solution = _____ g in 100 ml.
b. Epinephrine 1:1000 solution = _____ g in 1000 ml.
c. Magnesium sulfate 10% solution = _____ g in 100 ml.
d. Epinephrine 1:10,000 solution = _____ g in 10,000 ml.
e. Lidocaine 0.4% solution = _____ g in 100 ml.
f. Mannitol 25% solution = _____ g in 100 ml.
g. Dextrose 50% solution = _____ g in 100 ml.

73. Calculate the concentration per milliliter of the following drugs using the formula: Concentration = Total dose of drug (mg) ÷ Total volume (ml). For example, a 10-ml vial of lidocaine contains 100 mg of the drug. Concentration = 100 mg ÷ 10 ml = 10 mg/ml.
a. A 40-mg vial of furosemide is in a 4-ml vial. Concentration = _____.
b. A 10-ml vial of epinephrine contains 1 mg of the drug. Concentration = _____.
c. You have 25 g of D50W in 50 ml. Concentration = _____.
d. A 2-ml vial of diphenhydramine contains 50 mg of the drug. Concentration = _____.
e. There is 1 g of lidocaine in a 250-ml bag. Concentration = _____.

74. Calculate the total dose of a drug to be administered:
a. Lidocaine 1 mg/kg is ordered for a 100-kg patient who is having many premature ventricular contractions each minute. Dose = _____ mg.
b. Give bretylium 5 mg/kg to a 70-kg man in ventricular fibrillation. Dose = _____ mg.
c. Push sodium bicarbonate 1 mEq/kg during a lengthy cardiac arrest. The patient weighs 80 kg. Dose = _____ mEq.
d. Hang a dopamine drip at 5 mcg/kg/minute on a hypotensive patient who weighs 50 kg. Dose = _____ mcg/minute.
e. Give epinephrine 0.01 mg/kg to an 11-lb child who is in cardiopulmonary arrest. Dose = _____ mg.
f. Administer mannitol 1 g/kg to a 176-lb patient with rising intracranial pressure. Dose = _____ g.

75. Solve the following problems using the formula:

$$\text{Volume (x)} = \frac{\text{Desired dose (D)} \times \text{Volume on Hand (Q)}}{\text{Dose on hand (H)}.}$$

   a. You wish to give furosemide 20 mg. It is supplied in a 4-ml vial containing 40 mg of the drug. Volume = _____ ml.

   b. You wish to administer morphine 3 mg. You have a 1-ml Tubex containing 10 mg of the drug. Volume = _____ ml.

   c. You wish to give administer aminophylline 150 mg. You have a 10-ml vial containing 250 mg of the drug.7

   d. You must give 2.5 mg of diazepam. It is supplied in a 2-ml vial containing 10 mg. Volume = _____ ml.

   e. You have 50 mg of meperidine in a 1-ml Tubex. You need to give 12.5 mg of the drug. Volume = _____ ml.

   f. Your patient needs 0.3 mg of epinephrine (1:1000). You have a 1-ml vial containing 1 mg. Volume = _____ ml.

   g. Your patient needs 0.5 mg of dopamine. You have a 500-ml bag containing 400 mg of the drug. Volume = _____ ml.

76. Solve the following drug dose problems using the equation: Desired dose: Desired volume::Dosage on Hand:Volume on hand.

   Example: Give 50 mg of procainamide. It is supplied in a 10 ml-vial containing 1000 mg.

50 mg:x = 1000 mg:10 ml	Set up the ratio.
1000 mg × x = 50 mg × 10 ml	Multiply inside (means) and then outside (extremes) numbers.

$$\frac{1000 \text{ mg} \times x}{1000 \text{ mg}} = \frac{50 \text{ mg} \times 10 \text{ ml}}{1000 \text{ mg}}$$

$$x = \frac{50 \text{ mg} \times 10 \text{ ml}}{1000 \text{ mg}} \qquad \text{Solve for x.}$$

x = 0.5 ml

   a. Administer adenosine 6 mg. It is supplied in a 2-ml vial containing 6 mg of the drug. Desired volume = _____ ml.

   b. Administer diphenhydramine 25 mg. You have a 2-ml vial containing 50 mg of the drug. Desired volume = _____ ml.

   c. Give 2.5 mg of verapamil. It is supplied in a 2-ml vial containing 5 mg of the drug. Desired volume = _____ ml.

   d. Give 1000 mg of mannitol. You have a 20% solution. Desired volume = _____ ml.

77. Calculate the following problems using any of the methods demonstrated. Ensure that all units are compatible. If the dosage is given in mg/kg, make the appropriate calculation.

   a. You wish to give lidocaine 1 mg/kg to a 75-kg man. It is supplied in a 10-ml syringe containing 100 mg of the drug. How many milliliters will you administer?

   b. You must give bretylium 10 mg/kg to a 60-kg woman. You have a 10-ml Tubex containing 500 mg of the drug. How much will you give?

   c. You must give 0.5 mg of glucagon to a 90-kg patient. When you mix it up you have 1 mg in 1 ml of solution. How much will you give?

   d. You have diluted your phenobarbital so that you have 130 mg in 10 ml. You need to give 100 mg. The patient weighs 100 kg. How much will you give?

   e. You must give 1 g/kg of mannitol. The patient weighs 70 kg. You have a 20% solution. How many milliliters will you give?

   f. You need to administer 150 mg of aminophylline. You have 500 ml in a 20 ml ampule. How many milliliters will you give?

   g. Your patient needs a dopamine drip at 5 mcg/kg/min. He weighs 100 kg. You have 400 mg of dopamine in 500 ml of D5W. How many milliliters per minute will you administer and at how many drops/minute will you set the microdrip intravenous line?

h. You wish to administer a bretylium drip at 2 mg/min. You have 1 g of bretylium in a 250-ml bag of D5W. How many milliliters will you give each minute and how fast will you regulate your microdrip tubing to deliver this rate?

i. You wish to administer a lidocaine drip at 2 mg/min. You have an intravenous bag containing a 0.4% solution of lidocaine. How many milliliters will you give each minute and how fast will you set your microdrip tubing to deliver this rate?

78. For each of the following situations, calculate the correct volume of solution to be administered using the drug package information illustrated.

a. Give 0.5 mg of atropine (Fig. 14-5). Desired volume = _____ ml.

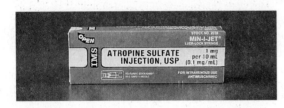

Figure 14-5

b. Give 0.3 mg of epinephrine (Fig. 14-6). Desired volume = _____ ml.

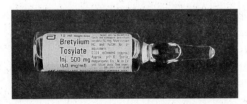

Figure 14-6

c. Give 5 mg/kg bretylium to a 70-kg patient (Fig. 14-7). Desired volume = _____ ml.

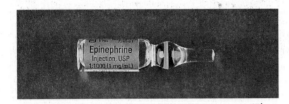

Figure 14-7

d. Give lidocaine 0.5 mg/kg to an 80-kg patient (Fig. 14-8). Desired volume = _____ ml.

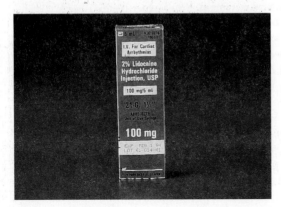

Figure 14-8

79. After determining the correct volume of drug to be administered in the following examples, shade the corresponding syringe in Fig. 14-9 to illustrate the proper amount to be given.

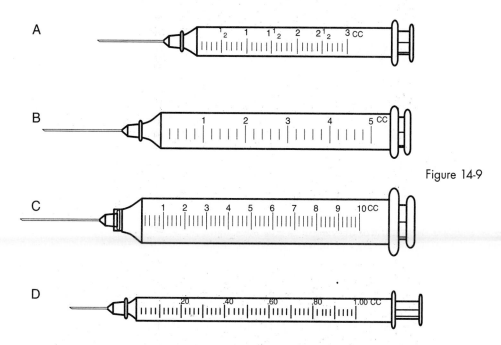

Figure 14-9

a. Adenosine 6 mg must be given to a patient with paroxysmal supraventricular tachycardia. You have a 2-ml vial containing 3 mg/ml of the drug. How many milliliters will you give?

b. Your patient has had a seizure and needs phenytoin 200 mg. You have a 5-ml vial containing 250 mg of the drug. How much will you give?

c. You have a 10-ml vial of bretylium containing 50 mg/ml of the drug. A total of 350 mg is indicated for your patient, who is in ventricular fibrillation. What volume will you administer?

d. You wish to administer epinephrine 0.3 mg to a patient experiencing an asthma attack. It is supplied in a 1-ml ampule containing 1 mg of a 1:1000 solution of the drug. How much will you give?

● DRUG ADMINISTRATION

80. List at least 10 general steps to be taken when administering *any* drug to avoid errors.

a.

b.

c.

d.

e.

f.

g.

h.

i.

j.

81. Complete the following sentences regarding drug administration routes: Oral medications should be given with the patient in the (a) _____ position. The drug should be swallowed

with (b) _____ ounces of fluid to ensure it reaches

the (c) _____. Sublingual medications should be

placed under the (d) _____ and allowed

to (e) _____. They should not be

(f) _____ because this will delay action of the drug.

Parenteral drug administration may cause (g) _____,

(h) _____, or (i) _____. The
correct needle length and size is important. For subcutaneous injections, a

(j) _____ -inch, (k) _____ -
gauge needle should be used. When administering an intramuscular shot, a

(l) _____ -inch, (m) _____
-gauge needle would be selected. To minimize the risk of needle stick injury,
the paramedic should understand that the use of two-handed needle recapping

is (n) _____. Also, all sharp items, including needles

should be placed in (o) _____. When withdrawing medica-
tion from a multidose vial, the paramedic should cleanse the stopper with alcohol

and then inject the same amount of (p) _____ as
drug to be withdrawn before aspirating the appropriate amount of medicine into
the syringe. To minimize the risk of glass particles entering the injection when

aspirating from a glass ampule, a (q) _____ needle
should be used. Subcutaneous injections should be administered at a

(r) _____ -degree angle. Sites of administration for this

route include (s) _____, _____,

and _____. Intramuscular injections should be ad-

ministered at a (t) _____ -degree angle. Administra-

tion sites for this route include the (u) _____,

_____, and _____. To prevent

drug effects on the rescuer, (v) _____ should always
be worn when administering transdermal medicines. To ensure maximal
absorption of drugs administered by the endotracheal route, dilution with

at least (w) _____ ml of fluid is

recommended. Two advantages of drugs administered by inhalation are

(x) _____ and fewer _____.

82. Circle the appropriate response regarding drug effects in children.

    a. The blood brain barrier in infants is *less/more* effective than in adults; therefore the central nervous system effects of drugs will be *less/more*.

    b. The newborn has a(n) *decreased/increased* ability to metabolize drugs; therefore drug toxicity is *less/more* likely to occur.

83. List three physiological factors that may result in altered drug absorption, distribution, biotransformation, or elimination in the older adult.

    a.

    b.

    c.

84. *You are called to a sparsely furnished, one-room apartment to care for a 79-year-old woman complaining of difficulty breathing. She states that she has a history of heart disease and "swelling," and she hands you a sack of empty medication bottles that contained furosemide, digoxin, and potassium. She thinks she last took them approximately 5 or 6 days ago.* Discuss three possible reasons for the patient's medication noncompliance.

    a.

    b.

    c.

● DRUG CLASSIFICATIONS

85. When given the following description and drug name, identify the *drug group* to which it belongs and give *one additional example* of another drug from the same group.

    a. *Your patient says he takes lorazepam (Ativan) to help him relax.*

        Drug group: _____   Example: _____

    b. *You arrive in the emergency department with a 65-year-old woman experiencing an acute myocardial infarction. Immediately, the emergency department staff administers tissue plasminogen activator in an attempt to dissolve the clot.*

        Drug group: _____   Example: _____

    c. *Before your Mediterranean cruise, you take dimenhydrinate (Dramamine) to prevent seasickness.*

        Drug group: _____   Example: _____

    d. *During a cardiopulmonary arrest or in selected cases of shock, drugs such as epinephrine (Adrenalin) may be used to stimulate the heart.*

        Drug group: _____   Example: _____

    e. *Your 45-year-old male patient is complaining of chest pain. His only home medications are minoxidil (Loniten) and hydrochlorothiazide (Hydrodiuril) for hypertension.*

        Drug group: _____   Example: _____

    f. *An older patient is taking digoxin (Lanoxin) for his "weak heart."*

        Drug group: _____   Example: _____

    g. *A 30-year-old patient with a seizure disorder is taking phenobarbital (Luminal).*

        Drug group: _____   Example: _____

    h. *A 52-year-old hospice patient is taking hydromorphone (Dilaudid) to control his pain.*

        Drug group: _____   Example: _____

i. *Diltiazem (Cardizem) is used by a patient who states that she takes it to control a fast heart rhythm.*

Drug group: _____   Example: _____

j. *A person at risk for developing clots that may cause heart attack or stroke may be prescribed dipyridamole (Persantine).*

Drug group: _____   Example: _____

k. *Asthmatics may have a large number of home medicines that may include isoetharine hydrochloride (Bronkosol) or theophylline (Bronkodyl).*

Drug group: _____   Example: _____

l. *All parents are advised to keep on hand a medicine that will induce vomiting in case their child ingests a harmful substance for which vomiting is indicated.*

Drug group: _____   Example: _____

m. *You will have increased vigilance for evidence of bleeding if a patient tells you he is taking warfarin sodium (Coumadin).*

Drug group: _____   Example: _____

n. *A 35-year-old patient is experiencing complications secondary to an outpatient surgical procedure. Her only home medication is pentazocine (Talwin).*

Drug group: _____   Example: _____

o. *Asthmatic patients may be on a variety of drugs besides bronchodilators in an attempt to control their disease. Examples of these include cromolyn sodium (Intal), beclomethasone dipropionate (Vanceril Inhaler), and ipratropium (Atrovent).*

Drug group: _____   Example: _____

● STUDENT SELF-EVALUATION

86. Any substance taken by mouth; injected into a muscle, blood vessel, or cavity of the body; or applied topically to treat or prevent a disease or condition is a(n):
  a. Antidote   **c.** Parenteral
  b. Drug   **d.** Vaccine

87. Meperidine is regulated under the Controlled Substance Act of 1970 and is a Schedule ___ drug.
  a. I   **c.** III
  b. II   **d.** IV

88. The blood-brain barrier and placental barrier will allow passage of only:
  a. Antibiotics   **c.** Undissociated drugs
  b. Lipid-soluble drugs   **d.** Water-soluble drugs

89. The measurement of the relative safety of a drug is the:
  a. Biological half-life   **c.** Lethal dose 50
  b. Effective dose 50   **d.** Therapeutic index

90. You wish to administer mannitol 500 mg/kg to a 100-kg woman. You have a 10% solution of the drug. How many milliliters will you give?
  a. 2   **c.** 20
  b. 5   **d.** 500

91. Which of the following drugs is *not* recommended for administration by endotracheal tube?
  a. Epinephrine   **c.** Lidocaine
  b. Hydroxyzine   **d.** Naloxone

92. Which of the following drug administration routes will deliver the most rapid effects?
  a. Oral   **c.** Subcutaneous
  b. Intramuscular   **d.** Transtracheal

93. *Your patient is in profound shock secondary to myocardial infarction.* The route of choice for drug administration will be:
    a. Intramuscular
    b. Intravenous
    c. By mouth
    d. Subcuteneous

94. Which of the following is an opioid antagonist:
    a. Butorphanol tartrate
    b. Naloxone hydrochloride
    c. Oxycodone hydrochloride
    d. Pentazocine hydrochloride

95. All of the following drugs have anticonvulsant properties, *except:*
    a. Diazepam
    b. Magnesium sulfate
    c. Nalbuphine
    d. Phenytoin

96. An indirect-acting cholinergic drug that may be used in the management of poisoning from atropine is:
    a. Glucagon
    b. Lorazepam
    c. Physostigmine
    d. Verapamil

97. What is the chief neurotransmittor for the parasympathetic nervous system?:
    a. Acetylcholine
    b. Adrenalin
    c. Aramine
    d. Norepinephrine

98. Stimulation of the beta$_2$ adrenergic receptors will cause:
    a. Negative inotropic effect on the heart
    b. Positive inotropic effect on the heart
    c. Bronchiolar dilation
    d. Peripheral vasoconstriction

99. Epinephrine has:
    a. Alpha effects only
    b. Beta effects only
    c. Alpha and beta effects
    d. Neither alpha nor beta effects

100. Drugs that increase the contractility of the heart have a positive _____ effect:
    a. Chronotropic
    b. Cholinergic
    c. Dromotropic
    d. Inotropic

101. *You are called to the home of an older man complaining of dizziness, nausea, vomiting, weakness, and yellow vision. When questioned about his home medications, he states that he takes a small tablet to help his "weak heart." His pulse is 45/min. You suspect he is suffering from:*
    a. Digoxin overdose
    b. Isopranolol overdose
    c. Tricyclic antidepressant overdose
    d. Verapamil overdose

102. Which of the following is a group IV antidysrhythmic drug?
    a. Bretylium tosylate
    b. Lidocaine
    c. Procainamide
    d. Verapamil

103. The primary mechanism by which antihypertensives reduce blood pressure is by decreasing:
    a. Cardiac output
    b. Intravascular blood volume
    c. Myocardial contractility
    d. Peripheral vascular resistance

104. Which of the following drugs acts by dissolving a clot that has already formed?
    a. Aspirin
    b. Coumadin
    c. Heparin
    d. Streptokinase

105. An example of a beta$_2$ specific bronchodilator is:
    a. Albuterol
    b. Aminophylline
    c. Ephedrine
    d. Isoproterenol

106. All of the following are indications for antihistamines, *except:*
    a. Allergic reactions
    b. Asthma
    c. Motion sickness
    d. Nausea and vomiting

107. Which of the following is true about insulin?
    a. It is secreted by the adrenal glands.
    b. It is secreted only during stress.
    c. It will increase the use of fat for fuel.
    d. It will move glucose into the cells.

108. Which of the following is an antiemetic?
  a. Bretylium tosylate (Bretylol)
  b. Hydroxyzine pamoate (Vistaril)
  c. Meperidine (Demerol)
  d. Syrup of ipecac

DIVISION TWO REVIEW TEST

1. Which of the following suffixes means "causing"?
   a. -asthenia   c. -pathy
   b. -genic   d. -phasia
2. The proper abbreviation for *chief complaint* is:
   a. cc   c. c/o
   b. CC   d. CHF
3. 1 g is equal to _____ mg.
   a. 0.001   c. 100
   b. 1   d. 1000
4. Which of the following is *not* part of the axial skeleton?
   a. Head   c. Pelvis
   b. Neck   d. Thorax
5. The cellular structure responsible for energy production in the cell is the:
   a. Lysosome   c. Nucleus
   b. Mitochondrion   d. Ribosome
6. The tissue type that forms blood, bone, and cartilage is _____ tissue.
   a. Connective   c. Muscular
   b. Epithelial   d. Nervous
7. Which of the following represents the correct number of vertebra per region of the spinal column?
   a. 5 cervical, 12 thoracic, 7 lumbar, 1 sacral, 1 coccygeal
   b. 7 cervical, 12 thoracic, 5 lumbar, 1 sacral, 1 coccygeal
   c. 5 cervical, 1 thoracic, 12 lumbar, 7 sacral, 1 coccygeal
   d. 12 cervical, 7 thoracic, 1 lumbar, 5 sacral, 1 coccygeal
8. The second rib joins the sternum laterally at the junction of the manubrium and body of the sternum. This junction is known as the:
   a. Jugular notch   c. Tragus
   b. Sternal angle   d. Xiphoid process
9. Joints that contain fluid that permits greater movement are known as _____ joints.
   a. Cartilaginous   c. Symphysis
   b. Fibrous   d. Synovial
10. A hockey player has sustained a shoulder injury that causes pain when the affected arm is moved toward the body. He has pain during _____ of the arm.
    a. Abduction   c. Pronation
    b. Adduction   d. Supination
11. The region of the brain stem responsible for regulation of heart rate, blood vessel diameter, breathing, and vomiting is the:
    a. Medulla   c. Pons
    b. Midbrain   d. Thalamus
12. Nerve pathways that transmit information away from the spinal cord are _____ nerves.
    a. Afferent   c. Dorsal
    b. Efferent   d. Ganglia
13. The division of the autonomic nervous system that prepares the body for vegetative functions such as digestion and urination is the _____ division.
    a. Adrenergic   c. Parasympathetic
    b. Cerebellar   d. Sympathetic
14. The bicuspid valve that separates the left atrium and ventricle is the _____ valve.
    a. Aortic   c. Pulmonic
    b. Mitral   d. Tricuspid

15. The lymphatic system performs all the following functions, *except:*
    a. Maintenance of fluid balance in tissues
    b. Absorption of fats from the digestive tract
    c. Infection defense system
    d. Carrying of nutrients from the blood to tissues
16. The apex of the lungs extends:
    a. To the sternal angle   c. Above the clavicle
    b. To the manubrium   d. Just below the second rib
17. The most inferior cartilage of the larynx is unpaired and forms a complete ring. It is the _____ cartilage.
    a. Arytenoid   c. Cuneiform
    b. Cricoid   d. Thyroid
18. Which of the following digestive juices is secreted in the stomach?
    a. Amylase   c. Bile
    b. Bicarbonate   d. Hydrochloric acid
19. The kidneys play a role in all of the following, *except:*
    a. Removal of wastes from the blood
    b. Control of red blood cell production
    c. Balance of body fluid volume
    d. Vitamin K metabolism
20. The inferior portion of the uterus is the:
    a. Cervix   c. Ovary
    b. Fundus   d. Vagina
21. Photoreceptor cells within the eye that receive visual impulses are in the:
    a. Cornea   c. Retina
    b. Iris   d. Sclera
22. Which of the following is *not* a component of the primary survey?
    a. Airway   c. Breathing
    b. Blood pressure   d. Level of consciousness
23. Physical findings that may indicate life-threatening breathing difficulties include all of the following, *except:*
    a. Asymmetrical chest movement
    b. Cyanosis of the lips
    c. Distended neck veins
    d. Muffled heart sounds
24. A heart rate of less than 60 per minute is defined as:
    a. Bradycardia   c. Normocardia
    b. Irregular   d. Tachycardia
25. *You are called to the scene of an automobile accident. You find a victim who was thrown from the car and who has a nearly amputated lower leg that is spurting bright red blood. Her respirations are absent.* Your priorities of care, in the proper order, will be to:
    a. Immobilize cervical spine, open airway, assess and establish respirations, and control bleeding.
    b. Open airway, assess and establish respirations, immobilize cervical spine, and control bleeding.
    c. Control bleeding, immobilize cervical spine, assess and establish respirations, and open airway.
    d. Control bleeding, immobilize cervical spine, open airway, and assess and establish respirations.
26. Skin color in a patient with advanced liver problems will typically be:
    a. Cyanotic   c. Red
    b. Pale   d. Yellow
27. Abnormally deep, very rapid sighing respirations characteristic of diabetic ketoacidosis are _____ respirations:
    a. Ataxic   c. Cheyne-Stokes
    b. Biot's   d. Kussmaul

28. High-pitched, musical airway noises caused by narrowing of the small airways are:
    a. Crackles   c. Rhonchi
    b. Rales   d. Wheezes
29. Which of the following organs is *not* located in the right upper quadrant of the abdomen?
    a. Duodenum   c. Gallbladder
    b. Liver   d. Stomach
30. What is the proper sequence for examination of the abdomen?
    a. Auscultation, inspection, palpation
    b. Inspection, palpation, auscultation
    c. Inspection, auscultation, palpation
    d. Auscultation, palpation, inspection
31. If deformity and point tenderness are noted on examination of the pelvis, the paramedic should consider:
    a. Appendicitis   c. Ruptured ectopic pregnancy
    b. Internal hemorrhage   d. Sudden precipitous delivery
32. To evaluate muscle strength in the lower extremities, the patient should be instructed to:
    a. Walk a straight line unassisted for 20 feet.
    b. Push the soles of his feet against the paramedic's palms.
    c. Flex and extend the feet and lower and upper legs.
    d. Lift and hold both legs in the air while lying supine.
33. Which of the following patient interview questions would be most likely to yield the best information?
    a. Is your pain pretty bad?
    b. Can you tell me about the pain?
    c. Does the pain go down your arm?
    d. Would you describe this as a sharp pain?
34. The mnemonic *AMPLE* used to obtain a patient history includes which of the following elements?
    a. Allergies, medicines, past history, last meal, events before the incident
    b. Alternative problems, medicines, past history, last meal, events before the incident
    c. Allergies, medical history, personal physician, last meal, events before the incident
    d. Allergies, medical history, personal physician, last medications, events before the illness
35. *You are called to care for a deaf patient with abdominal pain who is in obvious distress.* When obtaining the patient history, the paramedic should:
    a. Stay in full view of the patient when speaking.
    b. Transport because no communication will be possible.
    c. Obtain the history from the family rather than the patient.
    d. Shout loudly into the patient's ear.
36. Movement of gas into the lungs is due to:
    a. An increase in atmospheric pressure
    b. A decrease in atmospheric pressure
    c. An increase in intrapulmonic pressure
    d. A decrease in intrapulmonic pressure
37. All of the following are accessory muscles that aid in labored breathing, *except*:
    a. Abdominal muscles
    b. Posterior neck and back muscles
    c. Sternocleidomastoid muscles
    d. Gluteus maximus muscles

38. The partial pressure of oxygen at sea level is:
a. 21%   c. 160 torr
b. 79%   d. 600 torr

39. Oxygen and carbon dioxide pass from the alveoli to capillaries by:
a. Active transport   c. Filtration
b. Diffusion   d. Osmosis

40. Which of the following fluids is *most* acidic?
a. Beer, pH 3.0   c. Blood, pH 7.4
b. Coffee, pH 5.0   d. Ammonia, pH 11.0

41. All of the following are situations in which carbon dioxide production will increase, *except:*
a. Exercise   c. Anaerobic metabolism
b. Sleep   d. Fever

42. The area of the brain responsible for "quiet, unlabored" involuntary respiration is the:
a. Hypothalamus   c. Midbrain
b. Medulla   d. Pons

43. Each of the following modified respiratory patterns protects the respiratory system, *except:*
a. Coughing   c. Sighing
b. Hiccoughing   d. Sneezing

44. What maneuver may be used to minimize the risk of aspiration?
a. Place the patient on pulse oximetry.
b. Bag mask vigorously with high volumes of air.
c. Place the patient in a lateral recumbent position.
d. Sedate the patient with diazepam.

45. *A nursing home aide states that she found her patient unconscious with very slow, snoring respirations.* What is the first intervention?
a. Insert an oropharyngeal airway if there is no gag reflex.
b. Nasotracheally intubate with a 7.0 tube.
c. Hyperventilate with a bag-valve-mask for 2 minutes.
d. Perform the chin-lift/head-tilt airway maneuver.

46. If the endotracheal tube advances too far, it may be positioned in the:
a. Esophagus   c. Left mainstem bronchus
b. Trachea   d. Right mainstem bronchus

47. Which of the following complications may occur with endotracheal intubation?
a. Bradycardia   c. Esophageal intubation
b. Tachycardia   d. All of the above

48. Nasotracheal intubation is best performed on the patient who:
a. Is apneic   c. Has acute epiglottitis
b. Has basilar skull fractures d. Has oral trauma

49. When intubating an infant or young child's trachea, the paramedic should remember that:
a. An uncuffed tube will be necessary.
b. The child's epiglottis is shorter and fatter than the adult's.
c. The smaller tongue will make intubation easier.
d. Right mainstem intubation is uncommon.

50. Which of the following physiological factors increases the likelihood that an older patient will develop respiratory failure?
a. Decreased thoracic rigidity   c. Greater alveolar surface
b. Increased pCO_2 d. Decreased elastic recoil

51. Anaerobic metabolism results in the production of:
a. Greater energy than aerobic metabolism
b. Water and carbon dioxide
c. Lactic acid
d. Enzymes destructive to the cell

52. A decrease in peripheral vascular resistance causes the container size of the body to _____ and the blood pressure to _____.
   a. Decrease, decrease
   c. Increase, increase
   b. Decrease, increase
   d. Increase, decrease
53. The blood cells responsible for transportation of approximately 99% of the oxygen carried to the body tissues are the:
   a. Erythrocytes
   c. Plasma proteins
   b. Leukocytes
   d. Platelets
54. Which of the following electrolytes is found predominantly in the *intracellular* fluid?
   a. Bicarbonate
   c. Potassium
   b. Chloride
   d. Sodium
55. One thousandth of the molecular weight divided by the charges on an ion is expressed as:
   a. mEq
   c. ml
   b. mg
   d. moles
56. *Your patient is a 65-year-old woman who has had vomiting and diarrhea for 3 days. Skin turgor is poor, and the patient states that she has lost 10 pounds and has not urinated in 12 hours.* The fluid of choice for this patient would be:
   a. D5W
   c. 0.45% normal saline
   b. 0.9% normal saline
   d. D50W
57. *You are called to transport a 56-year-old patient with a history of renal failure who missed his last dialysis session. He is complaining of nausea, abdominal distention, weakness, and irritability.* You suspect:
   a. Hypercalcemia
   c. Hypernatremia
   b. Hyperkalemia
   d. Hyperuria
58. Prolonged diarrhea may result in all of the following electrolyte disturbances, *except:*
   a. Hypocalcemia
   c. Hypomagnesemia
   b. Hypokalemia
   d. Hypernatremia
59. The patient with metabolic acidosis and adequate spontaneous ventilations will typically have:
   a. Decreased pH and decreased pCO_2
   b. Decreased pH and increased pCO_2
   c. Increased pH and decreased pCO_2
   d. Increased pH and increased pCO_2
60. Sympathetic vasoconstriction during shock will result in:
   a. Tachycardia
   c. Increased container size
   b. Pupil dilation
   d. Pale, cool skin
61. Which of the following hormonal mechanisms increases urine production?
   a. Adrenal medullary mechanism
   b. Atrial natriuretic mechanism
   c. Renin-angiotensin-aldosterone mechanism
   d. Vasopressin mechanism
62. *Your patient was stabbed in the abdomen 20 minutes ago. Vital signs are blood pressure, 80/50 mm Hg; pulse, 136/min; and respirations, 26/min. He is anxious and very pale.* He is probably in which stage of shock?
   a. Compensated
   c. Transitional
   b. Irreversible
   d. Uncompensated
63. Which of the following fluids is a colloid solution?
   a. Dextran
   c. Lactated Ringer's solution
   b. 0.45% sodium chloride
   d. Normal saline
64. Which of the following blood recipients could safely be given type AB blood?
   a. Type A
   c. Type AB
   b. Type B
   d. Type O

65. *Your patient has fallen 30 feet from scaffolding and is anxious and confused and in obvious shock.* Which of the following indicates your priorities of care, in the proper order?
    a. Rapid transport, oxygen, and intravenous therapy
    b. Oxygen, intravenous therapy, and rapid transport
    c. Intravenous therapy, rapid transport, and oxygen
    d. Oxygen, rapid transport, and intravenous therapy
66. A 200-ml fluid challenge is to be infused over 20 minutes. The drop factor is 10 drops/ml. How fast will you run it?
    a. 1 drop/min   c. 100 drops/min
    b. 33 drops/min   d. 400 drops/min
67. Tylenol is the _____ name of a drug.
    a. Chemical   c. Official
    b. Generic   d. Trade
68. A warning on a drug label that administration of the drug in pregnancy will be very harmful is a(n):
    a. Antagonism   c. Side effect
    b. Contraindication   d. Untoward effect
69. 1 kg = _____ lb
    a. 0.45   c. 2.5
    b. 2.2   d. 4.5
70. 1 g = _____ mg
    a. 0.001   c. 100
    b. 0.01   d. 1000
71. *You want to give aminophylline 350 mg to your asthmatic patient. You have a 10 cc vial containing 500 mg of the drug.* How many cc will you give?
    a. 5   c. 10
    b. 7   d. 14
72. *You wish to give dopamine 10 mcg/kg/min. to your 80-kg patient. You have 400 mg of dopamine in 250 cc D5W.* How fast will you regulate the drip rate on your microdrip?
    a. 3 drops/min   c. 30 drops/min
    b. 8 drops/min   d. 77 drops/min
73. Which of the following is true regarding intramuscular injections?
    a. They should be given at a 45-degree angle.
    b. They should be given into the fatty tissue.
    c. Up to 5 cc may be given by this route.
    d. The preferred site is the abdomen.
74. Benzodiazepines have all of the following actions, *except:*
    a. Analgesic   c. Muscle relaxant
    b. Anticonvulsant   d. Sedative-hypnotic
75. An example of a cholinergic blocking agent is:
    a. Atropine   c. Propranolol
    b. Naloxone   d. Succinylcholine
76. The vagus nerve has its primary effect on:
    a. The parasympathetic nervous system
    b. The sympathetic nervous system
    c. The blood vessels
    d. The cerebrum and cerebellum
77. Stimulation of the adrenergic receptors will result in:
    a. Increased heart rate, increased gastrointestinal activity, and increased urination
    b. Decreased heart rate, increased gastrointestinal activity, and pupil constriction
    c. Increased heart rate, decreased gastrointestinal activity, and pupil dilation

    d. Decreased heart rate, decreased gastrointestinal activity, and pupil dilation

78. Because propranolol is a beta antagonist, it may cause:
    a. Bronchial dilation   **c.** Ventricular tachycardia
    b. Hypertension   **d.** Bradycardia

79. An example of a diuretic drug is:
    a. Aldactone   **c.** Hydralazine hydrochloride
    b. Captopril   **d.** Metoprolol

80. Nonspecific beta-adrenergic agents used to treat asthma are likely to cause what side effect?
    a. Bronchodilation
    b. Central nervous system depression
    c. Heart rate increase
    d. Skeletal muscle relaxation

DIVISION THREE
TRAUMA

CHAPTER 15
TRAUMA

● READING ASSIGNMENT
Chapter 15, pp. 398-483, in *Mosby's Paramedic Textbook*

● OBJECTIVES
As a paramedic, you should be able to:
1. Describe the immediate, early, and late distribution of trauma deaths.
2. Correlate the mechanism of injury with patient assessment based on an understanding of the kinematics of trauma.
3. List the critical steps in assessing a multiple-systems trauma patient.
4. Describe the pathophysiology, assessment, and management of patients with maxillofacial trauma.
5. Describe the pathophysiology, assessment, and management of patients with trauma to the skull and brain.
6. Describe the pathophysiology, assessment, and management of patients with anterior neck or spinal trauma.
7. Describe spinal immobilization techniques for trauma patients.
8. Discuss considerations for spinal immobilization of pediatric patients.
9. Describe the pathophysiology, assessment, and management of patients who have thoracic trauma.
10. Describe the pathophysiology, assessment, and management of patients who have abdominal trauma.
11. Describe the pathophysiology, assessment, and management of patients who have pelvic trauma.
12. Describe the pathophysiology, assessment, and management of patients with upper or lower extremity trauma.
13. Identify specific interventions for selected extremity injuries.
14. Given a specific patient scenario, calculate a trauma score, a revised trauma score, or a pediatric trauma score.
15. List priorities of emergency care for the trauma patient.

● REVIEW QUESTIONS
Match the appropriate energy law listed in Column 2 with its description in Column 1.

Column 1	Column 2
_____ 1. Force is equal to mass times acceleration or deceleration.	a. Newton's first law of motion
_____ 2. Equal to $\frac{1}{2}$ mass $\times$ velocity^2.	b. Newton's second law of motion
_____ 3. An object at rest or in motion remains in that state unless force is applied.	c. Conservation of energy law
_____ 4. Energy can neither be created nor destroyed; it can only change form.	d. Joules law
	e. Kinetic energy law

Match the type of skull fracture listed in Column 2 with the appropriate description in Column 1. Use each answer only once.

Column 1

_____ 5. Associated with Battle's sign and raccoon's eyes

_____ 6. Most common skull fracture, has low complication rate

_____ 7. Direct communication between scalp laceration and brain tissue

_____ 8. Fracture when bone is pushed downward often associated with scalp laceration

Column 2

a. Basilar
b. Depressed
c. Linear
d. Open vault

Select *all* of the appropriate immobilization devices from Column 2 to treat the fractures in Column 1. You may use each choice from Column 2 more than once.

_____ 9. Shoulder
_____ 10. Humerus
_____ 11. Elbow
_____ 12. Forearm
_____ 13. Wrist
_____ 14. Hand
_____ 15. Finger
_____ 16. Pelvis
_____ 17. Hip
_____ 18. Femur
_____ 19. Knee or patella
_____ 20. Tibia/fibula
_____ 21. Ankle or foot
_____ 22. Toes

a. Buddy splint
b. Formable splint
c. Long spine board
d. Rigid splint
e. Pneumatic antishock garment
f. Sling
g. Swathe
h. Traction splint

23. Sternal fractures are injuries frequently associated with improperly applied lap belts. True/false. If this is false, why is it false?

_____

24. Ejection from a vehicle is associated with a high number of spinal injuries. True/false. If this is false, why is it false?

_____

25. A full-face helmet should never be removed in the prehospital setting unless intubation is necessary. True/false. If this is false, why is it false?

_____

26. A pneumothorax may occur in the absence of a rib fracture. True/false. If this is false, why is it false?

_____

27. A strain is an injury to a muscle from overexertion or overextension. True/false. If this is false, why is it false?

_____

28. Identify three causes of death for each of the periods of the trimodal distribution of death, and for each period, identify prehospital interventions that may increase patient survival.

a. Immediate:

_____

b. Early:

_____

c. Late:

_____

29. *A 17-year-old female falls asleep at the wheel, rides the median for 50 feet, and then strikes a concrete bridge embankment head-on.*
   a. Identify the three collisions that will occur in this situation.

_____

   b. Assuming that this passenger took the down-and-under pathway during the collision, what injuries should you anticipate?

_____

30. Aside from speed and size, what factor will affect the injury pattern found in a lateral impact collision?

_____

31. In which of the following rear-end collisions will damage be greater, assuming that mass and other factors are equal? Why?
   a. *A vehicle traveling 50 mph is struck by a vehicle traveling 70 mph*
   b. *A vehicle traveling 5 mph is struck by a vehicle traveling 40 mph*

_____

32. For each of the body regions, list the injury or injuries that may occur during sudden rapid deceleration.
   a. Head/neck injuries:

_____

   b. Thoracic injuries:

_____

   c. Abdominal injuries:

_____

33. *You are called to the scene of a high-speed frontal crash caused by a cross-over accident. The driver of one of the vehicles complains of severe dyspnea and has a large, circular bruise on her chest. You note markedly decreased lung sounds on the right side of the chest and suspect a pneumothorax.*
   a. What traumatic mechanism can cause a pneumothorax in this example?

_____

   b. *The driver of the other vehicle has severe abdominal pain and is exhibiting signs of hypovolemic shock.* Which abdominal organs or structures can be injured from sudden compression of the abdomen?

_____

34. Identify the type of motorcycle collision most frequently associated with the pattern of injuries listed:

a. *A seasoned biker has a severely angulated fracture of the right forearm and extensive abrasions to the right side of the body.*

_____

b. *A 47-year-old executive has bilateral fractured femurs and facial injuries.*

_____

c. *A traffic officer has a severe crush injury to the left lower leg.*

_____

35. Identify the injuries to be anticipated in the following situations:
    a. *A motorist jogs across the highway and is struck by an oncoming vehicle.*

_____

   b. *As a young child hurries to avoid being late to school, he is struck by a full-size automobile.*

_____

36. When evaluating a sports injury, what principles of kinematics must be considered to determine probable areas of injury?

_____

37. *A suitcase filled with plastic explosives detonates in a locker at a busy urban airport.* Describe the type of injuries seen in each of the following categories:
    a. Primary blast injuries:

_____

   b. Secondary blast injuries:

_____

   c. Tertiary blast injuries:

_____

38. Briefly describe how each of the following ballistic properties influences injury patterns in penetrating trauma:
    a. Character of the penetrating object:

_____

_____

   b. Speed of penetration:

_____

_____

   c. Distance from patient that a bullet is fired:

_____

_____

39. *A 6-year-old unrestrained child strikes his face on the stick shift of a truck in a head-on collision. On arrival, you find him seated in the cab of the truck, alert, crying, and complaining of pain in his face. Blood is oozing from his mouth.*

a. Describe your evaluation of his head and face (assume that the primary survey is completed).

_____

b. _On physical examination, you note that he has difficultly closing his mouth and there is an apparent space between the two lower front teeth as well as a laceration that extends down through the gums. The bleeding continues, and there are excessive oral secretions. Vital signs are stable._ Describe how you will transport and manage this child.

_____

40. Briefly describe assessment of the patient who has a suspected eye injury.

_____

41. For each of the following patients, identify the injury you suspect and list prehospital management techniques:

a. _A 10-year-old complains of severe pain in the right eye after he was struck in the face with a handful of sand. The right eye is reddened and tearing._

_____

b. _A 35-year-old has sustained a partially avulsed right upper lid._

_____

c. _A fish hook is embedded in the eye of a 42-year-old woman._

_____

d. _A handball player is struck directly in the eye by the ball. He is having difficulty seeing out of the injured eye. You note blood in the anterior chamber of the eye._

_____

e. _During the National Hockey League playoffs, a high stick strikes a player in the eye. You note an irregular pupil on the affected side. There is a jellylike substance extruding from an apparent laceration to the globe._

_____

42. Briefly list the signs and symptoms associated with the following brain injuries:

a. Concussion:

_____

b. Contusion:

_____

c. Subdural hematoma:

_____

d. Epidural hematoma:

_____

43. *Your patient has been struck on the head with a baseball bat during a barroom brawl. He is alert and oriented, with an obvious depression and laceration at the right temporal area.* Describe the signs and symptoms you will see if his intracranial pressure progressively rises en route to the hospital.

_____

_____

44. *You are transporting by air a patient who has sustained an isolated head injury in a motorcycle accident. Initially, he was awake and talking, but over the past 10 minutes, his condition has rapidly deteriorated. He now has a fixed, dilated right pupil; irregular respirations; a blood pressure of 170/100 mm Hg; and a pulse of 64.* Identify treatment modalities you would provide for this patient.

_____

_____

45. *You are en route to a domestic disturbance in which a 45-year-old man has reportedly been stabbed in the neck with an ice pick.* Identify possible signs and symptoms of penetrating neck trauma.

_____

46. List the steps in patient management of a significant vascular injury to the neck.

_____

_____

47. List 4 criteria that would indicate a patient should be assumed to have a spinal injury.
   a.
   b.
   c.
   d.

48. Spinal sprains and strains usually result from (a) _____

   and (b) _____ forces. A hyperflexion sprain occurs

   when there is a tear of the posterior (c) _____

   _____ and _____

   _____, which allows partial

   (d)_____ of the intervertebral joints. Hyperextension
   strains are common with low-velocity, rear-end automobile collisions and

   are commonly known as (e) _____.

   The most frequently injured spinal regions, in descending order are

   (f)_____ to _____,

(g)_____ to _____, and

(h)_____ to _____.

The most common are wedge-shaped (i) _____ fractures.

49. *A cyclist was thrown from his bike and has severe pain in the back between his scapulae.* List signs and symptoms that can indicate a complete cord lesion as a result of this injury.

_____

50. Identify four situations involving suspected cervical spine injury when the head should not be moved to a neutral in-line position with manual immobilization.

a.　　　　　　　　　　c.

b.　　　　　　　　　　d.

51. Identify the steps involved in rolling a supine patient (Fig. 15-1), including positioning of rescuers.

a.

b.

c.

d.

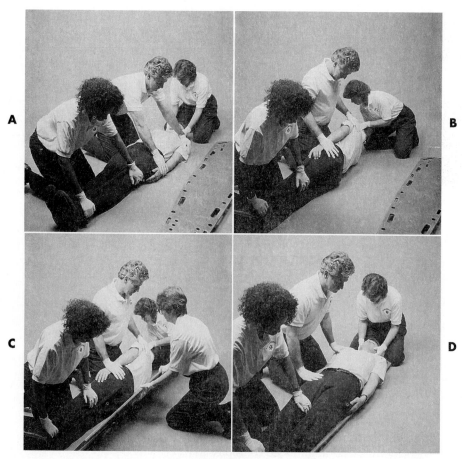

Figure 15-1

Questions 52 through 54 pertain to the following scenario: *You are transferring a 26-year-old woman who was a passenger in a car struck laterally on her door. She has a fractured right humerus and multiple fractures of ribs 3 to 8. En route to the trauma center, you note paradoxical movement of her chest.*

52. What chest injury do you suspect?

_____

53. Why is the patient likely to become hypoxic secondary to this injury?

_____

54. What patient care measures should you use to improve ventilation?

_____

_____

55. Identify three symptoms common to all types of pneumothorax.
   a.
   b.
   c.

56. _A deer hunter is accidently shot with a 30:30 shell from a rifle. There is an open wound inferior to the right nipple, and you cannot find an exit wound._
   a. Why is this patient likely to become hypoxic?

_____

_____

   b. What interventions must be taken immediately to correct the hypoxia?

_____

_____

57. _A patient from a motor vehicle crash has sustained severe blunt chest trauma. There are diminished breath sounds on the right side of the chest. He is anxious and dyspneic._
   a. What additional signs and symptoms would indicate that he has developed a tension pneumothorax?

_____

   b. Describe the prehospital intervention for tension pneumothorax.

_____

_____

58. What two life-threatening conditions may be caused by hemothorax?
   a.
   b.

59. _You are called to care for a worker who was momentarily crushed between a truck and a loading dock. His face and head are a bright, reddish-purple color, and his jugular veins are markedly distended._
   a. What injury do you suspect?

_____

   b. What treatment would you provide?

_____

60. _A 28-year-old woman was involved in a frontal collision during which her chest struck the steering wheel. She is complaining of crushing substernal chest pain and palpitations. Her blood pressure is normal, her pulse is 110 and irregular, and her lungs are clear._
   a. What injury do you suspect?

_____

b. What treatment measures should be instituted for this patient?

---

61. *A 27-year-old was splitting wood when a splinter of metal flew off the axe and penetrated his chest. On your arrival, he is confused, with a systolic blood pressure of 80, a narrow pulse pressure, muffled heart sounds, and distended neck veins.*
  a. What chest injury do you suspect?

b. What prehospital care should be rendered?

---

62. What signs should be anticipated in a patient with an aortic rupture secondary to a rapid deceleration injury?

---

63. *A 12-year-old boy recovering from mononucleosis is hit on the left side by another child. He is complaining of severe left upper quadrant abdominal pain and left shoulder pain. He has signs of shock.*
  a. What solid organ is most likely injured in this situation?

b. Why would his shoulder be hurting?

---

64. Describe complications that may result when hollow organs of the abdomen are injured.

---

65. Describe evaluation of an injured extremity before and after splinting.

---

66. Identify five general principles of splinting.
  a.
  b.
  c.
  d.
  e.

67. Calculate a Glasgow coma score and a revised trauma score for each of the following patient examples:
  a. *Your patient opens her eyes to voice, is confused, and pulls her hand away when you start intravenous therapy. Her vital signs are blood pressure, 90/70; pulse, 120; and respirations, 24 and unlabored. Capillary refill is 1 second. GCS = _____. RTS = _____.*
  b. *Your patient opens his eyes to deep pain, moans some unrecognizable sounds, and withdraws slightly from pain. His vital signs are blood pressure, 70 mm Hg by palpation; pulse, 136; and respirations, 30 and very shallow. His capillary refill is 4 seconds. GCS = _____. RTS = _____.*

● **STUDENT SELF-EVALUATION**

68. Air bags are designed to reduce injuries in:
  a. Frontal collisions   **c.** Roll-over collisions
  b. Lateral collisions   **d.** All of the above

69. A roofer falls from the top of a second story residence. What type of injuries will you anticipate?
   a. Minor injuries to the feet and spine
   b. Severe injuries to the feet and spine
   c. Minor injuries to the head and neck
   d. Major injuries to the head and neck

70. Which of the following is a high-energy weapon with the potential to cause the greatest injury to tissues?
   a. M-16   c. 12-gauge shotgun
   b. 357 magnum   d. Knife

71. The first steps in primary assessment of a multiple-system trauma patient include all of the following, *except:*
   a. Airway assessment and control
   b. Cervical spine immobilization
   c. Evaluation of carotid and radial pulse
   d. Eye opening and pupil response

72. *Your patient has been struck in the eye with a ball. She has diplopia, subconjunctival ecchymosis, enophthalmos, and numbness in the cheek.* What bone fracture is consistent with these findings?
   a. Mandible   c. Orbit
   b. Maxilla   d. Zygoma

73. Which of the following would be an acceptable way to transport an avulsed tooth?
   a. In a mild soap solution   c. In a dry gauze dressing
   b. In sterile water   d. In fresh whole milk

74. Your patient has a basilar skull fracture that has injured cranial nerve VIII. What sign or symptom is associated with this injury?
   a. Loss of smell   c. Deafness
   b. Blindness in one eye   d. Facial paralysis

75. The most reliable indicator of increasing intracranial pressure is:
   a. Deteriorating level of consciousness
   b. Nausea and vomiting
   c. Increased blood pressure and decreased pulse
   d. Unilateral dilated pupil

76. Which of the following breathing patterns is *not* likely to be exhibited by the patient with a brain injury?
   a. Ataxic breathing   c. Hypoventilation
   b. Cheyne-Stokes respirations   d. Kussmaul respirations

77. What is the most rapid and effective intervention to decrease intracranial pressure in a patient with a severe head injury and a Glasgow coma score of 6?
   a. Elevation of the head of the bed
   b. Intravenous administration of mannitol
   c. Intubation and hyperventilation
   d. Massive doses of steroids

78. *You wish to given 40 g of mannitol to a patient who has a head injury. You have a 20% solution of the drug.* How many milliliters will you give?
   a. 8   c. 80
   b. 50   d. 200

79. Paralysis and loss of sensation below the umbilicus indicates an injury at the level of:
   a. C4   c. T10
   b. T4   d. S1

80. When immobilizing a patient on a long spine board, what body region should be secured first?
   a. Arms   c. Legs
   b. Head   d. Torso

81. Which of the following is true regarding rib fractures?
    a. They are more common in children.
    b. The first rib is frequently fractured.
    c. They are associated with pancreatic injury.
    d. Ribs 3 to 8 are most commonly fractured.
82. Sternal injuries are frequently associated with:
    a. Airway compromise   c. Myocardial injury
    b. Flail chest   d. Spleen injury
83. *Your patient was in a motorcycle crash and has dyspnea and bowel sounds at the nipple line on the left side of the chest.* You suspect:
    a. Pericardial tamponade   c. Diaphragmatic rupture
    b. Liver rupture   d. Kidney injury

Questions 84 to 86 pertain to the following case study: *Your patient is a 50-year-old who was stabbed in the right upper quadrant of the abdomen. The patient is pale and restless, with cool, clammy skin. Vital signs are blood pressure, 106/88; pulse, 128; and respirations, 28.*

84. You would suspect injury to the:
    i. Chest   a. i and ii
    ii. Liver   b. i and iii
    iii. Spleen   c. ii and iv
    iv. Urinary bladder   d. iii and iv
85. Interventions for this patient would include:
    a. Oxygen 4 L/min via nasal cannula and intravenous lactated Ringer's solution to keep the vein open
    b. Oxygen 10 L/min via mask and intravenous lactated Ringer's solution to keep the vein open
    c. Oxygen 4 L/min via nasal cannula and intravenous lactated Ringer's solution via rapid infusion
    d. Oxygen 10 L/min via mask and intravenous lactated Ringer's solution via rapid infusion
86. Your *first* priority on arrival to this call would be:
    a. Airway   c. Scene safety
    b. Application of oxygen   d. Stop the bleeding
87. A traction splint may be helpful for the patient with:
    a. Femur fracture   c. Tibial fracture
    b. Humerus fracture   d. Pelvic fracture
88. Which of the following is true regarding sprains?
    a. It means injury to a tendon.
    b. No tissue disruption occurs, but bruising does.
    c. Severe hemorrhage can occur.
    d. Joint instability and dislocation may result.

SOFT TISSUE INJURIES AND BURNS

● READING ASSIGNMENT
Chapter 16, pp. 484-517, in *Mosby's Paramedic Textbook*

● OBJECTIVES
As a paramedic, you should be able to:
1. Describe the normal structure and function of the integumentary system.
2. Describe the pathophysiology of soft tissue injury.
3. Describe in the correct sequence patient-management techniques for control of hemorrhage.
4. Discuss pathophysiology as a basis for key signs and symptoms and describe the mechanism of injury, assessment, and management of specific soft tissue injuries.
5. Identify sources of burn injury.
6. Describe the pathophysiology of burn injury in local and systemic responses.
7. Classify burn injury according to depth, extent, and severity based on established standards.
8. Describe the assessment of the burn-injured patient.
9. Outline the prehospital management of the burn-injured patient.
10. Discuss pathophysiology as a basis for key signs, symptoms, and management of the patient with an inhalation injury.
11. Outline the general assessment and management of the patient who has a chemical injury.
12. Describe the specific complications and management techniques for selected chemical injuries.
13. Describe the physiological effects of electrical injury as they relate to each body system based on an understanding of key principles of electricity.
14. Outline assessment and management of the patient with electrical injury.
15. Describe the distinguishing features of radiation injury.

● REVIEW QUESTIONS
Match the chemicals listed in Column 2 with the appropriate description in Column 1.

Column 1	Column 2
_____ 1. Used in cleaning fabric and metal, can cause hypocalcemia and severe burns.	a. Alkali metal
_____ 2. Noxious gas that, when in solution, can cause blindness if it contaminates the eye.	b. Ammonia
	c. Hydrofluoric acid
_____ 3. Causes burns after prolonged exposure, also may result in lead poisoning.	d. Petroleum
_____ 4. Produces heat if exposed to water, should remove or cover with oil.	e. Phenol
_____ 5. Exposure may be painless and result in dysrhythmias and central nervous system depression.	

6. List at least six structures or tissues located in the dermis.
   a.
   b.
   c.
   d.
   e.
   f.
7. Identify three functions of the integumentary system.
   a.
   b.
   c.
8. Identify the three critical steps in the clotting mechanism.
   a.
   b.
   c.
9. Why are redness, swelling, warmth, and pain found at the site of an inflammatory response?

_____

_____

10. *You are called to a rural farm, where a 17-year-old has sustained a partial amputation of his left lower arm after tangling it in a corn picker. There is extensive soft tissue damage and deformity of the extremity, and it is squirting bright red blood. Your estimated time of arrival to the nearest hospital is 30 minutes. Describe in the proper sequence five measures that you could use to control the bleeding in this patient and briefly describe the proper technique for using each skill.*
   a.

_____

_____

   b.

_____

_____

   c.

_____

_____

   d.

_____

_____

   e.

_____

_____

11. For each of the following scenarios, list the soft tissue injury described and key prehospital interventions to manage the trauma.
   a. *You are called to a private residence to evaluate an electrician who shows you some burns on his right hand about the size of a quarter. He states he had been running some line yesterday and received an electrical shock but had not thought*

it serious enough to seek care. The right forearm is tense and tender to palpation. When you attempt to passively move the fingers on that hand, the patient screams in pain. A weak pulse is palpable distal to the injury, and the affected hand is pale when compared with the other side.

Injury:

Interventions:

---

b. *A 45-year-old woman is being transported for care after her husband repeatedly struck her head and face with his fist. You note multiple swollen, ecchymotic areas on the face and head.*

Injury:

Interventions:

---

c. *Rescuers have just removed a victim who had been trapped in a concrete structure for 2 days. The patient's lower torso had been pinned under a concrete piling. During the rescue phase, the patient was alert but somewhat confused. Vital signs were within normal limits. Shortly after extrication, the patient's physiological status begins to deteriorate.*

Injury:

Interventions:

---

d. *A wallpaper hanger has sustained a deep linear wound after cutting himself with an Exacto knife. The wound is oozing dark red blood, and fatty tissue is visible at the edges of the injury.*

Injury:

Interventions:

---

e. *A motorcyclist wearing only her swimming suit had to lay the bike down to avoid a collision. The patient states that the bike slid approximately 100 feet along the asphalt road. There are huge scrape-type injuries on her entire left side. She denies pain or tenderness anywhere else.*

Injury:

Interventions:

---

f. *Neighbors direct you to a yard where a young child has been attacked by a large dog. No one is sure of the dog's present location. The child is screaming, and his left arm has many puncture wounds and lacerations.*

Injury:

Interventions:

---

g. *A hunter has been impaled with an arrow. The arrow has penetrated the right upper quadrant of the abdomen. She is pale and cool.*

Injury:

Interventions:

---

h. *A mechanic reports an injury to his right hand while working with a high-pressure grease gun. You note a small puncture wound with a drop of grease on it at the distal end of the left thumb.*
   Injury:
   Interventions:

i. *A butcher slices off the distal tip of his index finger.*
   Injury:
   Interventions:

j. *A factory employee catches his hair in some large machinery and avulses a large portion of the posterior aspect of his scalp.*
   Injury:
   Interventions:

k. *A weekend handyman severs his right index finger with a skill saw. He drives himself to a nearby firehouse but does not have the digit with him.*
   Injury:
   Interventions:

12. List three factors that may increase the likelihood of infection or other complications during wound healing.
   a.
   b.
   c.

13. *You are called to the scene of a construction site, where a 57-year-old workman has lacerated his left hand.* Describe your assessment of this patient, including history and physical examination.

14. Identify the four major sources of burn injury.
   a.
   b.
   c.
   d.

15. Label the three zones of burn injury on Fig. 16-1 and briefly describe the characteristics of the tissue in each.

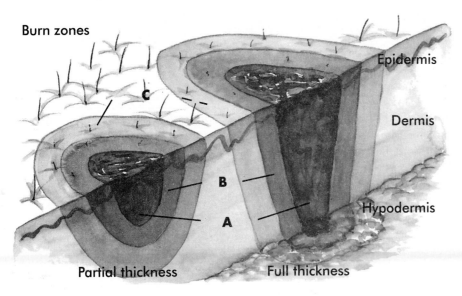

Burn zones

Epidermis

Dermis

Hypodermis

Figure 16-1

C

B

A

Partial thickness

Full thickness

a.

_____

_____

b.

_____

_____

c.

_____

_____

16. Explain two mechanisms that cause swelling in the burned tissue.
   a.
   b.

17. Describe the response in each of the following body systems to a major burn injury.
   a. Cardiovascular:

_____

   b. Pulmonary:

_____

   c. Gastrointestinal:

_____

   d. Musculoskeletal:

_____

   e. Neuroendocrine:

_____

f. Metabolic:

g. Immune:

h. Emotional:

18. For each of the following situations, classify the burn according to depth (first, second, or third degree), extent (body surface area), and severity (according to American Burn Association). Identify those patients who meet the American Burn Association criteria for referral to a burn center.

    a. *A chef at a local restaurant has spilled hot grease down the anterior surface of his body. The wound is exquisitely painful and is moist and red, with many blisters. The burns cover the anterior surface of his chest, abdomen, arms, and left leg.*
      Depth:
      Extent:
      Severity:
      Referral:

    b. *On a hot summer day a young motorist opens his radiator cap and sprays hot steam and fluid over the upper half of his torso. The wounds are painful, moist, and red, with some blistering, and they blanch to touch. The burns cover his face, anterior chest, and abdomen.*
      Depth:
      Extent:
      Severity:
      Referral:

    c. *An 80-year-old woman steps into a tub of excessively hot water. Because of severe arthritis, it takes a long time for her to get out of the water. She has circumferential burns around the right lower extremity up to the knee. The burn wound appears white and leathery and has no capillary refill.*
      Depth:
      Extent:
      Severity:
      Referral:

    Questions 19 to 22 pertain to the following scenario: *A 13-year-old boy starts a bonfire using gasoline and ignites his clothing. As he attempts to pull his flaming jacket over his head, it gets stuck while continuing to burn. On your arrival, he is alert after an initial brief loss of consciousness. He has extensive burns on his face, neck, and chest. The burns are white and dry, with charred patches. They do not blanch when touched. His nasal hair is singed, and he is coughing up black, sooty sputum.*

19. What aspects of the mechanism of injury and history of the event lead you to believe that this patient may have an inhalation injury?

20. What physical findings suggest inhalation injury?

21. At what point would you consider intubation?

22. Do you suspect an inhalation injury above or below the glottis and why?

23. *As you arrive at the scene of a residential fire, rescue workers carry out an approximately 40-year-old, 80-kg man who is unconscious and has white, leathery burns.*

The burns cover the entire body surface except the posterior surface of both legs. He has shallow respirations at a rate of 24/min, and his blood pressure is 106/70 mm Hg. Patchy pieces of his smouldering clothing remain.

a. Describe your initial assessment of this patient, including depth, extent, and severity of burns.

_____

_____

b. Describe the prehospital care, including airway and fluid resuscitation with type of fluid and rate.

_____

_____

24. Describe the specific interventions to be used when the following third-degree burns are present:

a. Burns to the face:

_____

b. Extremity burns:

_____

c. Circumferential burns:

_____

25. Identify two examples of chemicals that can cause burn injury in each of the following categories:

a. Acids:

_____

b. Alkalis:

_____

c. Organic compounds:

_____

26. *You are responding to a call for a person who has a chemical burn. En route to the industrial complex, you review the questions you will ask to determine the potential seriousness of the burn.*

a. Give two examples of these questions.

_____

_____

b. *You find your patient covered with a powder known to cause chemical burns to the skin.* Describe patient decontamination techniques.

_____

_____

27. The amount of tissue damage caused by electrical current depends on six

factors: (a) _____, _____,

_____, _____,

_____, and _____. Amperage

is the measure of current (b) _____ per unit time. Volt-

age is a continuous (c) _____ applied to any electrical
circuit causing a flow of electricity. High-voltage electrical injuries result

from contact with an electrical source of (d) _____

or greater. Resistance to electricity depends on four factors: (e) _____

_____, _____,

_____, and _____. Resistance

to electrical flow in the body is greatest in the (f) _____

tissue. The two types of current commonly used are (g) _____

and _____. Direct current flows in

(h) _____ direction. It is used in (i)

_____. Alternating current periodically reverses (j)

_____ of flow. This may cause muscle contractions

that may (k) _____ the patient to the source.
In general, the current pathway in low-voltage current follows the path of

(l) _____ _____, and high

voltage current follows the (m) _____ path. As the
duration of contact with the patient increases, tissue damage will (n)

_____.

28. Name the three burn patterns that can result from electrical current.
    a.
    b.
    c.
29. Briefly describe the potential effects of electrical injury on each of the following body regions.
    a. Cutaneous:

_____

    b. Cardiovascular:

_____

    c. Neurological:

_____

    d. Vascular:

_____

    e. Muscular:

_____

f. Renal:

_____

g. Pulmonary:

_____

h. Orthopedic:

_____

i. Ocular and otic:

_____

30. _A homeowner was trimming his trees when he came into contact with overhead electrical wires. On your arrival, he is still in contact with the electrical source._
    a. What must be done before treatment commences?

_____

   The patient is conscious and alert. You note multiple small, round, white burns on his right hand. When his clothing is removed, you discover significant burns and tissue injury to both feet.
    b. Describe your history and physical examination of this patient.

_____

_____

_____

    c. Describe treatment, including fluid resuscitation (rate and type).

_____

_____

31. Describe the appearance of wounds characteristically associated with lightning burns.

_____

32. For each of the following classes of lightning injury, list two physical signs.
    a. Minor:

_____

    b. Moderate:

_____

    c. Severe:

_____

● **STUDENT SELF-EVALUATION**

33. The avascular layer of the skin is the:
    a. Dermis   **c.** Sebaceous
    b. Epidermis   **d.** Subcutaneous tissue
34. Which of the following does _not_ play a role in normal hemostasis?
    a. Activation of platelets   **c.** Thrombin formation
    b. Aldosterone synthesis   **d.** Vasoconstriction

35. Which of the following is an early finding in crush injury?
    a. Paralysis
    c. Paresthesia
    b. Paresis
    d. Pulselessness
36. Compartment syndrome is likely to be found in the:
    a. Abdomen
    c. Head
    b. Upper arm
    d. Thorax
37. What is the appropriate prehospital care for avulsed body tissue?
    a. Placing it directly on ice
    b. Sealing it in a plastic bag
    c. Soaking it in a cup of lactated Ringer's solution
    d. Debridement of all dirt
38. Which of the following risk factors is associated with a high incidence of burn fatality?
    a. Female gender
    c. Industrial setting
    b. Child
    d. High-income family
39. The most common source of burn injury is:
    a. Chemical
    c. Radiation
    b. Electrical
    d. Thermal
40. Hypovolemia in burn injury occurs secondary to:
    a. Blood loss
    b. Condensation of tissue fluid
    c. Increased capillary permeability
    d. Decrease in fluid intake
41. Which of the following is a systemic response to burn injury?
    a. Hypoventilation
    b. Hyperactive gastrointestinal tract
    c. Decreased metabolic rate
    d. Depressed inflammatory response
42. To cool the burn of a patient with a burn on 50% of the body surface area, the paramedic should:
    a. Apply ice intermittently in 15-minute cycles.
    b. Leave the patient exposed to air and apply a fan.
    c. Apply cool water and then cover the patient with sheets and blankets.
    d. Continuously apply cool water while en route.
43. Which of the following statements is true regarding carbon monoxide poisoning?
    a. Oxygen saturation on the pulse oximeter will be 80 or less.
    b. Skin color will be cyanotic and often mottled.
    c. Respiratory rate will be depressed in early stages.
    d. Oxygen administration will reduce the half-life of carbon dioxide.
44. What is the treatment of choice for almost all chemical injuries?
    a. Vigorous drying of the chemical
    b. Application of a chemical antidote
    c. Copious irrigation with water
    d. Delayed treatment until arrival at the hospital
45. Calcium gluconate gel and solution are used to treat which of the following chemical injuries?
    a. Ammonia
    c. Petroleum
    b. Hydrofluoric acid
    d. Phenol
46. Electrical burns that result when the heat of the electric current ignites the patient's clothing are _____ burns:
    a. Alternating
    c. Direct
    b. Arc
    d. Flash
47. Death in lightning injury most frequently results from:
    a. Cardiac or respiratory arrest
    c. Coagulation of the blood
    b. Central nervous system injury
    d. Severe burn shock

DIVISION THREE REVIEW TEST

1. Kinetic energy will be increased most by:
   a. Increasing speed 10 miles/hr
   b. Increasing the weight of the occupant 10 lb
   c. Increasing the stopping distance
   d. Increasing the deceleration time

2. The primary concern with facial fractures is:
   a. Airway   c. Disfigurement
   b. Bleeding   d. Edema

3. How should foreign bodies in the eye be removed?
   a. Irrigation with normal saline   c. With small splinter forceps
   b. With a Q-tip swab   d. Should not be removed

4. An early sign of basilar skull fracture that may be evident at the scene of injury is:
   a. Mastoid ecchymosis   c. Periorbital ecchymosis
   b. Cerebrospinal fluid drainage   d. Unilateral pupil dilation

5. The cerebral injury caused by structural damage to the brain that typically heals spontaneously is:
   a. Concussion   c. Epidural hematoma
   b. Contusion   d. Increased intracranial pressure

6. A 72-year-old patient's family states he has had a progressive deterioration in his level of consciousness over the past 3 days after a fall from bed. He arouses only to voice and has a large contusion on the forehead. You suspect:
   a. Concussion   c. Intracerebral bleed
   b. Epidural hematoma   d. Subdural hematoma

7. Which of the following spinal injuries can result in permanent neurological dysfunction?
   a. Fractures   c. Sprains and strains
   b. Dislocation   d. All of the above

8. Signs and symptoms consistent with a high-level spinal cord lesion include all of the following, *except:*
   a. Loss of bladder control   c. Poikilothermy
   b. Priapism   d. Tachycardia

9. When a patient with a suspected spinal injury is log-rolled, the patient's arms should be placed:
   a. Extended above the head
   b. Flexed and folded across the chest
   c. Extended with palms on the lateral thighs
   d. Rotated behind the back

10. What is the most effective way to improve ventilation in a patient with a flail chest and significant respiratory distress?
    a. Application of a pillow to the flail segment
    b. Use of the patient's arm to splint the flail segment
    c. Application of pressure with tape to the flail segment
    d. Initiation of positive-pressure ventilation

11. After application of an occlusive Vaseline gauze dressing (sealed on four sides) to treat an open chest wound, the patient begins to develop signs of tension pneumothorax. What is your *first* action?
    a. Increase inspired oxygen concentration.
    b. Loosen one side of the dressing.
    c. Insert a needle in the second intercostal space.
    d. Intubate the patient's lung and hyperventilate.

12. *Your patient has a large chest contusion after a high-speed frontal collision. Vital signs are blood pressure, 140/100; pulse, 120; and respirations, 20. Femoral pulses are difficult to obtain, and there is obvious trauma to the chest.* You suspect:
    a. Aortic injury
    b. Myocardial contusion
    c. Neurogenic shock
    d. Tension pneumothorax
13. Beck's triad of signs for pericardial tamponade is:
    a. Tracheal deviation, widened pulse pressure, and muffled heart sounds
    b. Jugular venous distention, muffled heart sounds, and rising blood pressure
    c. Jugular venous distention, muffled heart sounds, and narrowed pulse pressure
    d. Tracheal deviation, muffled heart sounds, and falling blood pressure
14. *Your patient has a splenic injury and severe left shoulder pain.* This sign is called:
    a. Battle's sign
    b. Cullen's sign
    c. Kehr's sign
    d. Kernig's sign
15. Flank tenderness and pain in the costrovertebral angle after blunt trauma to the lower back may indicate injury to the:
    a. Liver
    b. Kidney
    c. Pelvis
    d. Spleen
16. Which of the following statements is true with regard to femur fracture?
    a. It is best stabilized with a long leg splint.
    b. It can result in hypovolemia.
    c. Traction should not be applied.
    d. It is rarely painful.
17. A patient who is awake, alert, and oriented, with a blood pressure of 120/80 and respirations of 16 will have a Revised Trauma Score of:
    a. 10
    b. 12
    c. 16
    d. 20
18. Which of the following is a normal function of the integumentary system?
    a. Transportation of nutrients
    b. Regulation of temperature
    c. Interpretation of sensory input
    d. Production of hormones
19. The inflammatory response is characterized by:
    a. Local vasoconstriction
    b. Decreased local capillary permeability
    c. Accumulation of plasma and plasma proteins in the intravascular space
    d. Transport of white blood cells to the affected area
20. Techniques for the control of hemorrhage should be used in the following order:
    a. Elevation, direct pressure, tourniquet, and pressure points
    b. Tourniquet, pressure points, elevation, and direct pressure
    c. Direct pressure, elevation, pressure points, and tourniquet
    d. Pressure points, direct pressure, elevation, and tourniquet
21. Emergency intervention for the patient suffering from crush syndrome should include:
    a. High-volume fluid resuscitation
    b. Potassium administration
    c. Lowering of body temperature
    d. Application of pneumatic antishock garments
22. Bite injuries can result in the transmission of all of the following infectious diseases, *except:*
    a. Gonorrhea
    b. Hepatitis
    c. Tetanus
    d. Rabies
23. During resuscitative efforts of the patient with a burn injury, care is directed to promoting optimal conditions for salvage of the skin in the zone of _____:
    a. Coagulation
    b. Hyperemia
    c. Necrosis
    d. Stasis

24. A burn characterized by a moist, red appearance with blisters is probably _____ degree.
   - **a.** First
   - **b.** Second
   - **c.** Third
   - **d.** Fourth

25. A 5-year-old patient with third-degree burns of the anterior and posterior surfaces of both legs has approximately a(n) _____% burn.
   - **a.** 18
   - **b.** 24
   - **c.** 28
   - **d.** 36

26. Using the consensus formula, calculate the minimum fluid requirement during the first hour for a 100-kg patient who has 60% third-degree burns covering his body.
   - **a.** 250 ml
   - **b.** 500 ml
   - **c.** 750 ml
   - **d.** 6000 ml

27. Which of the following is *not* a reason to suspect inhalation injury?
   - **a.** Burns involving petroleum products
   - **b.** Documented loss of consciousness
   - **c.** Hoarseness or stridor
   - **d.** Burns in an enclosed space

28. Severity of chemical injury is related to all of the following, *except:*
   - **a.** Chemical concentration
   - **b.** Duration of contact
   - **c.** External environment
   - **d.** Type of chemical agent

29. Electrical current flows through the body most easily through _____ tissue.
   - **a.** Bone
   - **b.** Blood
   - **c.** Muscle
   - **d.** Nerve

DIVISION FOUR
MEDICAL

CHAPTER 17
RESPIRATORY DISORDERS

● **READING ASSIGNMENT**

Chapter 17, pp. 520-537, in *Mosby's Paramedic Textbook*

● **OBJECTIVES**

As a paramedic, you should be able to:

1. Describe pathophysiology, assessment, and management of the following noninfectious respiratory disorders:
   a. Adult respiratory distress syndrome
   b. Obstructive airway disease
   c. Chronic obstructive pulmonary disease
   d. Asthma
   e. Cystic fibrosis
   f. Pulmonary embolism
   g. Pickwickian syndrome
   h. Central nervous system dysfunction
2. Describe pathophysiology as a basis for key signs and symptoms, patient assessment, and management of the following infectious respiratory disorders:
   a. Pleurisy
   b. Influenza
   c. Pneumonia
   d. Legionnaires' Disease
   e. Tuberculosis

● **REVIEW QUESTIONS**

Match the description in Column 1 with the correct *noninfectious* pulmonary disease in Column 2. Use each answer only once.

Column 1	Column 2
_____ 1. Chronic production of excessive mucus, hypoxia, and inflammation of bronchi	a. Adult respiratory distress syndrome
_____ 2. Pulmonary edema secondary to trauma, inhaled toxins, or metabolic disorders	b. Asthma c. Chronic bronchitis d. Cor pulmonale e. Cystic fibrosis
_____ 3. Exocrine gland disorder causing abnormal secretion of thick mucus	f. Emphysema g. Guillain-Barré syndrome
_____ 4. Impaired oxygenation resulting from blockage of a pulmonary artery by a clot	h. Myasthenia gravis i. Pickwickian syndrome j. Pulmonary embolism
_____ 5. Bronchiolar smooth muscle spasm and excess mucus production resulting from allergy	

_____ 6. Ascending postinfectious paralysis
involving the respiratory muscles

_____ 7. Somnolence and periods of apnea
in an extremely obese patient

_____ 8. Chronic disease resulting in
decreased alveolar membrane
surface area and polycythemia

_____ 9. Poor inspiratory effort resulting
from impaired nervous transmission
to the muscle cells

10. _You are transporting a 56-year-old male from a small rural hospital to a trauma center 70 miles away. Some 24 hours ago, he was involved in a head-on motor vehicle collision. He has been diagnosed with bilateral pulmonary contusions and two fractured ribs. Early in his care, he received a large volume of normal saline intravenously. He has been increasingly short of breath, was intubated before your arrival, and is very difficult to ventilate._
   a. What problem do you suspect?

   _____

   b. Describe the measures you will use during transport to assess and care
   for this patient.

   _____

   _____

   _____

11. Briefly describe the following two complications of chronic obstructive pulmonary disease:
   a. Pulmonary hypertension:

   _____

   _____

   b. Cor pulmonale:

   _____

   _____

12. Differentiate the signs and symptoms of chronic bronchitis and emphysema.
   a. Chronic bronchitis:

   _____

   b. Emphysema:

   _____

   Questions 13 to 15 pertain to the following scenario: _Your 65-year-old patient has a history of chronic bronchitis and emphysema. She states that she has become acutely short of breath today and cannot complete a sentence without gasping for air. Loud wheezing is audible without a stethoscope._

13. How much oxygen should you administer to this type of patient?

   _____

   _____

14. List two drugs (other than oxygen) that may be administered to alleviate this patient's dyspnea if not contraindicated by history or physical findings.

_____

15. Describe any additional patient care to be given en route to the hospital.

_____

_____

Questions 16 to 19 pertain to the following scenario: _You are called to a junior college to evaluate a 19-year-old who became acutely short of breath during a soccer game. He states that he has a history of asthma. On examination, you note inspiratory and expiratory wheezes throughout the lungs. Vital signs are blood pressure, 130/80; pulse, 136; and respirations, 30. There is a pulsus paradoxis of 30._

16. Other than oxygen, what two drugs can be administered to treat this patient (include correct dose and route)?

_____

17. Describe how you will reassess the patient after the medication has been administered and what you will find if the patient's condition is improving.

_____

_____

_____

18. If therapy is unsuccessful and the patient continues to deteriorate despite aggressive medication therapy, what condition might exist?

_____

19. What additional treatment measures will you use?

_____

20. List five pathological causes of wheezing.
   a.
   b.
   c.
   d.
   e.

21. _A 16-year-old girl with cystic fibrosis is in severe respiratory distress. She has markedly diminished breath sounds with slight wheezing. Vital signs monitoring reveals tachypnea and tachycardia. Describe the prehospital care for this patient._

_____

_____

22. List eight factors that increase the risk of pulmonary emboli.
   a.
   b.
   c.
   d.
   e.
   f.
   g.
   h.

23. List the signs and symptoms of pulmonary embolism.

_____

24. Briefly describe the prehospital care appropriate for dyspneic patients with myasthenia gravis or Guillain-Barré syndrome.

_____

_____

25. List six factors that increase the risk of contracting an infectious respiratory disease.
  a.
  b.
  c.
  d.
  e.
  f.

26. Pleurisy is a(n) (a) _____ of the visceral and parietal pleura of the lungs. It may occur secondary to several respiratory diseases,

including, (b) _____, _____, or

_____. The pain of pleurisy is described as (c)

_____. It is located in the (d)

_____ _____ or

_____ and may radiate to the (e)

_____.

27. Influenza is characterized by the following symptoms: (a) _____

_____, _____,

_____, and _____. This infec-

tion is spread by (b) _____

_____. A frequent respiratory complication of

influenza is (c) _____ _____.

28. Legionnaires' disease is a(n) (a) _____
infection that results from _Legionella pneumophila,_ which is found in

(b) _____. Signs and symptoms of this disease are sim-

ilar to (c) _____ _____. Compli-

cations of Legionnaires' disease include (d) _____,

_____, and _____.

29. List four types of pneumonia.

a.

b.

c.

d.

30. List the signs and symptoms of bacterial pneumonia.

_____

31. Describe the prehospital care for patients with known or suspected pneumonia.

_____

_____

_____

32. What patient groups are at high risk for tuberculosis?

_____

33. List signs and symptoms of tuberculosis.

_____

_____

34. What classic symptom of tuberculosis should alert paramedics to take personal protective measures?

_____

● STUDENT SELF-EVALUATION

35. Pulmonary hypertension can lead to:

a. Heart failure

b. Pulmonary edema

c. Pulmonary embolism

d. Renal failure

36. Signs and symptoms of an acute asthma attack are due to all of the following, _except:_

a. Bronchial muscle contraction

b. Bronchial inflammation

c. Mucus hypersecretion

d. Pulmonary hypertension

37. Which of the following is evidence of chronic emphysema on physical examination?

a. Decreased heart rate

b. Decreased capillary refill

c. Diminished breath sounds

d. Decreased blood pressure

38. The hypoxia, hypercapnia, and acidosis found in an acutely ill patient with cystic fibrosis are due to:

a. Alveolar wall destruction

b. Bronchiolar spasm

c. Thick pulmonary mucous plugs

d. Excess secretion of norepinephrine

39. Patients with myasthenia gravis or Guillain-Barré syndrome experience respiratory failure resulting from:
  a. Obstructed lower airways
  b. Muscle paralysis
  c. Shock lung syndrome
  d. Ventilation perfusion mismatch
40. Inflammation of the visceral and parietal pleura is known as:
  a. Atelectasis
  b. Bronchitis
  c. Pleurisy
  d. Pneumonia
41. Influenza can be prevented by:
  a. Antibiotic therapy
  b. Immunization
  c. Regular exercise
  d. Vitamin therapy
42. Which of the following statements is true regarding tuberculosis?
  a. It is found only in the lung.
  b. The causative agent is always a bacterium.
  c. Hemoptysis is always present.
  d. Symptoms are always present 5 days after exposure.

CARDIOVASCULAR EMERGENCIES

● READING ASSIGNMENT
Chapter 18, pp. 538-665, in *Mosby's Paramedic Textbook*

● OBJECTIVES
As a paramedic, you should be able to:
1. Describe the normal physiology of the heart and vascular system.
2. Discuss electrophysiology as it relates to the normal electrical events in the cardiac cycle.
3. Describe the mechanical activity of the cardiac cells.
4. Detail in the correct sequence the electrical conduction system in the heart.
5. Describe basic monitoring techniques that permit clear electrocardiogram interpretation.
6. Explain the relationship of the electrocardiogram tracing to the heart's electrical activity.
7. Describe in sequence the steps in electrocardiogram interpretation.
8. Identify the characteristics of normal sinus rhythm in lead II.
9. Interpret electrocardiogram tracings.
10. Given a dysrhythmia, identify the site of origin, discuss its possible causes, recognize its critical features in monitoring lead II, interpret a selected rhythm tracing, describe prehospital management, and describe treatment.
11. Assess a patient who may be suffering from a cardiovascular disorder.
12. Describe patient assessment and management of selected cardiovascular diseases based on knowledge of the pathophysiology of the illness.
13. List indications, contraindications, mechanism of action for pharmacological agents for cardiovascular disease.
14. Identify critical patient care measures for a person in cardiac arrest.
15. Given a scenario, state correct interventions according to the American Heart Association.

● REVIEW QUESTIONS
Match each term in Column 2 with its definition in column 1. Use each term only once.

Column 1	Column 2
_____ 1. Heart rate × stroke volume	a. Afterload
_____ 2. Volume available for ventricles to pump each contraction	b. Blood pressure
_____ 3. Peripheral vascular resistance produces this pressure	c. Cardiac output
_____ 4. Ventricular relaxation	d. Contractility
_____ 5. Cardiac output × peripheral vascular resistance	e. Diastole
_____ 6. Increased myocardial contractility in response to increased preload	f. Preload
_____ 7. Ventricular ejection per heartbeat	g. Starling's Law
	h. Stroke volume
	i. Systole

8. When viewing an electrocardiogram (ECG) strip, the paramedic can determine the patient's heart rate and strength of contractions. True/false. If this is false, why is it false?

9. Explain how the sympathetic and parasympathetic divisions of the autonomic nervous system influence cardiac function in the following areas:

	Sympathetic	Parasympathetic

   a. Heart rate
   b. Myocardial contractility
   c. Lungs
   d. Blood vessels (peripheral)

10. Name the two adrenal hormones and describe the effects of each on the cardiovascular system.

Name	Function

   a.
   b.

11. Fill in the blanks in the following sentences about electrophysiology: Within the body, separated charged particles with opposite charges have a (a)

   _____ force of attraction that gives them (b)

   _____ energy. This energy is released when the cell

   membrane becomes (c) _____ to the charged particles and allows the charges to come together. The electrical charge between the

   inside and outside of cells is the (d) _____ difference

   and is measured in (e) _____. Although there is a relatively equal number of positively and negatively charged ions inside and

   outside the cell, the intracellular area has a (f) _____

   charge because of the (g) _____ charged proteins that cannot move outside the cell. The electrical charge difference in the resting state has the potential to do work and is known as the resting membrane

   (h) _____ (RMP). In this phase the inside of the cell is

   (i) _____ relative to the outside of the cell (approxi-

   mately (j) _____ mV). The RMP is primarily due to the difference between the intracellular and extracellular (k)

   _____ ion level. Because of the chemical gradient, (more of these ions inside than outside of the cell), one would expect that the

   (l) _____ would move out of the cell in an attempt to achieve equilibrium. However, they remain in the cell because of the nega-

   tive intracellular charge generated by the (m) _____.
   In the RMP, sodium will not rush into the cell because the cell membrane is

not (n) _____ to sodium. The ability of nerve and muscle cells to produce action potentials is known as (o)

_____. If this action potential results in a decreased charge difference across the cell membrane, the RMP becomes less nega-

tive, and this is called (p) _____. If a stimulus is strong enough to cause depolarization of a cell membrane to a level called the (q)

_____ _____, a chain reaction

of permeability changes cause an (r) _____

_____ to spread over the entire cell membrane. Action

potentials have two phases: a (s) _____ phase and a

(t) _____ phase. During an action potential, the sodium ions rush into the cell, and RMP becomes (u)

_____ on the inside and (v)

_____ on the outside of the cell membrane. This

occurs during the (w) _____ phase. The repolarization phase is due to potassium leakage out of the cell and the return of the cell

membrane to its normal resting (x) _____

_____ state.

12. Answer the following questions regarding the five phases of the cardiac action potential:
   a. During phase 0 (rapid depolarization), what causes the inside of the cell to become positive?

_____

   b. What is the membrane potential during phase 1 (early rapid repolarization)?

_____

   c. How is the the membrane potential held at 0 during phase 2 (plateau phase)?

_____

   d. What happens to the membrane potential of the cell during phase 3 (terminal phase of rapid repolarization)?

_____

   e. How is the balance of sodium and potassium restored during phase 4?

_____

   f. Why can cardiac pacemaker cells depolarize without an external stimulus to initiate an action potential?

_____

_____

● INTRODUCTION TO ECG MONITORING

13. Circle the correct response in each of the following statements: The ECG tracing represents an amplified view of the myocardial (a) *action potentials* or *contractions*. If the voltage displayed is positive, the ECG tracing will display a(n) (b) *upward, downward,* or *isoelectric* deflection. Cardiac pacemaker cells can spontaneously generate impulses, a property known as (c) *automaticity* or *conductivity*. This rhythmic activity occurs because these cells do not have a stable (d) *action* potential or *resting membrane* potential.

14. a. Label Fig. 18-1 illustrating the cardiac conduction system.

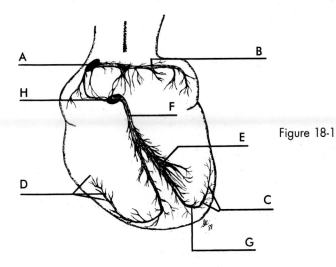

Figure 18-1

a.

b.

c.

d.

e.

f.

g.

h.

15. The sinoatrial node is the dominant pacemaker. If it fails to fire, what will happen?

_____

16. Briefly describe the mechanism for ectopic impulse formation by each of the following mechanisms:

   a. Enhanced automaticity:

_____

   b. Reentry:

_____

17. Place the positive (+) and negative (–) and electrodes for the four leads shown in Fig. 18-2.

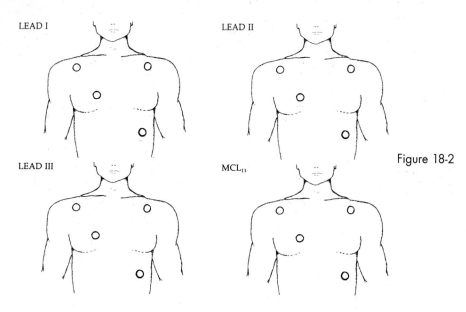

LEAD I

LEAD II

LEAD III

MCL₁₁

Figure 18-2

18. List three problems that may interfere with a clear ECG recording. For each problem, discuss a possible solution.

   a.

   b.

   c.

19. Label Fig. 18-3 with the appropriate measurement intervals.

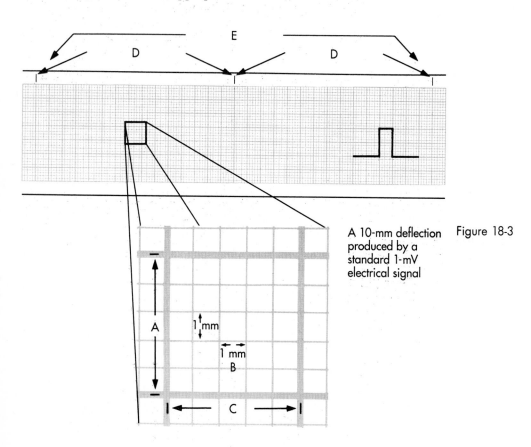

A 10-mm deflection produced by a standard 1-mV electrical signal

Figure 18-3

a. _____ mm
b. _____ sec
c. _____ sec
d. _____ sec
e. _____ sec

20. Label the sample ECG tracing in Fig. 18-4.

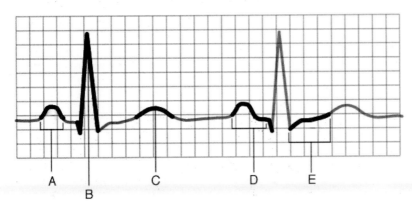

Figure 18-4

a.

b.

c.

d.

e.

21. List five causes of artifact.

a.

b.

c.

d.

e.

● ECG INTERPRETATION

22. List the five steps in ECG analysis.

a.

b.

c.

d.

e.

23. a. Calculate the rate of the ECG in Fig. 18-5 using four different methods, describing the steps you use in each method.

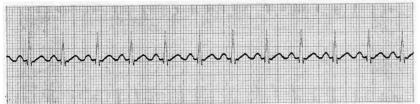

Figure 18-5

a.

_____

_____

b.

_____

_____

c.

_____

_____

d.

_____

_____

24. If the rate in Question 23 is within normal limits, can we assume that the patient is stable in this situation?

_____

25. Which method of calculation would be *most* accurate if the rhythm in Question 23 was:
   a. Regular:

_____

   b. Irregularly irregular:

_____

26. What criterion must be met when analyzing the ECG rhythm to determine that the rhythm is regular?

_____

27. What analysis can be made about conduction in each of the following examples?
   a. The QRS width is less than or equal to 0.12 second.

_____

   b. The QRS width is greater than 0.12 second.

_____

28. List the four criteria that must be evaluated when analyzing the P waves.
   a.
   b.
   c.
   d.

29. Briefly describe the significance of each of the following PR-interval findings.
   a. PR interval 0.08 sec:

_____

   b. PR interval 0.16 sec:

_____

   c. PR interval 0.24 sec:

_____

30. Analyze the ECG rhythm strip in Fig. 18-6 using the five steps described in Question 22, and give your interpretation.

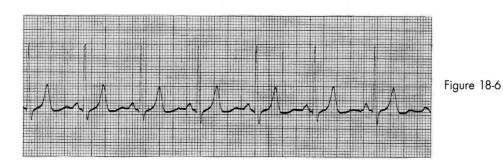

Figure 18-6

    a. Step 1:

_____

    b. Step 2:

_____

    c. Step 3:

_____

    d. Step 4:

_____

    e. Step 5:

_____

    Interpretation:

_____

● INTRODUCTION TO DYSRHYTHMIAS

31. When a dysrhythmia is noted on the monitor, what factors must be considered to determine whether any intervention is necessary?

_____

32. **a.** Dysrhythmias originating in the sinoatrial node frequently result from

    increases or decreases in (a) _____

    _____. ECG features common to all
    sinoatrial node dysrhythmias are
    b. QRS complex:

_____

    c. P waves (lead II):

_____

    d. PR interval:

_____

33. List two causes of each bradycardic and tachycardic dysrhythmia that originates in the sinus node.

    a. Bradycardia:

_____

    b. Tachycardia:

_____

Complete the missing information on Flashcards 1 to 4 at the end of the text.

34. Complete Flashcard 1 (Fig. 18-7): Sinus bradycardia.

35. Complete Flashcard 2 (Fig. 18-8): Sinus tachycardia.

36. Complete Flashcard 3 (Fig. 18-9): Sinus dysrhythmia.

37. Complete Flashcard 4 (Fig. 18-10): Sinus arrest.

38. Atrial dysrhythmias originate in the (a) _____ of the

    (b) _____ or in the (c) _____
pathways.

39. Common features of atrial dysrhythmias are:

    a. QRS complex:

_____

    b. P waves (if present):

_____

    c. PR intervals:

_____

40. List four causes of dysrhythmias that originate in the atria.

    a.

    b.

    c.

    d.

Complete the missing information on Flashcards 5 to 9 showing dysrhythmias originating in the AV junction.

41. Complete Flashcard 5 (Fig. 18-11): Wandering pacemaker.

42. Complete Flashcard 6 (Fig. 18-12): Premature atrial contractions.

43. Complete Flashcard 7 (Fig. 18-13): Atrial tachycardia.

44. Complete Flashcard 8 (Fig. 18-14): Atrial flutter.

45. Complete Flashcard 9 (Fig. 18-15): Atrial fibrillation.

46. **a.** Rhythms that start in the atrioventricular node or junction are called (a)

    _____ rhythms. These rhythms share the following
common features:

    b. QRS complex:

_____

    c. P waves:

_____

    d. PR interval:

_____

47. List four causes of dysrhythmias that start in the atrioventricular junction.

　　a.

　　b.

　　c.

　　d.

Complete the missing information on Flashcards 10 to 12 showing dysrhythmias originating in the atrioventricular junction.

48. Complete Flashcard 10 (Fig. 18-16): Premature junctional contractions.

49. Complete Flashcard 11 (Fig. 18-17): Junctional escape rhythm.

50. Complete Flashcard 12 (Fig. 18-18): Accelerated junctional rhythm.

51. Rhythms originating from the ventricle have an intrinsic rate of (a)

_____ to _____ but can be

accelerated at rates up to (b) _____/min or tachy-

cardic at rates greater than (c) _____.

52. List five causes of dysrhythmias that originate in the ventricles.

　　a.

　　b.

　　c.

　　d.

　　e.

Complete the missing information on Flashcards 13 to 18 showing dysrhythmias originating in the ventricles.

53. Complete Flashcard 13 (Fig. 18-19): Ventricular escape rhythm.

54. Complete Flashcard 14 (Fig. 18-20): Premature ventricular contraction.

55. Complete Flashcard 15 (Fig. 18-21): Ventricular tachycardia.

56. Complete Flashcard 16 (Fig. 18-22): Ventricular fibrillation.

57. Complete Flashcard 17 (Fig. 18-23): Asystole.

58. Complete Flashcard 18 (Fig. 18-24): Artificial pacemaker rhythm.

59. Delays or interruptions in cardiac electrical conduction are called (a)

_____ _____. They may

be caused by disease of the (b) _____

_____.

60. List five causes of dysrhythmias caused by delays in cardiac electrical conduction.

　　a.

　　b.

　　c.

　　d.

　　e.

Complete the missing information on Flashcards 19 to 22 showing dysrhythmias originating from conduction disorders.

61. Complete Flashcard 19 (Fig. 18-25): First-degree atrioventricular block.

62. Complete Flashcard 20 (Fig. 18-26): Second-degree atrioventricular block (Mobitz I).

63. Complete Flashcard 21 (Fig. 18-27): Second-degree atrioventricular block (Mobitz II).

64. Complete Flashcard 22 (Fig. 18-28): Third-degree atrioventricular block.

● ASSESSMENT OF THE CARDIAC PATIENT

65. *A 62-year-old woman is complaining of chest pain.* What questions should you ask, using the PQRST mnemonic, to determine the nature and severity of her pain?

P—

Q—

R—

S—

T—

66. List three chief complaints that may lead you to believe a patient has a cardiovascular problem.

a.

b.

c.

67. *An older man experiences a syncopal episode at a local gym.* Write two questions you should ask in an attempt to determine the nature of his syncopal episode.

a.

b.

68. *A 34-year-old woman walks into your ambulance base complaining of a fluttering sensation in her chest.* What will your history and physical examination include to determine the cause of this sensation?

Questions 69 to 71 pertain to the following scenario: *An 87-year-old white woman calls you to her home complaining of weakness and nausea. On arrival, you find her seated on the commode. She is pale, cool, and diaphoretic. Her blood pressure is 70 mm Hg by palpation, and her ECG is shown in Fig. 18-29.*

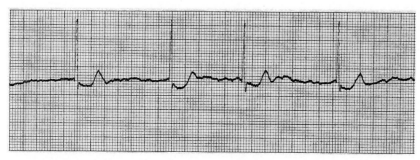

Figure 18-29

69. What information from this patient's past medical history will be important to elicit at this time?

70. What is your interpretation of her ECG?

71. *She tells you that she is taking digoxin, diltiazem, potassium, and furosemide.* Could any of her home medicines be playing a role in her problem? If yes, which ones and why?

72. *An older man is found unresponsive and bradycardic in a local park. A caretaker states that he complained of chest pain before collapsing. No one is available to give you any information regarding his history. Briefly outline specific findings you may encounter in your patient assessment if he has a cardiac history.*

_____

_____

73. Identify two risk factors each of atherosclerotic heart disease:
  a. That cannot be altered:

_____

  b. That can be altered:

_____

74. How can a paramedic distinguish between unstable angina and myocardial infarction in the prehospital environment?

_____

75. Briefly outline the sequence of pathophysiological events that occur from the time that a clot forms until cardiac tissue dies in acute myocardial infarction.

_____

_____

76. Identify four complications secondary to myocardial infarction.
  a.
  b.
  c.
  d.

Questions 77 to 84 pertain to the following scenario: *A 57-year-old, 80-kg man with a history of untreated hypertension is complaining of crushing midsternal chest pain that began 2 hours ago. He takes no medicines but admits to smoking two packs of cigarettes a day. His blood pressure is 162/102 mm Hg. His ECG strip is shown in Fig. 18-30.*

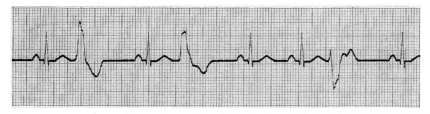

Figure 18-30

77. What other associated signs or symptoms may be present if the patient is experiencing a myocardial infarction?

_____

78. What is your interpretation of his ECG?

_____

79. Describe general treatment measures you will use for this patient.

_____

_____

80. List two drugs (excluding oxygen) with the appropriate dosage that you can administer to this patient for relief of pain that will also decrease the cardiac workload.

   a.

   b.

81. *In consultation with medical direction, you elect to treat the dysrhythmias with lidocaine 1.5 mg/kg. It is supplied in 10-ml syringes, which contain 100 mg of the drug.* How many milliliters will you administer? _____ ml.

82. If this dose of lidocaine fails to correct the dysrhythmia, what will your next dose be? _____ mg/kg.

83. How many milliliters of lidocaine will you push for this second dose? _____ ml.

84. If the second dose of lidocaine successfully abolishes the dysrhythmia, what action should you take?

Questions 85 to 89 pertain to the following scenario: *A 72-year-old, 70-kg woman calls you to her home complaining of a sudden onset of severe dyspnea without chest pain. You find her anxious, sitting upright, with diaphoretic skin and circumoral cyanosis. Her only home medicine is a diuretic. Vital signs are blood pressure, 170/106 mm Hg; pulse, 124; and respirations, 28 and labored. Rales are audible to the level of the scapulae. SaO$_2$ is 86%. Her ECG is shown in Fig. 18-31.*

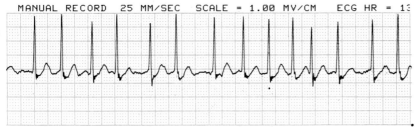

MANUAL RECORD   25 MM/SEC   SCALE = 1.00 MV/CM   ECG HR = 1⁞

Figure 18-31

85. What medical condition or conditions do you suspect?

---

86. What other physical findings would help confirm this diagnosis?

---

87. What is your interpretation of her ECG?

---

88. *You have placed the patient on oxygen and wish to administer other pharmacological agents to improve her oxygenation.* List three drugs that you would consider as well as the correct dose and desired effect of each.

   a.

   b.

   c.

89. *You decide to administer furosemide 0.5 mg/kg. It is supplied in a 4-ml ampule that contains 40 mg of the drug.* How many milliliters will you give? _____ ml.

90. List causes and signs and symptoms of right-sided heart failure.

   a. Causes:

---

   b. Signs and symptoms:

Questions 91 to 94 pertain to the following scenario: *You are evaluating a 67-year-old man who has a history of two myocardial infarctions. His wife states that he had chest pain that began 4 hours ago, but he stubbornly refused to let her call EMS until he passed out. He is conscious but confused and is pale and diaphoretic. His blood pressure is 80/50 mm Hg, and his SaO₂ is 90%. His only home medicines are nitroglycerine paste, which he has on his left chest. This patient's ECG is shown in Fig. 18-32.*

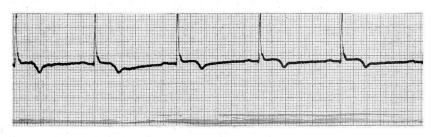

Figure 18-32

91. What is your interpretation of his ECG?

_____

92. What drug and what dosage will you administer in consultation with medical direction to correct this dysrhythmia?

_____

After administering the first dose of this drug, the heart rate accelerates to 70/min; however, the patient's other physical findings remain unchanged.
93. What do you suspect this patient is suffering from?

_____

94. List critical interventions that you should use, including drug therapy, assuming that your estimated time of arrival to the hospital is 30 minutes.

_____

_____

Questions 95 to 98 pertain to the following scenario: *A 70-year-old man experiences a sudden onset of a "tearing" abdominal pain at the area of the umbilicus that radiates to his back. He is pale and complains of the urge to defecate. His only history is hypertension, for which he takes captopril. Vital signs are blood pressure, 106/70 mm Hg; pulse 100; and respirations, 20. On physical examination, you auscultate a bruit over the periumbilical area.*
95. What illness do you suspect?

_____

96. Should you palpate this patient's abdomen?

_____

97. Should you allow this patient to go to the toilet and defecate?

_____

98. Briefly outline your management of this patient.

_____

_____

Questions 99 to 101 pertain to the following scenario: *An older man complains of a severe "ripping" pain between his scapulae that extends down to his legs. He is pale and diaphoretic and has the following vital signs: blood pressure 170/110 mm Hg in the right arm and 130/80 mm Hg in the left arm.*

99. What medical emergency do you suspect?

100. Describe other physical findings that may confirm your suspicions.

101. Outline your management of this patient in the prehospital phase.

102. Differentiate between the following characteristics of embolic arterial occlusion and thrombotic arterial occlusion.

	Embolic	Thrombotic
Causes:		
Onset:		
Signs and symptoms		

103. *An older woman calls you to her home because she bumped her leg and a varicose vein is bleeding.* What care should be rendered to this patient?

104. List three signs or symptoms of acute deep vein thrombosis.

a.

b.

c.

Questions 105 to 108 pertain to the following scenario: *A 60-year-old man is complaining of a severe headache, blurred vision, and vomiting. He states that he has a history of hypertension but has not been taking his medicine because the cost is too much. His vital signs are blood pressure, 190/128 mm Hg; pulse, 88; and respirations, 20.*

105. What medical emergency do you suspect?

106. If this man is not treated promptly, what other symptoms may result?

107. Outline general management principles for this patient.

108. If your transport time is delayed, list one drug (with the appropriate dose) that medical direction may order to lower this patient's blood pressure.

● **TECHNIQUES OF MANAGEMENT FOR CARDIAC EMERGENCIES**

109. *You are at a friend's home playing tennis. After retrieving the ball, you turn around see that your friend has collapsed on the court.* Outline the steps you must take from this moment until EMS arrives if he has had a cardiac arrest (assume that no one else is nearby to help).

110. *A basic life-support unit is caring for a patient who is in cardiac arrest when your advanced life-support unit arrives on the scene. An automated external defibrillator that does not have a display is attached to the patient, and five shocks have already been delivered.*

   a. When should you cardiovert this patient?

   b. If a rescuer is in contact with the patient when the automated external defibrillator fires, will an injury occur?

Questions 111 to 114 pertain to the following scenario: *You arrive on the scene to care for a patient who is pulseless and apneic. The monitor displays the rhythm shown in Fig. 18-33.*

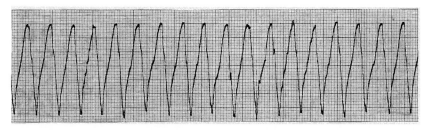

Figure 18-33

111. What is your interpretation of the ECG?

112. What is your first intervention, after rhythm determination and pulselessness are verified?

113. List two factors that will improve the success rate of this treatment.
   a.
   b.

114. List the steps in performing this intervention.

115. *You are at the home of a patient whose wife states that he was experiencing severe chest pain. Moments after you hook up the patient to your monitor, he loses consciousness, and the rhythm shown in Fig. 18-34 is displayed. Blood pressure is*

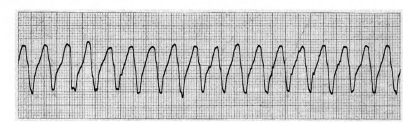

Figure 18-34

60 mm Hg by palpation, and ventilations are adequate. Another paramedic applies oxygen by nonrebreather mask at 12 L/min. State the appropriate therapy for this patient up to and including administration of the first drug.

_____

116. What is the advantage of synchronized cardioversion?

117. Briefly outline the steps in synchronized cardioversion that are different from unsynchronized cardioversion.

_____

118. *A 69-year-old patient has a blood pressure of 76/50 mm Hg and the ECG shown in Fig. 18-35.*

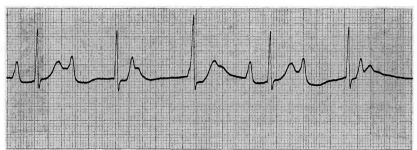

Figure 18-35

   a. What is your interpretation of the ECG?

_____

   b. Assuming that no drugs are readily available, list the steps you would take to initiate transcutaneous pacing on this patient.

_____

_____

_____

_____

119. *An approximately 50-year-old man is found unconscious in a parking lot downtown. He is pulseless and apneic. The attendant is sure that he has been there fewer than 5 minutes but does not know what happened. The patient's ECG is shown in Fig. 18-36.*

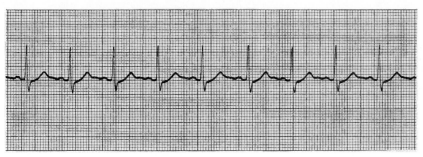

Figure 18-36

a. You identify the rhythm as:

_____

b. Outline the appropriate interventions for this patient based on current treatment guidelines by the American Heart Association.

_____

120. *An older man is found unresponsive, apneic, and pulseless in the busy bathroom of a shopping mall. A quick examination reveals the monitor pattern shown in Fig. 18-37.*

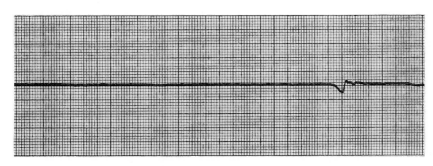

Figure 18-37

a. You interpret the rhythm as:

_____

b. What drugs (with appropriate doses) should be administered?

_____

c. What electrical therapy would be appropriate for this patient?

_____

121. *You are en route to the hospital with a 55-year-old man whom you suspect is having an acute myocardial infarction. Suddenly, the patient gasps and becomes pulseless and apneic. As you look at the monitor, you note the ECG shown in Fig. 18-38.*

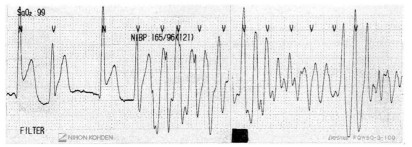

Figure 18-38

177

a. You identify the rhythm as:

b. What single treatment modality is most likely to restore circulation in this patient?

c. List the appropriate drugs (in the proper order) with correct doses that may be given to this patient if the answer in b is unsuccessful.

● STUDENT SELF-EVALUATION

122. *You are treating a 60-year-old woman with atrial fibrillation at a rate of 168/min. Her blood pressure is 80 by palpation, and she feels very faint.* The appropriate intervention would be:
   a. Adenosine 6 mg via rapid intravenous administration
   b. Verapamil 2.5 mg intravenously over 2 min
   c. Procainamide 30 mg/min intravenously
   d. Synchronized cardioversion at 100 joules

123. Blood pressure is equal to:
   a. Heart rate × Stroke volume × Cardiac output
   b. Stroke volume × Peripheral vascular resistance
   c. Heart rate × Stroke volume × Peripheral vascular resistance
   d. Heart rate × Contractility × Stroke volume

124. The valve that separates the left atrium from the left ventricle is the _____ valve:
   a. Aortic   c. Pulmonic
   b. Mitral   d. Tricuspid

125. When evaluating a patient for jugular venous distention, the paramedic should:
   a. Raise the head of the bed 90 degrees.
   b. Raise the head of the bed 45 degrees.
   c. Lay the patient in the supine position.
   d. Have the patient stand with assistance.

126. Death secondary to myocardial infarction is *most commonly* due to:
   a. Dysrhythmias   c. Pulmonary embolism
   b. Low blood pressure   d. Cardiac rupture

127. Appropriate care for a stable patient with acute myocardial infarction would include all of the following, *except:*
   a. Placing the patient in a semi-Fowler position
   b. Administering lactated Ringer's solution at 500 ml/hr intravenously
   c. Administering oxygen by nasal cannula
   d. Documenting and reporting all intravenous sticks

128. Medications that may help in the management of a patient with cardiac pulmonary edema include all of the following, *except:*
   a. Epinephrine   c. Nifedipine
   b. Furosemide   d. Nitroglycerin

129. When a patient suffers from right-sided heart failure, blood backs up into the:
   a. Aorta   c. Pulmonary veins
   b. Pulmonary arteries   d. Venae cavae

130. Cardiogenic shock is:
  a. Fatal in only 10% to 15% of patients
  b. Caused by extensive myocardial damage
  c. Due to an intravascular electrolyte imbalance
  d. Caused by obstruction of the renal vessels

131. Which of the following drugs is used in treating asystole?
  a. Atropine   **c.** Calcium chloride
  b. Bretylium   **d.** Lidocaine

132. Acute arterial occlusion may result in:
  a. Absent distal pulses   **c.** Pulmonary congestion
  b. Hypertension   **d.** Torsades de pointes

133. Which of the following is an ectopic rhythm?
  a. Atrial tachycardia   **c.** Normal sinus rhythm
  b. Junctional tachycardia   **d.** Sinus bradycardia

134. Which of the following will *not* cause sinus bradycardia?
  a. Digoxin   **c.** Isoproterenol
  b. Increased vagal tone   **d.** Sleep

135. Which of the following is a side effect from bretylium tosylate?
  a. Drowsiness   **c.** Hypotension
  b. Headache   **d.** Hypothermia

136. Which of the following is an action of morphine sulfate?
  a. Dilation of peripheral vasculature
  b. Increase in cardiac preload
  c. Calming of the patient with a head injury
  d. Bronchodilation

137. Which of the following is true of digoxin?
  a. It increases the force of ventricular contraction.
  b. It is a first line drug in the management of bradycardia.
  c. It causes decreased cardiac output.
  d. It increases impulse conduction through the atrioventricular node.

138. Which of the following drugs stimulates the beta receptors?
  a. Amyl nitrite   **c.** Epinephrine
  b. Atropine   **d.** Propranolol

139. *A 60-year-old, 100-kg woman has a blood pressure of 80/50 mm Hg. The ECG is shown in Fig. 18-39. Which of the following would* not *be appropriate to correct this?*

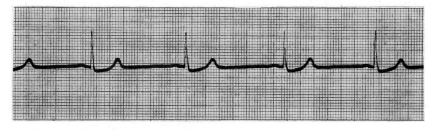

Figure 18-39

  a. Atropine 0.5 to 1.0 mg intravenously
  b. Dopamine 5 to 20 mcg/kg/min
  c. Epinephrine 2 to 10 mcg/kg/min
  d. Isoproterenol 2 to 10 mcg/min

140. *You suspect that your patient has an arterial occlusion affecting the lower leg. Which of the following treatment measures would be appropriate?*
  a. Initiate intravenous fluid therapy and administer a fluid challenge.
  b. Massage the affected extremity to encourage circulation.
  c. Immobilize the affected extremity and protect it from injury.
  d. Administer furosemide 40 mg intravenously to flush out the embolus.

141. Chronic, uncontrolled hypertension puts a patient at risk for all of the following, *except:*
   a. Cerebral hemorrhage   c. Myocardial infarction
   b. Diabetes mellitus   d. Renal failure

142. Which of the following statements is *true* with regard to synchronized cardioversion?
   a. It is faster than unsynchronized cardioversion.
   b. It is not as safe as unsynchronized cardioversion.
   c. It is indicated for pulseless ventricular tachycardia.
   d. It is indicated for unstable PSVT.

143. When attempting to initiate transcutaneous pacing on a conscious patient, the current should be set at:
   a. 70/min and increased until patient is stable
   b. Minimum and increased until capture occurs
   c. 70/min and decreased until the patient becomes unstable
   d. Maximum and decreased until capture is lost

144. Identify the ECG tracing in Fig. 18-40.

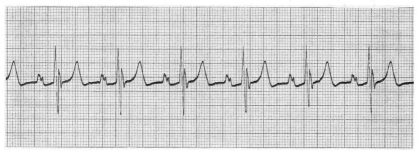

Figure 18-40

   a. Normal sinus rhythm
   b. Sinus rhythm with first-degree atrioventricular block
   c. Second-degree heart block type II
   d. Ventricular demand pacer with capture

145. Identify the ECG tracing in Fig. 18-41.

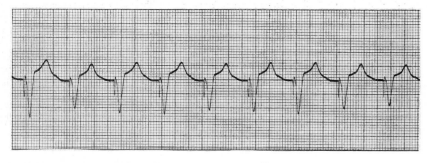

Figure 18-41

   a. Accelerated idioventricular rhythm
   b. Junctional tachycardia
   c. Ventricular pacemaker
   d. Ventricular tachycardia

146. Identify the ECG tracing in Fig. 18-42.

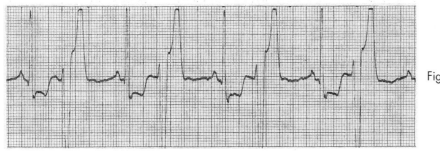

Figure 18-42

    a. Multifocal premature ventricular contractions
    b. Salvo of premature ventricular contractions
    c. Ventricular bigeminy
    d. Ventricular escape rhythm

147. Identify the ECG tracing in Fig. 18-43.

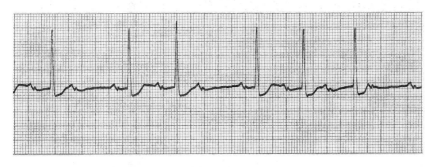

Figure 18-43

    a. Second-degree atrioventricular block type I
    b. Second-degree atrioventricular block type II
    c. Sinus arrest
    d. Sinus arrythmia

148. Identify the ECG tracing in Fig. 18-44.

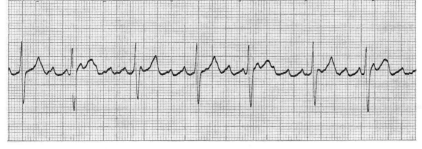

Figure 18-44

    a. Atrial fibrillation
    b. Atrial flutter
    c. Junctional tachycardia
    d. Third-degree atrioventricular block

149. Identify the ECG tracing in Fig. 18-45.

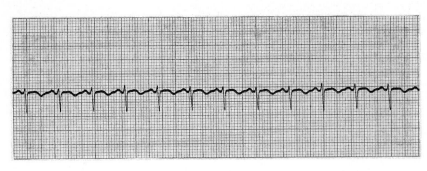

Figure 18-45

    a. Atrial fibrillation   **c.** Atrial tachycardia
    b. Atrial flutter   **d.** Sinus tachycardia

150. Identify the ECG tracing in Fig. 18-46.

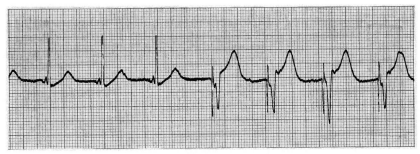

Figure 18-46

    a. Accelerated junctional rhythm followed by pacemaker
    b. Junctional rhythm followed by pacemaker
    c. Junctional rhythm followed by idioventricular
    d. Second-degree atrioventricular block type II followed by idioventricular

DIABETIC EMERGENCIES

● READING ASSIGNMENT

Chapter 19, pp. 666-679, in *Mosby's Paramedic Textbook*

● OBJECTIVES

As a paramedic, you should be able to:

1. Discuss the role of the pancreas in maintaining normal blood glucose.
2. Describe the mechanism of action of insulin and glucagon.
3. Outline how the process of digestion influences serum glucose levels.
4. Discuss the pathophysiology of diabetes as a basis for key signs and symptoms.
5. Describe the role of insulin and oral hypoglycemics in managing diabetes.
6. Discuss pathophysiology as a basis for key signs and symptoms, patient assessment, and patient management for the diabetic emergencies of hypoglycemia, diabetic ketoacidosis, and hyperosmolar hyperglycemic nonketotic coma.

● REVIEW QUESTIONS

Match the signs or symptoms listed in Column 2 with the appropriate diabetic emergencies listed in Column 1. Signs or symptoms can be used more than once.

Column 1	Column 2
_____ **1.** Diabetic ketoacidosis	**a.** Abdominal pain
	b. Coma
_____ **2.** Hyperosmolar hyperglycemic	**c.** Cool, clammy skin
nonketotic coma	**d.** Fruity breath odor
_____ **3.** Hypoglycemia	**e.** Kussmaul respirations
	f. Polyuria
	g. Psychotic behavior
	h. Seizures
	i. Tachycardia
	j. Warm, dry skin
	k. Vomiting

4. Name the hormone secreted from each of these cells in the pancreas.
   a. Alpha cells:
   b. Beta cells:
   c. Delta cells:
5. When food is ingested, it is broken down into smaller units and used or stored. Name the breakdown products and storage sites of the following food types:

Food	Breakdown Products	Storage
a. Carbohydrates		
b. Proteins		
c. Fats		

6. **a.** How is excess glucose stored in the liver?

_____

   b. How are glucose stores released from the liver?

_____

7. Briefly explain the role of glucagon in the metabolism of food.

_____

8. Why does a patient develop cerebral signs and symptoms of hypoglycemia rapidly?

_____

9. List three medical illness associated with long-term diabetes.
   a.
   b.
   c.

10. _You arrive on the scene of a suspected diabetic emergency. On arrival you find a 35-year-old man whose wife says that he took his insulin 2 hours ago and has not eaten. He arouses only to pain and has noisy, snoring respirations. He has no other medical history._ Outline the steps in your patient management.

_____

_____

_____

_____

● STUDENT SELF-EVALUATION

11. The primary action of insulin is to:
    a. Reduce the glucose needs of the cells
    b. Increase blood glucose levels
    c. Transport glucose into the cells
    d. Manufacture amino acids

12. Oral hypoglycemic agents include all of the following, _except:_
    a. Diabinese   **c.** Insulin
    b. Dymelor   **d.** Orinase

13. Type II diabetes mellitus is most likely to:
    a. Require insulin injections
    b. Develop after 40 years of age
    c. Have a sudden onset of symptoms
    d. Result in life-threatening complications

14. The breakdown of glucose stores in the liver is known as:
    a. Glucogenesis   **c.** Gluconeogenesis
    b. Glucolysis   **d.** Glucogenolysis

15. Before administration of D50W in a lethargic patient with diabetes, the paramedic should do all of the following, _except:_
    a. Initiate intravenous fluids.   **c.** Draw a blood sample.
    b. Administer glucagon.   **d.** Determine blood glucose.

16. When giving D50W to a diabetic who is also a known alcoholic, the paramedic should administer:
    a. Glucagon   **c.** Insulin
    b. Half the usual dose **d.** Thiamine

CHAPTER 20
NERVOUS SYSTEM DISORDERS

● **READING ASSIGNMENT**

Chapter 20, pp. 680-699, in *Mosby's Paramedic Textbook*

● **OBJECTIVES**

As a paramedic, you should be able to:
1. Discuss the anatomy and function of nerve cells.
2. Describe impulse transmission in the nervous system.
3. Label a diagram of the brain and discuss the normal physiological functions of the blood vessels supplying the brain and the divisions and areas of specialization of the brain.
4. Describe the general assessment of a patient who has a nervous system disorder.
5. Discuss the specific neurological patient evaluation.
6. Describe the pathophysiology, assessment, and specific management techniques for each of the following neurological disorders: coma, seizure, and cerebrovascular accident.

● **REVIEW QUESTIONS**

For each of the etiologies listed in Column 1, identify the appropriate general cause of coma in Column 2. You may use each answer more than once.

Column 1	Column 2
_____ 1. Hypertensive encephalopathy	a. Cardiovascular system
	b. Drugs
_____ 2. Chronic obstructive pulmonary disease	c. Infectious
	d. Metabolic system
_____ 3. Kidney failure	e. Respiratory system
	f. Structural
_____ 4. Alcohol	
_____ 5. Hypoglycemia	
_____ 6. Brain tumor	
_____ 7. Meningitis	

8. Complete the following sentences: The cells of the nervous system that

protect the neurons are called (a) _____. Each neuron has three main parts: the area that contains the nucleus is the

(b) _____ _____, one or more branching projections that receive impulses are known as the

(c) _____, and a single, elongated projection that

transmits impulses is called the (d) _____. In the

peripheral nervous system, bundles of axons and their sheaths are called

(e) _____ _____. Neurons are classified by the direction in which they transmit impulses. The neurons that transmit impulses to the spinal cord and brain from the body are

(f) _____ neurons. Neurons that transmit impulses away from the brain to muscle and glandular tissue are

(g) _____ neurons. Neurons that conduct impulses from sensory neurons directly to motor neurons are

(h) _____ neurons. In its resting state the charge inside the

neuron is (i) _____, and the charge outside the

neuron is (j) _____. When the neuron is stimu-

lated while the outside is positively charged, (k) _____ ions

rush into the cell and begin a wave of (l) _____ that travels down the cell. Myelinated axons have interruptions in the myelin

sheaths called (m) _____ _____

_____ that cause the action potential to be conducted

more (n) _____ than unmyelinated axons. The space between the nerve endings of two adjacent neurons is known as a

(o) _____. Impulses are transmitted across these

spaces by neurotransmitters such as (p) _____

or _____
9. List the basic anatomical components of a reflex.

_____

10. Name the two paired arteries that supply blood to the brain.
    a.
    b.
11. State whether the following factors will *increase, decrease,* or *not change* the cerebral blood flow.
    a. Intracranial pressure of 30 mm Hg:
    b. Mean arterial pressure of 40 mm Hg:
    c. Expanding tumor in the brain:
    d. Hypovolemic shock:
12. Describe your assessment of the eyes for a patient with a suspected stroke.

_____

_____

13. List two causes of coma for each of the following six general classifications.

   a. Structural:

   _____

   b. Metabolic:

   _____

   c. Drug induced:

   _____

   d. Cardiovascular:

   _____

   e. Respiratory:

   _____

   f. Infection:

   _____

14. How would you differentiate between hysterical coma and coma of organic cause?

_____

15. For each of the following features of coma, state whether it is most likely to be found in structural or toxic-metabolic coma.

   a. Asymmetric neurologic findings:

   b. Slow onset:

   c. Unilateral fixed dilated pupil:

16. *You arrive at a private residence to evaluate a 65-year-old woman whose neighbors found her unresponsive. She has snoring respirations at a rate of 8/min, and an oral airway is easily placed. Carotid and radial pulses are present and rapid. Blood pressure is 110/70 mm Hg. She flexes to painful stimuli. No history is available. Outline your assessment and management of this patient, including drugs with appropriate dose and route.*

_____

_____

_____

17. List five causes of seizures:

   a.

   b.

   c.

   d.

   e.

18. State the type of seizure for each of the following signs and symptoms:
  a. Numbness of the body or unusual visual, auditory, or taste symptoms:

  b. Brief loss of consciousness in a child without loss of posture lasting less than 15 sec:

  c. Partial seizure activity that spreads in an orderly fashion to surrounding areas:

  d. Preceding aura followed by loss of consciousness and tonic-clonic motor activity followed by a postictal state:

  e. Aura followed by automatisms such as lip smacking and chewing during which time the patient is amnesic:

19. What history should be obtained from the family of a patient who has had a grand mal seizure?

20. List two findings suggesting that the seizure is hysterical versus grand mal.
  a.
  b.

21. State whether each of the following characteristics is more suggestive of seizure or syncope.
  a. It starts in a standing position.

  b. It is preceded by lightheadedness.

  c. The patient remains unconscious for minutes to hours.

  d. Tachycardia occurs.

22. List two anticonvulsants with the appropriate doses that may be given to the adult patient who is having a seizure.
  a.
  b.

23. List five risk factors for cerebrovascular accident.
  a.
  b.
  c.
  d.
  e.

24. List six signs and symptoms of cerebrovascular accident that are common to embolic and thrombotic strokes.

a.

b.

c.

d.

e.

f.

25. Describe the typical progression of signs and symptoms of hemorrhagic stroke.

_____

_____

● **STUDENT SELF-EVALUATION**

26. Which of the following will cause a decrease in the cerebral blood flow?
   a. Blood pressure of 70/50 mm Hg
   b. Intracranial pressure of 15 mm Hg
   c. Decreased levels of intraocular fluid
   d. Body temperature of 102° F (38.9°C)

27. Respiratory patterns associated with neurological disorders include all of the following, *except:*
   a. Ataxic respirations   c. Diaphragmatic breathing
   b. Cheyne-Stokes respirations   d. Kussmaul respirations

28. Posturing caused by structural impairment of the subcortical regions of the brain is known as:
   a. Decerebrate rigidity   c. Dysconjugate rigidity
   b. Decorticate rigidity   d. Flaccidity

29. Your comatose patient's pupils are 2 mm wide and round and are reactive to light. This is suggests:
   a. Barbiturate overdose   c. Opiate overdose
   b. Medullary injury   d. Temporal herniation

30. Management of the postictal patient who arouses only to pain includes:
   a. Administration of naloxone 2 mg intravenously
   b. Administration of diazepam 5 mg intravenously
   c. Intravenous fluid therapy of normal saline 100 ml/hr
   d. Recumbent positioning of patient

31. Significant findings in the past medical history of a patient you suspect is having a cerebrovascular accident include all of the following, *except:*
   a. Cigarette smoking   c. Oral contraceptive use
   b. Obesity   d. Sickle cell disease

ACUTE ABDOMINAL PAIN AND RENAL FAILURE

● READING ASSIGNMENT
Chapter 21, pp. 700-719, in *Mosby's Paramedic Textbook*

● OBJECTIVES
As a paramedic, you should be able to:
1. List the solid and hollow organs of the abdomen and retroperitoneal space.
2. Identify the location of abdominal organs by quadrant.
3. Label diagrams of female and male genitourinary anatomy.
4. Distinguish hemorrhagic and nonhemorrhagic gastrointestinal disorders.
5. Identify precipitating factors, signs and symptoms, and patient management techniques for selected gastrointestinal and genitourinary disorders.
6. Outline specific assessment techniques for evaluating the patient with acute abdominal pain.
7. Distinguish the following types of pain: visceral, somatic, and referred.
8. Outline general management techniques for care of the patient with acute abdominal pain.
9. Discuss the etiology of renal failure.
10. Distinguish between acute and chronic renal failure.
11. List the signs and symptoms of acute and chronic renal failure.
12. Describe hemodialysis.
13. Describe peritoneal dialysis.
14. Discuss the prehospital implications of emergencies that may be encountered in the dialysis patient.

● REVIEW QUESTIONS
Match the gastrointestinal disorder in Column 2 with its description in Column 1. Use each disorder only once.

	Column 1		Column 2
_____	1. Occlusion of the intestinal lumen	a.	Appendicitis
		b.	Arteriovenous malformation
_____	2. Increased pain after ethyl alchohol ingestion, may have fever and signs of sepsis and shock	c.	Cholecystitis
		d.	Diverticulitis
_____	3. Protrusion of viscus from normal position through opening in groin or abdominal wall	e.	Diverticulosis
		f.	Esophageal varices
		g.	Esophagitis
_____	4. Pain most intense at McBurney's point	h.	Gastritis
		i.	Hemorrhoids
_____	5. Most common cause of massive rectal bleeding in older adults	j.	Hernia
		k.	Intestinal obstruction
_____	6. Open erosion wound in digestive system that may bleed	l.	Pancreatitis
_____	7. Characterized by blood dripping into toilet after normal bowel movement	m.	Peptic ulcer
_____	8. Left lower quadrant abdominal pain resulting from pouch in colon wall		

_____ 9. Painless bleeding resulting from vascular abnormality in gastrointestinal tract

_____ 10. Bright red hematemesis caused by rupture of vessels distended by portal hypertension

_____ 11. Inflammation of the gallbladder

_____ 12. Inflammation of the gastric mucosa

13. Identify the genitourinary disorder you suspect in each of the following situations:
    a. _A 35-year-old afebrile man complains of a sudden onset of severe flank pain that radiates into his testicle._

    b. _Your 21-year-old patient is complaining of painful swelling in the scrotal sac unrelieved by elevation. He is in acute distress and has vomited twice._

    c. _A 35-year-old woman with a recent history of recurrent urinary infections is complaining of fever, chills, and severe flank pain._

    d. _A 27-year-old woman complains of having burning on urination and says that she feels she must urinate every 20 minutes._

14. _Your patient is a 72-year-old man complaining of left lower quadrant abdominal pain._ For each of the following abdominal disorders, state whether you would or would not expect this patient to be suffering from each and why.
    a. Pancreatitis:

    b. Cholecystitis:

    c. Diverticulitis:

    d. Urinary calculus:

    e. Testicular torsion:

15. Name the type of pain described in each of the statements below.
    a. _Your patient is supine on his back with his legs flexed and complains of a constant, sharp stabbing pain._

    b. _A 40-year-old woman complains of a severe cramping pain at the umbilicus that peaks and then subsides. She is nauseated and has vomited twice._

    c. _A 30-year-old man complains of severe flank pain that goes into his groin._

16. *A 65-year-old man complains of severe epigastric pain.*

    a. List specific questions you must ask of this patient's past and present medical history to determine whether this is a gastrointestinal problem.

_____

_____

_____

    b. What other significant medical problems must you try to rule out by this line of questioning?

_____

17. *A 17-year-old boy states that he had severe right lower quadrant pain that diminished several hours ago and is now generalized.*

    a. What signs and symptoms would indicate that this patient has an acute abdominal condition and may be developing peritonitis?

_____

    b. Describe the prehospital treatment for this patient.

_____

_____

18. Identify three causes of each of the following:

    a. Acute renal failure

_____

    b. Chronic renal failure

_____

19. *You are called to a dialysis center for a "person in shock."*

    a. What types of patient problems should you anticipate en route to this call?

_____

    b. If the patient is hypotensive and needs fluid resuscitation, describe how you will initiate fluid therapy and the volume you will infuse.

_____

_____

20. What physiological problem suffered by a patient in renal failure makes him or her more susceptible to hypoxia?

_____

_____

21. *During dialysis, a large amount of air is introduced into a patient because of a problem with the machine. The patient is dyspneic and hypotensive. Describe management of this patient en route to the medical center.*

_____

_____

_____

22. The cause of acute abdominal pain is most accurately assessed in the pre-hospital setting by:
    a. Abdominal examination   **c.** Secondary survey
    b. Patient history   **d.** Vital sign assessment

23. Which of the following is *most* suggestive of a hemorrhagic gastrointestinal problem?
    a. Anorexia   **c.** Melena
    b. Fever   **d.** Tachycardia

24. *A 78-year-old man states that he has been unable to have a bowel movement for a week and has been vomiting profusely.* You suspect:
    a. Appendicitis   **c.** Diverticulosis
    b. Bowel obstruction   **d.** Peptic ulcer

25. Prehospital management of the patient with severe right lower quadrant abdominal pain and nausea and vomiting will include:
    a. Meperidine 25 to 50 mg intramuscularly
    b. Morphine 2 to 5 mg intravenously
    c. Nitrous oxide self-administered
    d. Rapid and gentle transport for physician evaluation

26. Which of the following represents a genitourinary emergency that requires treatment within 4 hours or irreversible consequences may ensue?
    a. Epididymitis   **c.** Testicular torsion
    b. Pyelonephritis   **d.** Urinary calculus

27. *You are caring for a patient with a temperature of 102.5° F (39.2° C) who is on continuous peritoneal dialysis.* What is a common cause of fever in this patient group?
    a. Dehydration   **c.** Peritonitis
    b. Infected fistula   **d.** Pneumonia

28. Which of the following vascular access sites may be used routinely by the paramedic to administer medications with a standard 21-gauge needle?
    a. AV fistula   **c.** Port-a-cath
    b. Heparin lock   **d.** Tenckhoff catheter

29. *You are called to the home of an unconscious person in chronic renal failure. The ECG tracing is shown in Fig. 21-1.* What electrolyte imbalance do you suspect?

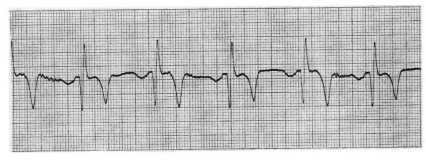

Figure 21-1

    a. Hyperkalemia   **c.** Hypercalcemia
    b. Hypokalemia   **d.** Hypocalcemia

30. What drug may be ordered by medical direction to correct the underlying electrolyte imbalance illustrated in Question 29?
    a. Atropine sulfate 1.0 mg intravenously
    b. Sodium bicarbonate 1.0 mEq/kg intravenously
    c. Magnesium sulfate 1.0 to 2.0 g intravenously
    d. Verapamil 2.5 mg intravenously

CHAPTER 22

ANAPHYLAXIS

● READING ASSIGNMENT

Chapter 22, pp. 720-729, in *Mosby's Paramedic Textbook*

● OBJECTIVES

As a paramedic, you should be able to:
1. Describe how the lymphatic system, leukocytes, lymphocytes, immunoglobulins, and mediators work with other factors to provide the immune response.
2. Differentiate between an allergic reaction and a normal immune response.
3. Define *anaphylaxis*.
4. Identify allergens associated with anaphylaxis.
5. Describe signs and symptoms of anaphylaxis.
6. Describe the pathophysiology, assessment, and management of anaphylaxis.

● REVIEW QUESTIONS

Match the terms in Column 2 with their description in Column 1. Use each term only once.

Column 1
_____ 1. Body's defense system against antigens
_____ 2. Immunity present at birth
_____ 3. Antibody responsible for anaphylaxis
_____ 4. Cell that releases histamine in anaphylaxis
_____ 5. Foreign protein that triggers an allergic response
_____ 6. Immunity resulting from exposure to an antigen
_____ 7. Bind to antigens, allowing white blood cells to destroy them

Column 2
a. Acquired immunity
b. Antibody
c. Antigen
d. Bone marrow cells
e. IgE immunoglobulin
f. Immunity
g. Mast cells
h. Natural immunity
i. Passive immunity

8. Briefly describe the function of the lymphatic system.

_____

9. List the signs and symptoms associated with each of the following chemical mediators released from basophils and mast cells in an anaphylactic reaction:
   a. Histamines:

_____

   b. Leukotrienes:

_____

   c. Eosinophil chemotactic factor:

_____

10. List three agents in each of the following groups that can cause anaphylaxis:
    a. Drugs:

    _____

    b. Insects:

    _____

    c. Foods:

    _____

11. *You are called to a church picnic to care for a 30-year-old woman with wheezing and dyspnea.*
    a. What other illness or injury may produce these symptoms?

    _____

    b. List two home medicines that may influence your care of this patient.

    _____

    Questions 12 through 14 pertain to the following scenario: *You are at a Chinese restaurant caring for a 25-year-old patient experiencing an anaphylactic reaction. He is in acute respiratory distress with wheezing and has a blood pressure of 90/70 mm Hg.*
12. What are some causative agents that may be found at this restaurant to trigger this person's anaphylaxis?

    _____

13. *After a rapid primary survey and vital sign assessment, you determine that immediate pharmacological therapy is indicated.* Identify two drugs, with appropriate dose and route, that may be indicated for this patient.
    a.
    b.
14. Describe other signs or symptoms that this patient may exhibit.

    _____

15. *You arrive at a dental office, where you find a 35-year-old woman who rapidly developed hives, angioedema, and stridor after an injection of a local anesthetic. She is unconscious, with labored, stridorous respirations: no radial pulse; and a rapid, irregular, barely palpable carotid pulse. No medicines have been administered to treat her.* Describe your priorities of care for this patient, including the appropriate drugs, doses, and routes.

    _____

    _____

    _____

● **STUDENT SELF-EVALUATION**

16. Neutrophils, eosinophils, and basophils are all:
    a. Antigens   c. Lymphocytes
    b. Leukocytes   d. Monocytes
17. Which immunoglobulin (antibody) is responsible for anaphylaxis?
    a. IgA   c. IgG
    b. IgE   d. IgM
18. Mediators that cause blood vessels to dilate are known as:
    a. Chemotactic substances   c. Opsonins
    b. Leukotactic substances   d. Vasoactive substances

19. Which of the following agents is *not* commonly associated with anaphylaxis?
    a. Aspirin   c. Fire ants
    b. Bananas   d. Peanuts
20. What is the most likely cause of death in anaphylaxis?
    a. Upper airway obstruction
    b. Hypoxia resulting from bronchospasm
    c. Hypotension resulting from fluid leak
    d. Vasogenic shock resulting from histamines
21. All of the following are signs or symptoms associated with anaphylaxis, *except:*
    a. Abdominal cramps   c. Rhinorrhea
    b. Cool, pale skin   d. Urticaria
22. Diphenhydramine is a(n):
    a. Anticholinergic   c. Bronchodilator
    b. Antihistamine   d. Sedative-hypnotic

TOXICOLOGY, DRUG ABUSE, AND ALCOHOLISM

● READING ASSIGNMENT

Chapter 23, pp. 730-777, in *Mosby's Paramedic Textbook*

● OBJECTIVES

As a paramedic, you should be able to:

1. Define *poisoning*.
2. Discuss poison control centers.
3. Describe general principles of patient assessment and management of ingested poisons.
4. Describe the causative agents and pathophysiology of selected ingested poisons and management of patients who have taken them.
5. Distinguish among the three categories of inhaled toxins: simple asphyxiants, chemical asphyxiants and systemic poisons, and irritants or corrosives.
6. Describe general principles of managing the patient who has inhaled poison.
7. Describe the signs, symptoms, and management of patients who have inhaled ammonia or hydrocarbon.
8. Describe the signs, symptoms, and management of patients with organophosphate or carbamate poisoning.
9. Describe the signs, symptoms, and management of patients injected with poison by insects, reptiles, and hazardous aquatic creatures.
10. List factors associated with drug and alcohol abuse.
11. Describe the common characteristics of drug and alcohol abuse.
12. Outline the general principles of managing patients with drug overdose.
13. Describe methods of administration, street names, signs, symptoms, and management for drug overdoses.
14. Describe the short- and long-term physiological effects of ethanol ingestion.
15. Describe signs, symptoms, and management of alcohol-related emergencies.

● REVIEW QUESTIONS

Match the poisons in Column 2 with their descriptions in Column 1. Use each poison only once.

	Column 1		Column 2
_____	1. It originated the expression "blind drunk" due to toxic visual effects.		**a.** Acid
_____	2. Ingestion of odorless, sweet liquid in antifreeze causes central nervous system depression.		**b.** Alkali
			c. Ammonia
_____	3. Inhalation, ingestion, absorption, prevents oxygen from reaching cells.		**d.** Carbamate
			e. Cyanide
_____	4. Inhalation produces lacrimation, dyspnea, and inflammation of the airway.		**f.** Ethylene glycol
			g. Hydrocarbon
_____	5. Vomiting should not be induced for phenol and others in this group.		**h.** Isopropanol
			i. Methanol
_____	6. These chemicals include lye and cause immediate damage to the mucosa.		**j.** Organophosphate

_____ 7. The long duration of action
requires treatment with atropine
and pralidoxime.

Match the drugs in Column 2 with the appropriate overdose description in Column 1. Use each drug only once.

Column 1

_____ 8. Central nervous system stimulant
and depressant properties can
produce violent, unpredictable
behavior.

_____ 9. It causes visual disturbances, dry
mouth, seizures, and tachycardia
with wide QRS complex.

_____ 10. It causes tachypnea, central nervous system depression, gastrointestinal irritation, and tinnitus.

_____ 11. Mild influenza-like symptoms are
followed by latent liver failure.

_____ 12. This stimulant can cause dysrhythmias, myocardial infarction, and
hyperthermia.

Column 2

a. Acetaminophen
b. Cocaine
c. Heroin
d. Iron
e. Phencyclidine
f. Salicylate
g. Tricyclic
    antidepressant

13. The severity of tricyclic antidepressant overdose can be determined in the prehospital phase of care. True/false. If this is false, why is it false?

14. Delirium tremens can be a life-threatening complication of alcohol with-drawal. True/false. If this is false, why is it false?

15. The effects of ingestion or overdose will be evident within 30 minutes of in-gestion. True/false. If this is false, why is it false?

16. Poisoning secondary to ingestion of toxic plants is rare in the United States. True/false. It this is false, why is it false?

17. Ice should *not* be applied to a snake bite wound. True/false. If this is false, why is it false?

18. *You are called to the home of a young child whose family states that he ingested some bleach.* After a rapid assessment of the patient, you contact the Regional Poison Control Center. What information should you be prepared to give them?

19. List the five signs of major toxicity that point to serious poisoning.
   a.
   b.
   c.
   d.
   e.

Questions 20 through 22 pertain to the following scenario: *A 32-year-old woman has ingested an overdose of sleeping pills.*

20. What information regarding the poisoning is critical to the care of this patient?

_____

_____

21. If you determine that it is safe to administer syrup of ipecac, write the appropriate dose and method of administration.

_____

22. What dose of activated charcoal should be given?

_____

23. For each of the following ingested poisons, indicate by *Yes* or *No* whether activated charcoal or ipecac is indicated. List other interventions specifically indicated in this situation.

Poison/Overdose	Ipecac?	Charcoal?	Other Interventions
a. Bleach			
b. Ammonia			
c. Gasoline			
d. Methanol			
e. Ethylene glycol			
f. Isopropanol			
g. Cyanide			
h. Aspirin			
i. Acetaminophen			
j. Iron			

24. *A 65-year-old woman complains of food poisoning after eating at a local seafood restaurant 2 hours earlier.*
   a. What is the typical time onset for signs of food poisoning?

_____

   b. What treatment should be provided for the patient with food poisoning?

_____

_____

25. When inserting an orogastric tube:
   a. What position should the patient be in?

_____

   b. What precaution should be taken for the unconscious patient?

_____

   c. How should irrigation be performed?

_____

_____

26. Briefly explain how each of the following gases causes harm to the body.

   a. Carbon monoxide and cyanide:

   b. Methane and propane:

   c. Chlorine and ammonia:

27. *A worker in a chemical plant is exposed to ammonia gas and is dyspneic, choking, and wheezing.* What treatment should be provided for this patient?

Questions 28 through 31 pertain to the following scenario: *A farmer calls you to his ranch after spraying pesticide on a windy day. On your arrival, he is coming out of the bathroom complaining of severe diarrhea and says he cannot stop urinating. Tears are running down his face, and he is coughing up copious amounts of phlegm. His ECG is shown in Fig. 23-1.*

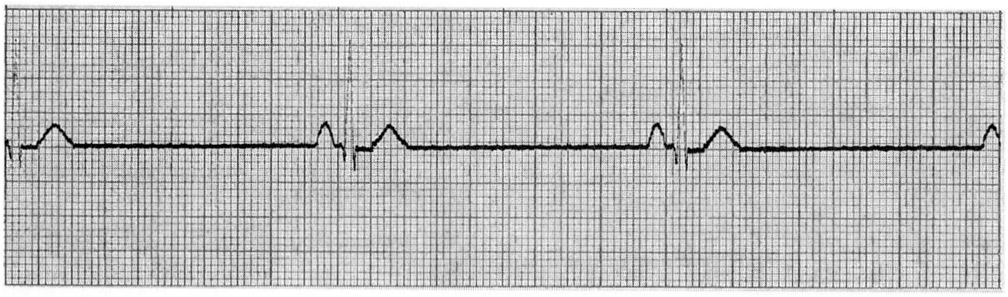

Figure 23-1

28. What poisoning do you suspect?

29. What other signs or symptoms might be present?

30. What is your interpretation of the ECG?

31. List specific interventions to be used in his care.

32. *You are at the first aid station for a church picnic. A 16-year-old comes to the station complaining of a "bee sting." No signs of anaphylaxis are present.*

   a. List general care measures for this person.

   b. Describe the method for removing the stinger.

33. List two diseases produced by ticks and possible signs and symptoms for each.

   a.

   b.

34. Describe the proper technique for removing a tick.

_____

_____

35. *A hysterical 20-year-old male camper states that he has just been bitten by a copperhead snake.*

   a. List signs and symptoms that would be present if a moderate envenomation had occured.

_____

   b. Describe the appropriate prehospital management of this patient.

_____

36. For each of the following marine animal classifications, list one example and outline general management principles for envenomation.

   a. Coelenterates:

_____

_____

   b. Echinoderms:

_____

_____

   c. Stingrays:

_____

_____

37. Give two examples of drugs commonly abused in each of the following categories:

   a. Narcotics:

_____

   b. Central nervous system depressants:

_____

   c. Central nervous system stimulants:

_____

   d. Hallucinogens:

_____

38. Interpret the following historical information presented to you at the scene of a potential drug overdose.

   a. *"He main-lined some China white."*

_____

   b. *"She was space basing angel dust and candy."*

_____

c. *"They were freebasing a rock."*

d. *"He was skin popping some M."*

e. *"She snorted some PCP before she went crazy."*

Questions 39 through 41 pertain to the following scenario: *Your patient injected heroin intravenously and arouses only to pain. He has pinpoint pupils and slow, snoring respirations.*

39. What is the primary life threat that must be immediately managed in this patient?

40. List the appropriate drug and dose used to improve this patient's condition.

41. If this person is a chronic heroin abuser and the drug listed above is administered, what signs and symptoms of narcotic withdrawal will you anticipate?

Questions 42 through 44 pertain to the following scenario: *A 17-year-old has taken approximately 50 tablets of chlordiazepoxide and is comatose, with slow, irregular respirations.*

42. What is the pupil response likely to be in this person?

43. What drug may be given to this patient on arrival to the emergency department to antagonize the effects of this ingestion?

44. Before administration of this antidote, careful history and scene assessment must be done to ensure that the patient has not taken what additional medication?

45. *Local college students call you to a party, where it is determined that participants have been freebasing cocaine. One of the participants has lost consciousness.* What life-threatening effects of this drug may have caused loss of consciousness in this patient?

Questions 46 through 48 pertain to the following scenario: *The Head Bangers are playing at a local club. Security calls you to the parking lot to care for a patient who has reportedly taken PCP.*

46. What should be your primary concern when caring for this patient?

47. Describe the appropriate initial approach to this patient, who is alert and quiet.

48. List signs and symptoms that may be displayed by this patient.

Questions 49 through 52 pertain to the following scenario: *An 18-year-old woman took approximately 20 tablets of amitriptyline approximately 1 hour before your arrival at her home. She is drowsy and confused, has a dry mouth, and complains of blurred vision. Her ECG is shown in Fig. 23-2.*

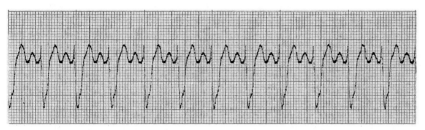

Figure 23-2

49. Should you administer syrup of ipecac to this patient? Why or why not?

_____

50. What is your interpretation of the ECG?

_____

51. What drug (with appropriate dose) may be given to prevent deterioration of this patient's cardiac status?

_____

52. What additional signs and symptoms do you anticipate as this patient's condition deteriorates?

_____

Questions 53 and 54 pertain to the following scenario: *Your unit is on the scene of a two-car accident. You are caring for a 47-year-old man who appears to be intoxicated. His friend says that he is an alcoholic. The patient states that he drank three beers in the past 5 hours.*

53. Should you accept this history of the number of drinks as reliable?

_____

54. If the patient is an alcoholic, what *chronic* physiological changes in the following areas will make it more difficult to assess his condition and more likely for severe injury to occur?
   a. Neurological changes:

_____

   b. Nutritional problems:

_____

   c. Fluid and electrolyte imbalances:

_____

   d. Coagulation disorders:

_____

55. Describe the management of a comatose patient suspected to be severely intoxicated by alcohol.

_____

_____

_____

56. Describe the management of a patient experiencing alcohol withdrawal accompanied by severe seizures.

_____

_____

_____

57. List signs and symptoms of delirium tremens.

_____

_____

● **STUDENT SELF-EVALUATION**

58. _An alert 4-year-old child ingested approximately 10 of his grandmother's blood pressure tablets 20 minutes ago._ What drug should be administered in this situation?
  a. Syrup of ipecac 15 ml   **c.** Syrup of ipecac 30 ml
  b. Syrup of ipecac 15 mg   **d.** Syrup of ipecac 30 mg
59. Charcoal is effective in treating specific overdoses because it:
  a. Reverses the effects of the ingested drug
  b. Binds the drug and prevents absorption
  c. Causes severe nausea and vomiting
  d. Makes the drug speed through the intestine
60. What should be the paramedic's primary concern when caring for a patient who has ingested hydrocarbon?
  a. Aspiration   **c.** Dysrhythmias
  b. Central nervous system effects   **d.** Hypotension
61. Medical direction may advise administration of sodium bicarbonate in all of the following poisoning and overdose situations, _except:_
  a. Ethylene glycol   **c.** Isopropanol
  b. Methanol   **d.** Tricyclic antidepressant
62. Symptoms commonly associated with poisonous mushroom ingestion are likely to include:
  a. Bradycardia   **c.** Hypertension
  b. Dry mouth   **d.** Hyperthermia
63. Which of the following overdose or poisonings will typically lead to bradycardia?
  a. Carbamates   **c.** Isopropanol
  b. Cocaine   **d.** Methanol
64. When evaluating a patient contaminated with organophosphates, the paramedic's first priority should be to:
  a. Administer atropine.   **c.** Put on protective gear.
  b. Establish intravenous therapy.   **d.** Suction excess secretions.
65. _Atropine is supplied in a 10-ml syringe that contains 1 mg of the drug. You wish to administer 2 mg._ How many milliters will you give?
  a. 1 ml   **c.** 10 ml
  b. 2 ml   **d.** 20 ml

66. *An 18-year-old who attempts to extract honey from a beehive on a dare sustains approximately 20 to 30 stings. He has a headache, fever, and involuntary muscle spasms and reports a syncopal episode.* What type of reaction do you suspect?
    a. Anaphylactic
    c. Local
    b. Delayed
    d. Toxic

67. *A 52-year-old man states that he was bitten by a spider at a woodpile. He is now complaining of back, chest, and abdominal pain and has a severe headache.* What type of spider envenomation would produce these symptoms?
    a. Black widow
    c. Tarantula
    b. Brown recluse
    d. Wolf

68. *A hiker states that he was bitten by a red and yellow snake and is now complaining of slurred speech and dysphagia. His pupils are dilated.* You suspect envenomation by what kind of snake?
    a. Copperhead
    c. Coral
    b. Cottonmouth moccasin
    d. Massasauga

69. Naloxone will antagonize the effects of all of the following drugs, *except:*
    a. Diazepam
    c. Morphine
    b. Meperidine
    d. Propoxyphene

70. The patient who has taken an overdose of oil of wintergreen will most likely present with:
    a. Bradycardia, hyperglycemia, and nystagmus
    b. Seizures, hyperglycemia, and ventricular tachycardia
    c. Hypoglycemia, tachypnea, and tinnitus
    d. Hematemesis, metabolic alkalosis, and coma

71. Typical findings within the first 24 hours of acetaminophen overdose include:
    a. Dysrhythmias
    b. Hypoglycemia
    c. No symptoms
    d. Right upper quadrant abdominal pain

72. When ingestion of multivitamins is suspected in a child, it is critical to determine whether the preparation contains:
    a. Ascorbic acid
    c. Iron
    b. Folic acid
    d. Thiamine

73. Intravenous therapy in the alcoholic with depleted thiamine stores may lead to:
    a. Disulfiram-ethanol reaction
    c. Mallory Weiss tears
    b. Guillain-Barré syndrome
    d. Wernicke-Korsakoff syndrome

INFECTIOUS DISEASES

● READING ASSIGNMENT

Chapter 24, pp. 778-803, in *Mosby's Paramedic Textbook*

● OBJECTIVES

As a paramedic, you should be able to:
1. Describe the chain of elements necessary for an infectious disease to occur.
2. Explain how internal and external barriers decrease susceptibility to infection.
3. Outline the inflammatory response.
4. Distinguish among the four stages of infectious disease: the latent period, the incubation period, the communicability period, and the disease period.
5. Given specific patient scenarios, describe the Centers for Disease Control recommendations for personal protection.
6. Describe the mode of transmission, pathophysiology, prehospital interventions, and personal protective measures to be taken for selected infectious diseases.
7. List the signs, symptoms, and potential secondary complications of selected childhood infectious diseases.

● REVIEW QUESTIONS

Match the infectious diseases listed in Column 2 with their descriptions in Column 1. Use each disease only once.

Column 1

_____ 1. Infection that produces influenza-like symptoms, dark colored urine, and light colored stools
_____ 2. Macular rash that can cause severe birth defects if a susceptible mother is exposed in pregnancy
_____ 3. Bacterial pulmonary infection spread by airborne droplets
_____ 4. Viral infection that impairs the body's ability to fight other infectious disease
_____ 5. Sexually transmitted disease characterized in the early stage by a painless chancre
_____ 6. Inflammation of lining of the central nervous system that may produce headache, stiff neck, seizures, and coma
_____ 7. Bacterial infection that produces mucopurulent discharge but rarely causes septicemia
_____ 8. Generalized illness accompanied by vesicular lesions, fever, and malaise

Column 2

a. Chlamydia
b. Gonorrhea
c. Hepatitis
d. Herpes simplex
e. Acquired immunodeficiency syndrome
f. Meningitis
g. Rubella
h. Syphilis
i. Tuberculosis
j. Varicella

9. Patients with chickenpox, influenza, or herpes simplex are typically treated with antibiotics. True/false. If this is false, why is it false?

10. The Occuational Safety and Health Administration requires that all employees at high risk for exposure to infectious diseases be offered the hepatitis vaccine to prevent infection by HBV. True/false. If this is false, why is it false?

11. Bacterial meningitis is more serious than viral meningitis. True/false. If this is false, why is it false?

12. List the five components of the "chain of elements" that must be present for an infectious disease to occur.
    a.
    b.
    c.
    d.
    e.

13. Describe two situations that interfere with the external barriers to infection, thereby increasing the risk of infection.
    a.
    b.

14. Name two factors that can affect the ability of the internal barriers to fight infectious disease.
    a.
    b.

15. For each of the following patient care scenarios, describe the personal protective measures that should be taken by the paramedic attending the patient:
    a. *A 23-year-old woman is about to deliver her fourth child. The baby's head is crowning, and you are preparing for delivery.*

    b. *A 50-year-old man is complaining of severe substernal chest pain. You are preparing to initiate an intravenous line to administer medications.*

    c. *You are preparing to administer epinephrine subcutaneously to a 25-year-old patient with dyspnea due to asthma.*

    d. *A 17-year-old ingested a large amount of alcohol and barbiturates, has vomited, and rapidly lost consciousness. You elect to intubate her trachea.*

    e. *A 55-year-old man attempted to commit suicide by holding a shotgun under his chin and firing. He is very combative and thrashes about as you try to control the large amount of bleeding and secure his airway.*

    f. *A butcher sustained a laceration to her hand at work. The wound is oozing a small amount of blood.*

Questions 16 through 19 pertain to the following scenario: *While caring for a 40-year-old man who had nausea, vomiting, right upper quadrant abdominal pain, and jaundice, you puncture your finger with a needle contaminated with the patient's blood. The hospital notifies you the next day that he tested positive for hepatitis.*

16. What type or types of hepatitis can produce the symptoms experienced by this patient?

_____

17. What are the most effective measures you can take to prevent exposure to hepatitis at work?

_____

18. Describe the modes of transmission for hepatitis B.

_____

_____

19. Is there anything you can do now that you have received this exposure so that you will not get hepatitis?

_____

_____

20. What signs and symptoms may be evident on the prehospital examination of a patient in each of the following stages of infection from the human immunodeficiency virus?
   a. Acute retroviral infection:

_____

   b. Asymptomatic infection:

_____

   c. Early symptomatic infection:

_____

   d. Late symptomatic infection from the human immunodeficiency virus:

_____

21. *You are transporting a patient with human immunodeficiency virus to the hospital after he sustained a sprained ankle at a volleyball game. No other injuries are evident.*
   a. What personal protective measures should you take while caring for this patient?

_____

   b. How should the ambulance be cleaned before transport of the next patient?

_____

22. What is the best way for emergency care workers to monitor whether they have been exposed to a patient with tuberculosis?

_____

23. *A 3-year-old child has a severe headache and a temperature of 102° F (38.9° C) and complained to his mother earlier of a stiff neck. Now he is limp and arouses only to a loud voice. You suspect meningitis.*
   a. What personal protective measures should you use on this call? (You plan to initiate an intravenous line and apply oxygen by mask).

_____

b. If the emergency department contacts you later to inform you that the child has bacterial meningitis, is there anything you can do to minimize your risk of becoming infected?

---

24. List three chronic signs or symptoms that may develop if syphilis is untreated for a number of years.
    a.
    b.
    c.

25. What personal protective measures should be taken when examining the mouth of a child with an outbreak of herpes simplex on the lips?

---

26. For each of the following, list the signs and symptoms and site of infestation:
    a. Pubic lice:

---

    b. Head lice:

---

    c. Scabies:

Questions 27 through 29 pertain to the following scenario: *You transport a child who has a temperature of 101° F (38.3° C) and a skin rash that began the previous day. The rash is generalized. Some lesions are flat and red, some are raised blisters, and others have scabbed. On arrival to the emergency department, the pediatrician confirms that the child has chickenpox.*

27. Is this disease communicable at this stage? _____

28. If you have never had chickenpox, how long would you expect to wait before symptoms appear?

---

29. Are you contagious during this entire time?

● STUDENT SELF-EVALUATION

30. All of the following drugs have analgesic, antipyretic, and antiinflammatory properties, *except:*
    a. Acetaminophen   **c.** Ibuprofen
    b. Aspirin   **d.** Ketorolac

31. The infectious disease phase that begins when the agent invades the body and ends when the disease process begins is the _____ period.
    a. Communicability   **c.** Incubation
    b. Disease   **d.** Latent

32. The risk of death is greatest from:
    a. Hepatitis A
    b. Hepatitis B
    c. Hepatitis C
    d. There is no risk of death from hepatitis.

33. *A patient has a headache, malaise, fever, lymphadenopathy, and a symmetrical rash that involves the palms and soles. He states that an ulcerated sore on his penis 3 weeks earlier healed spontaneously.* Which infectious disease do you suspect?

    a. Chlamydia   **c.** Herpes

    b. Gonnorrhea   **d.** Syphilis

34. What is the primary mode of transmission for rubella, mumps, and varicella?

    a. Blood-to-blood contact   **c.** Lesion contact

    b. Fecal contamination   **d.** Respiratory droplets

35. Complications of varicella may include all of the following, *except:*

    a. Bacterial infection   **c.** Meningitis

    b. Croup   **d.** Reye syndrome

ENVIRONMENTAL EMERGENCIES

● READING ASSIGNMENT

Chapter 25, pp. 804-823, in *Mosby's Paramedic Textbook*

● OBJECTIVES

As a paramedic, you should be able to:
1. Describe the physiology of thermoregulation.
2. Discuss the pathophysiology, assessment findings, and management of specific hyperthermic conditions, hypothermia, and frostbite.
3. Distinguish between hyperthermia syndrome and fever.
4. Describe patient management of fever.
5. Identify patients at increased risk for hypothermia.
6. List factors that predispose to frostbite.
7. Distinguish between drowning and near-drowning.
8. Discuss the pathophysiology, assessment, and prehospital management of near-drowning and pressure-related diving emergencies.
9. Identify factors that influence patient survival of a near-drowning episode.
10. Differentiate the pathophysiology of saltwater and fresh-water drowning.
11. Outline properties of gas that affect pressure-related diving emergencies.
12. Discuss the pathophysiology, assessment, and prehospital management of high-altitude illness.

● REVIEW QUESTIONS

1. Patients who have drowned in fresh water may have hemolysis, hyperkalemia, and anemia. True/false. If this is false, why is it false?

2. As a diver descends, the pressure on gases in the body increases. True/false. If this is false, why is it false?

3. Briefly describe how each of the following contributes to heat production in the body:
   a. Chemical control;

   b. Musculoskeletal:

   c. Endocrine:

4. For each of the following situations, select the mechanisms of heat loss that apply. (conduction, convection, evaporation, radiation). You may use each answer more than once.
   a. *On a windy autumn evening, you remove the clothing of a trauma patient to assess his injuries more accurately. On arrival to the emergency department, his temperature is 94° F (34.4° C).* _____.

b. *During a multiple patient situation, you extricate a partially clothed patient onto a cold metal backboard. On arrival to the emergency department, her*

temperature is 96° F (35.6° C). _____.

c. *On a dry, cool spring evening you transport a wet patient who injured her neck after diving into a swimming pool. On arrival to the the emergency department,*

her temperature is 94.6° F (34.8° C). _____.

d. *A burn patient with a 40% BSA burn is continuously cooled with iced normal saline en route to the hospital. On arrival to the emergency department, his*

temperature is 93.5° F (34.2° C). _____.

5. *You are on the scene of a multiple-car collision on a very hot July day.* List 4 ways your body will compensate to prevent your temperature from rising.

   a.

   b.

   c.

   d.

6. *You are assisting with a search-and-rescue effort after a hurricane. It is cold, wet, and very windy.* List 4 ways your body will attempt to maintain a normal temperature.

   a.

   b.

   c.

   d.

7. For each of the following examples of heat illness, identify the type of heat illness and briefly describe the appropriate prehospital patient care.

   a. *You are working at an amusement park on a 95° F (35° C) humid day. A hot, sweaty 45-year-old woman comes to your aid station complaining of severe cramping in her calves. Her vital signs are blood pressure, 116/72 mm Hg; pulse, 116; and temperature, 98.6° F (37° C).*

      Illness:

      Management:

   b. *A 55-year-old man is complaining of dizziness, nausea, and vomiting while participating in a long-distance walk fund-raiser. His vital signs are blood pressure, 104/70 mm Hg, and pulse, 108, while lying down and blood pressure, 86/50 mm Hg, and pulse, 128, while standing. His temperature is 101° F (38.3° C).*

      Illness:

      Management:

   c. *On a 100° F (37.8° C) day, an 80-year-old woman becomes confused and agitated and then has a seizure in her apartment, which does not have air conditioning. She is responsive to pain, has jugular venous distention and profuse sweating, and her vital signs are: blood pressure, 92/70 mm Hg; pulse, 120/min; respirations, 24; and temperature 106° F (41.1° C).*

      Illness:

      Management:

8. Why is the increased metabolic rate that is produced in mild hypothermia undesirable for a patient who already has an injury or medical illness?

_____

_____

Questions 9 to 11 pertain to the following scenario: *You are caring for a snow-mobiler whose rig broke through the ice 30 minutes ago. He pulled himself out of the water and collapsed before rescuers reached him 20 minutes later. He has been moved to a safe area.*

9. Describe general measures of care to be initiated immediately on this patient.

_____

_____

10. *You determine that he is apneic and pulseless. His ECG displays the rhythm shown in Fig. 25-1.* What actions should be taken if:

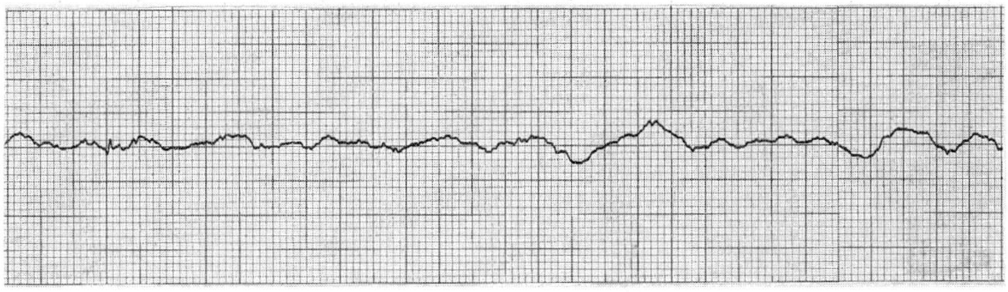

Figure 25-1

a. His core temperature is less than 86° F (30° C).

_____

_____

b. His core temperature is greater than 86° F (30° C).

_____

_____

11. When should resuscitation efforts be terminated?

_____

12. *You are transporting a hiker who became lost on a trail. He is shivering and hungry and has a temperature of 97° F (36.1° C).* How would you treat this patient?

_____

_____

13. *A firefighter dives into an ice-covered pond to rescue a child who has fallen through the ice on a windy, cold January evening. On the 10-minute walk back to the firetruck, he develops slurred speech and ataxia and complains that his heart is*

pounding. At the ambulance, his temperature is 89.5° F (31.9° C), and his ECG is shown in Fig. 25-2.

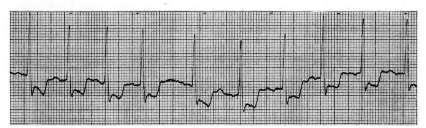

Figure 25-2

    a. What is your interpretation of the ECG tracing?

_____

    b. Describe your management of this patient.

_____

_____

_____

    Questions 14 to 16 pertain to the following scenario: *During a cross-country ski meet, a participant complains of coldness, numbness, and extreme pain in the fingers of his right hand.*

14. Differentiate between superficial frostbite and deep frostbite.

_____

_____

15. List four factors that increase susceptibility to frostbite.
    a.
    b.
    c.
    d.

16. How would you treat frostbite in this patient ?

_____

_____

    Questions 17 to 19 pertain to the following scenario: *A 2-year-old child pulled from a backyard pool is apneic and pulseless.*

17. Identify four factors that will influence this patient's clinical outcome.
    a.
    b.
    c.
    d.

18. What complications do you anticipate if the patient is resuscitated?

_____

_____

19. Describe prehospital management of this child.

_____

_____

20. List five body areas that may experience pain resulting from SQUEEZE.
   a.
   b.
   c.
   d.
   e.

21. *A diver experiences acute distress immediately after rapidly surfacing from a deep dive.*
   a. List five signs or symptoms of air embolism
      a.
      b.
      c.
      d.
      e.
   b. Describe special considerations necessary in the care of this patient while providing advanced life support and transport.

_____

_____

22. *A tourist at a local resort complains of severe joint pain, fatigue, vertigo, and paraesthesia 12 hours after returning from his first dive.*
   a. What diving injury do you suspect?

_____

   b. Describe prehospital management of this patient.

_____

_____

23. *You respond to a mountain resort, where a participant in a cycling event has become ill.*
   a. List the three types of high-altitude illness.
      a.
      b.
      c.
   b. What single intervention is most critical to long-term improvement of the patient suffering from high altitude illness after the ABCs have been managed?

_____

● **STUDENT SELF-EVALUATION**

24. What is the most important organ for regulation of body temperature?
   a. Heart   **c.** Pituitary gland
   b. Lungs   **d.** Skin

25. Shock may develop in the patient with heat stroke because of:
   a. Fluid loss   **c.** Peripheral vasodilation
   b. Myocardial depression   **d.** All of the above

215

26. What is the most critical intervention for heat stroke?
    a. Fluid resuscitation
    c. Rapid cooling in transit
    b. Medication administration
    d. Rapid transport to a hospital
27. Shivering stops in a hypothermic patient when:
    a. The body temperature drops to 90° F (32.2° C).
    b. Glucose or glycogen is depleted.
    c. Excessive amounts of insulin are excreted.
    d. pCO_2 is increased to greater than 50 mm Hg.
28. Prehospital care of a frostbitten extremity should include:
    a. Application of a tourniquet
    b. Elevation of the affected extremity
    c. Rapid rewarming in hot water
    d. Refreezing of the injured extremity
29. All drownings are characterized by:
    a. Hypovolemia, hypoxia, and acidosis
    b. Hypoxia, acidosis, and hypothermia
    c. Hypoxia, acidosis, and hypercapnia
    d. Hypovolemia, acidosis, and hypercapnia
30. Which law of physics states that the volume of gas is inversely related to its pressure at a constant temperature?
    a. Boyle's law
    c. Henry's law
    b. Dalton's law
    d. Newton's law
31. *A diver is in respiratory distress after ascent. You palpate subcutaneous emphysema.* He is probably suffering from:
    a. Barotrauma of descent
    b. Decompression sickness
    c. Pulmonary air embolus
    d. Pulmonary overpressurization syndrome
32. What is the primary danger of nitrogen narcosis?
    a. Hypoxemia
    b. Impaired judgment
    c. Respiratory acidosis
    d. Shock resulting from hypovolemia
33. The critical sign or symptom that indicates deterioration of the patient with acute mountain sickness is:
    a. Ataxia
    c. Irritability
    b. Headache
    d. Vomiting

GERIATRICS

● **READING ASSIGNMENT**

Chapter 26, pp. 824-835, in *Mosby's Paramedic Textbook*

● **OBJECTIVES**

As a paramedic, you should be able to:

1. Describe the pathophysiology of the aging process as it relates to major body systems and homeostasis.
2. Describe physical assessment techniques specific to older adults.
3. Discuss the effects of aging as they relate to the physiological response to trauma.
4. Describe management techniques specific to older patients who have sustained trauma.
5. Discuss the incidence and unique features of selected medical problems in the older patient.
6. Distinguish between delirium and dementia.
7. Discuss the incidence and symptoms of depression in the geriatric population.
8. Identify factors that contribute to drug toxicity in the older adult.

● **REVIEW QUESTIONS**

1. *An 85-year-old woman falls down an escalator at a department store.* Explain how age-related changes in each of the following areas increase her risk of sustaining trauma or influence her body's response to a major injury.

    a. Respiratory system:

    _____

    _____

    b. Cardiovascular system:

    _____

    _____

    c. Renal system:

    _____

    _____

    d. Musculoskeletal system:

    _____

    _____

    e. Thermoregulation:

    _____

    _____

2. *A woman calls you to the home of her 70-year-old father who has fallen. He says he is just fine. On your arrival, she states that he has a history of diabetes, a heart attack, heart failure, and lung disease. His home medications include Lanoxin, insulin, Dyazide, Slow-K, Theo-Dur, and a number of vitamins and laxatives. He is on oxygen at 2 L/min by nasal cannula.*

    a. What factors will make it difficult to assess and determine the nature of his acute problem?

_____

_____

_____

_____

    b. List eight possible causes of his fall.

        a.

        b.

        c.

        d.

        e.

        f.

        g.

        h.

3. Why might the symptoms of increased intracranial pressure be delayed in an older patient?

_____

_____

    Questions 4 to 7 pertain to the following scenario: *You are on the scene of a single-car collision in which a compact car struck a bridge abutment at high speed. The driver is an anxious 75-year-old man complaining of mild abdominal discomfort. His blood pressure is 90/70 mm Hg, his pulse is 70, and his respirations are 24 and somewhat labored. His skin is pale and clammy, and his nailbeds are dusky.*

4. What vital sign assessment does *not* fit with this man's clinical picture?

_____

5. What aspect of his history may explain this discrepancy?

_____

6. Since he has just mild abdominal pain, should you be concerned?

_____

7. What prehospital treatment should be given after the cervical spine is appropriately immobilized?

_____

_____

_____

Questions 29 to 32 pertain to the following scenario: *An 80-year-old woman complains of chest pain and shortness of breath. Vital signs are blood pressure, 82/50 mm Hg; pulse, 50; and respirations, 24. Her ECG tracing is shown in Fig. 26-7.*

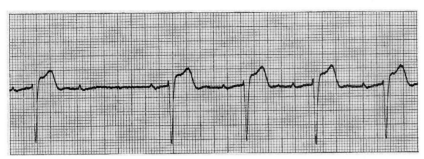

Figure 26-7

29. Identify the rhythm strip.

30. *Medical direction advises you to initiate transcutaneous pacing on this patient.* Where should the pacing pads be positioned?

31. How fast will you set the rate?

32. How will you know if the pacing has captured?

33. *A 67-year-old man describes the sudden onset of a pounding sensation in his chest. His vital signs are blood pressure, 118/70 mm Hg; pulse, 150; and respirations, 20. His ECG is shown in Fig. 26-8.*

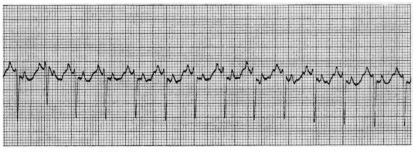

Figure 26-8

   a. Identify the rhythm.

   b. What drug, with the appropriate dose, is indicated to correct this dysrhythmia?

34. Of older patients with head trauma, two thirds who have which of the following signs will die?

   a. Blood pressure elevation   **c.** Bradycardia
   b. Irregular respirations   **d.** Unconsciousness

35. The most frequent trauma sustained from falls in the older adult is:

   a. Cardiac contusion   **c.** Subdural hematoma
   b. Fractured hip   **d.** Tension pneumothorax

36. Your primary concern when caring for a patient who is on chemotherapy will be to:

   a. Control bleeding from multiple sites.
   b. Fluid resuscitate aggressively for hypovolemia.
   c. Treat the ventricular dysrhythmias, which are common.
   d. Use aseptic technique for invasive techniques.

37. The most common psychiatric disorder in the older adult is:

   a. Bipolar disorder   **c.** Hysteria
   b. Depression   **d.** Schizophrenia

38. Which of the following is *not* a risk factor for elder abuse?

   a. Woman   **c.** Married
   b. Isolation   **d.** Poverty

PEDIATRICS

● READING ASSIGNMENT

Chapter 27, pp. 836-859, in *Mosby's Paramedic Textbook*

● OBJECTIVES

As a paramedic, you should be able to:
1. Distinguish among patient assessment techniques appropriate for patients at different developmental levels.
2. Identify common age-related illness in pediatric patients.
3. Discuss common historical and physical findings of the sudden infant death syndrome patient.
4. Describe common features in the profile of an abusive situation.
5. Describe abnormal physical findings that have a high index of suspicion for child abuse.
6. Discuss appropriate interventions in cases of suspected child abuse.
7. Discuss the pathophysiology, assessment, and management of seizures and dehydration in children.
8. Describe the pathophysiology, assessment, and management of children with selected respiratory illnesses.
9. Outline the correct pediatric drug dosage, cardioversion energy levels, and sequence for specific pediatric resuscitation situations.
10. Select the correct endotracheal blade and tube for a given age group.
11. Interpret vital sign values as normal or abnormal for selected age groups.
12. For a seriously injured child, identify considerations for blood volume, hypothermia, cardiac reserve, respiratory fatigue, and vital sign assessment.
13. Describe special considerations for intravenous fluid therapy and intraosseous infusion in children.

● REVIEW QUESTIONS

Match the drugs in Column 2 with their appropriate initial *pediatric* dose in Column 1. Use each drug only once.

Column 1	Column 2
_____ 1. 0.1 ml/kg	a. Adenosine
	b. Atropine sulfate
_____ 2. 2 to 20 mcg/kg/min	c. Bretylium
	d. Calcium chloride
_____ 3. 1 mEq/kg per dose	e. Dopamine hydrochloride
	f. Epinephrine (1:10,000)
_____ 4. 0.1 to 0.2 mg/kg	g. Lidocaine
	h. Sodium bicarbonate
_____ 5. 1 mg/kg	
_____ 6. 0.02 mg/kg	
_____ 7. 5 mg/kg	

8. In what pediatric age group(s) are you most likely to see the following illness or injuries?

   a. Sepsis:

   b. Febrile seizures:

   c. Jaundice:

   d. Ingestions:

   e. Falls:

   f. Child abuse:

   g. Drowning or near-drowning:

   h. Suicide gestures:

Questions 9 through 12 pertain to the following scenario: *A frightened mother tells you she put her 14-kg, 4-year-old child to bed and that he was complaining of a slight earache with a low-grade temperature. She heard a noise several hours later and found her child having a grand mal seizure, which stopped after approximately a minute. The child's temperature is 105.5° F (40.8° C). He appears to be postictal at this time.*

   9. After you have ensured that the child is stable, what history should you obtain from the mother?

10. What care should be provided en route to the hospital?

11. If the child has a seizure during transport, list two anticonvulsant drugs with the appropriate dose and route(s) that may be given.

   a.

   b.

12. You check a fingerstick glucose level and determine that this child's blood sugar is 50 mg/dl. What drug should you administer (include dose and route)?

Questions 13 through 17 pertain to the following scenario: *A limp, 14-month-old child is carried into the ambulance base by his mother. She states that he has had a fever with vomiting and diarrhea for 3 days. His eyes are sunken, his tongue is furrowed, and his lips are cracked. Physical examination reveals rapid respirations; cold, mottled extremities; and the electrocardiogram in Fig. 27-1.*

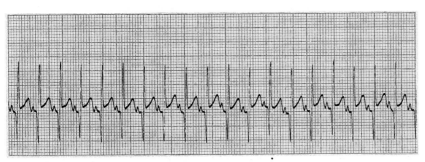

Figure 27-1

13. What is this child's problem?

_____

14. Interpret the electrocardiogram.

_____

15. Describe management of this child assuming a 45-minute transport time.

_____

_____

16. What are the appropriate vital signs for this child?

_____

17. Besides an improvement in vital signs, for what other clinical signs of improvement will you watch?

_____

Questions 18 to 21 pertain to the following scenario: *A 7-year-old is in acute respiratory distress after visiting a friend's home. He gives a history of asthma and allergy to dogs (his friend has three). His home medicines include an Atrovent inhaler, which he takes daily, and albuterol by nebulizer as necessary, which he hasn't had for a week. He has circumoral cyanosis, is working very hard to breath, and has faint inspiratory and expiratory wheezes.*

18. What interventions are appropriate for this child? Include two possible beta-agonist drugs you could administer (with appropriate doses).

_____

_____

19. What side effects do you anticipate from the administration of these drugs?

_____

20. In 15 minutes, you see no clinical improvement and your estimated arrival time is still 20 minutes. What do you do?

_____

21. What aspects of the physical examination will change when the patient improves?

_____

_____

22. List three characteristic signs or symptoms of epiglottitis.

a.

b.

c.

23. *A 20-month-old with croup is in mild respiratory distress on a cool October evening.*

a. What intervention should you use before entering the ambulance that may cause rapid improvement in the patient's signs and symptoms?

_____

b. When in the ambulance, how will you care for this child?

_____

_____

Questions 24 to 26 pertain to the following scenario: *At 1 AM on a cool February night, you are dispatched for a "baby choking." On arrival, you find a well-nourished 4-month-old baby boy apneic and pulseless in his crib. There is frothy sputum in the nose and mouth, and his diaper is wet and full of stool. The child is cold, and dependent lividity is present. The hysterical mother states that he and his older sister have both had a slight cold, but otherwise he was healthy.*

24. What characteristics of sudden infant death syndrome does this call meet?

_____

25. What other findings should you document in this situation?

_____

You spend some time on the scene comforting the family and making the appropriate notifications and then spend a quiet ride back to the firehouse with your normally talkative partner. You ask if he is OK, and he says, "Of course, I'm fine." Then he immediately rushes to the phone, where you hear him awaken his wife and ask her to check on their 6-month-old daughter.

26. Should you ignore your partner's unusual behavior, since he told you he is OK? If not, what action(s) can you take?

_____

_____

Questions 27 to 29 pertain to the following scenario: *A mother tells you that her 8-month-old fell off his tricycle early in the day and was acting fine. Later, she could not wake him from his nap. On physical examination, you find a dirty child who has agonal respirations, a slow pulse, and decerebrate posturing. No visible signs of trauma are present on the head, although small bruises are noted on the shoulders.*

27. What should your immediate interventions be for this child?

_____

_____

28. What findings might lead you to suspect child abuse?

_____

_____

29. After delivering the child to the appropriate medical center, what are your responsibilities?

_____

_____

30. What history and physical examination should be elicited on a child who is a victim of sexual abuse?

_____

_____

31. _Your 3-year-old patient weighs 17 kg. He was involved in a head-on motor vehicle collision and was restrained only by a lap belt. He says his "tummy hurts." The physical examination reveals an anxious, pale child with a rigid, tender abdomen. Discuss the significance of the following physiological differences in children and specifically how they will influence your care of this child:_

   a. Children have a greater percentage of circulating blood volume than adults.

_____

_____

   b. Children have a large body surface area in proportion to body weight.

_____

_____

   c. Children's hearts function at near-maximum performance in a normal, healthy state.

_____

_____

   d. Volume replacement in children is weight related.

_____

_____

_____

   e. Intravenous access is difficult to establish in children.

_____

_____

_____

32. How do you determine that an intraosseous needle is properly placed?

_____

Questions 33 to 36 pertain to the following scenario: _A 3-year-old, 35-kg child is found unconscious after suffocation with a plastic bag. On arrival, you find a dusky, pale child who is unresponsive and apneic. Occasionally you can palpate a faint pulse at the_ *carotid artery, but no blood pressure is obtainable. The electrocardiogram is shown in Fig. 27-2.*

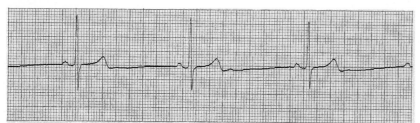

Figure 27-2

33. Interpret the electrocardiogram tracing.

34. What actions will you take immediately up to and including the first drug (with appropriate dose)?

35. If an intravenous line cannot be immediately established, what two actions can be taken?
   a.
   b.

36. After your initial interventions result in no patient improvement, what drug at what dose is indicated?

37. *A 3-week-old, 5-kg infant is found unconscious and not breathing at home in his crib. On arrival, you find him pulseless and apneic. Cardiopulmonary resuscitation is initiated, the child's trachea is intubated, and lactated Ringer's solution is initiated intravenously. The electrocardiogram tracing in Fig. 27-3 is noted.*

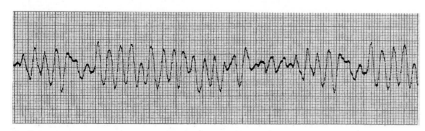

Figure 27-3

   a. Outline your continued care of this patient up to and including the first two drugs (including dose).

   b. If a repeat dose of epinephrine is necessary, what is the correct dose and concentration?

38. Which age group has a fear of bodily injury and mutilation and interprets words literally?
    a. Adolescents   c. School-agers
    b. Preschoolers   d. Toddlers
39. Which of the following is *not* likely to cause seizures?
    a. Central nervous system infection
    b. Metabolic abnormalities
    c. Prolonged dehydration
    d. Serious head trauma
40. After intravenous administration of diazepam, the paramedic should monitor closely for:
    a. Decreased pulse   c. Respiratory depression
    b. Increased blood pressure   d. Vomiting or nausea
41. Reye syndrome, a postviral illness, is characterized by liver dysfunction and presents with:
    a. Bradycardia and respiratory depression
    b. Stocking and glove paralysis
    c. Central nervous sytem depression and vomiting
    d. Dysrhythmias and dehydration
42. Poliomyelitis can lead to:
    a. Liver failure   c. Respiratory paralysis
    b. Renal failure   d. Vertebral degeneration
43. Which of the following may be indicated for the management of severe respiratory distress associated with bronchiolitis?
    a. Albuterol 0.15 mg/kg by inhalation
    b. Atropine 0.01 mg/kg by inhalation
    c. Epinephrine 0.1 mg/kg subcutaneously
    d. Terbutaline 0.2 mg/kg subcutaneously
44. Which of the following is an appropriate intervention for a child suspected of having epiglottitis?
    a. Lay the child supine on the mother's lap.
    b. See if the epiglottis is swollen.
    c. Infuse intravenous normal saline fluids at 20 ml/kg.
    d. Give humidified oxygen by mask.
45. A 5-year-old, 44-lb child is in ventricular fibrillation. The correct *initial* energy level for defibrillation is:
    a. 20 joules   c. 80 joules
    b. 40 joules   d. 88 joules
46. What is the maximum single dose of atropine that should be given to a 6-year-old?
    a. 0.05 mg   c. 0.1 mg
    b. 0.01 mg   d. 0.5 mg
47. The correct sequence of interventions for a bradycardic, hypotensive child after the airway has been secured, an intravenous established, and cardiopulmonary resuscitation initiated is:
    a. Atropine and epinephrine   c. Atropine only
    b. Epinephrine and atropine   d. Epinephrine only

DIVISION FOUR REVIEW TEST

1. Management of a 21-year-old asthmatic patient who is in acute distress with wheezing and diminished breath sounds may include:
   a. Aminophylline 25 mg/kg intravenously
   b. Diphenhydramine 25 mg intramuscularly
   c. Epinephrine 0.3 to 0.5 mg/kg intravenously
   d. Terbutaline 0.25 mg subcutaneously

2. A sign or symptom indicating deterioration in a patient with chronic bronchitis would be:
   a. Agitation and confusion
   b. Dyspnea on exertion
   c. Production of yellow sputum
   d. Spasmodic coughing

3. Signs and symptoms of a pulmonary embolism may include which of the following?
   a. Fever
   b. Green sputum
   c. Hypertension
   d. Stridor

4. Impaired oxygenation during pneumonia is due to:
   a. Poor blood flow to the affected lung
   b. Decreased minute volume
   c. Cellular hypoxia and hypercarbia
   d. Decreased ventilation-perfusion ratio

5. The process by which cardiac muscle fibers are stimulated to contract by alteration of the electrical charge of the cell is:
   a. Depolarization
   b. Repolarization
   c. Absolute refractory period
   d. Relative refractory period

6. Blood from the right ventricle is immediately propelled to the:
   a. Left ventricle
   b. Lungs
   c. Right atrium
   d. Superior vena cava

7. Which of the following patient statements regarding dyspnea is most suggestive of a cardiovascular problem?
   a. "I've been coughing up green sputum for 3 days."
   b. "I've needed three pillows to sleep the past 2 nights."
   c. "It started suddenly after my penicillin shot."
   d. "It hurts right in my ribs when I breathe in deeply."

8. When evaluating a patient whom you suspect may be having a myocardial infarction, which of the following home medicines would suggest that the patient is at high risk for heart disease?
   a. Ampicillin
   b. Amitriptyline
   c. Cimetidine
   d. Hydrochlorothiazide

9. When treating a patient with chest pain, what is the correct sequence for nitroglycerin administration?
   a. 0.4 mg sublingually, repeated every 5 min for up to 3 doses
   b. 1.0 mg sublingually, repeated every 5 min for up to 3 doses
   c. 0.4 mg sublingually, one dose only for angina
   d. Nitroglycerin is not indicated for angina.

10. Your goals in managing a patient with acute cardiogenic pulmonary edema will include:
    a. Decreasing venous return to the heart
    b. Increasing myocardial oxygen demand
    c. Increasing afterload with venodilators
    d. Sedating the patient with diazepam to slow respirations

11. Which of the following drugs is used in managing cardiogenic shock?
    a. Albuterol
    b. Dopamine
    c. Isoproterenol
    d. Phenytoin

12. What energy levels are used to cardiovert the heart of a patient in ventricular tachycardia with a blood pressure of 70 mm Hg by palpation?
    a. 50, 100, 200, and 360 joules
    c. 100, 200, 300, and 360 joules
    b. 75, 100, 200, 300, and 360 joules
    d. 100, 200, and 360 joules
13. *You want to give lidocaine 3 mg/min to a 50-kg man. You have a 250-ml bag of lidocaine with a 0.4% solution of the drug.* How fast will you run your microdrip tubing to administer the proper dose (gtts/min)?
    a. 15   c. 45
    b. 30   d. 60
14. The drug of choice for a stable patient on oxygen who has the rhythm in Fig. D-1 is:

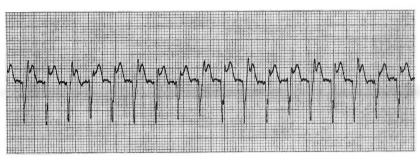

Figure D-1

    a. Adenosine 6 mg intravenously
    b. Diltiazem 0.25 mg/kg
    c. Lidocaine 1.5 mg/kg intravenously
    d. Verapamil 2.5 mg intravenously
15. Which of the following patients will be at greatest risk for developing a dissecting thoracic aortic aneurysm?
    a. A 60-year-old black man with a history of hypertension
    b. A 23-year-old white woman pregnant with her first child
    c. A 50-year-old black woman with adult-onset diabetes
    d. A 90-year-old white man with chronic lung disease
16. Identify the electrocardiogram tracing in Fig. D-2.

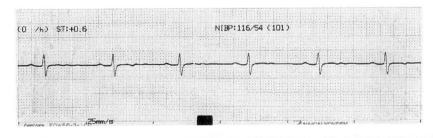

Figure D-2

    a. Junctional rhythm   c. Sinus bradycardia
    b. Mobitz II   d. Ventricular escape rhythm

17. Identify the electrocardiogram tracing in Fig. D-3.

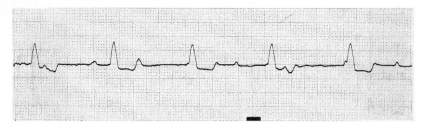

Figure D-3

    a. First-degree atrioventricular block
    b. Second-degree atrioventricular block type I
    c. Second-degree atrioventricular block type II
    d. Third-degree atrioventricular block

18. Identify the electrocardiogram tracing in Fig. D-4.

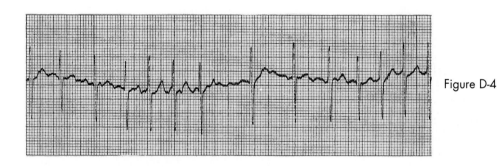

Figure D-4

    a. Atrial fibrillation
    b. Normal sinus rhythm with frequent premature atrial contractions
    c. Second-degree atrioventricular block type II
    d. Sinus arrest

19. Identify the electrocardiogram tracing in Fig. D-5.

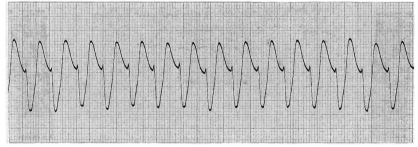

Figure D-5

    a. Atrial tachycardia   **c.** Sinus tachycardia
    b. Idioventricular rhythm   **d.** Ventricular tachycardia

20. The diabetic patient who has vomiting, dehydration, and hypotension will benefit most from administration of:
    a. D50W   **c.** Intravenous fluid
    b. Glucagon   **d.** Orange juice

21. Complications of status epilepticus may include:
    a. Brain damage   **c.** Fractures
    b. Dehydration   **d.** All of the above

22. Patients with cholecystitis, pancreatitis, and hepatitis are most likely to complain of pain in which of the following quadrants?
    a. Left lower
    b. Left upper
    c. Right lower
    d. Right upper
23. Complications of untreated renal failure include:
    a. Acidosis
    b. Cyanosis
    c. Hypercalcemia
    d. Polycythemia
24. What is the drug of choice for anaphylaxis?
    a. Cimetidine
    b. Dexamethasone
    c. Diphenhydramine
    d. Epinephrine
25. Which of the following patients may be given syrup of ipecac?
    a. A pregnant 17-year-old who took an aspirin overdose 15 minutes ago
    b. A 40-year-old who took 30 diuretic tablets 3 hours ago
    c. A 65-year-old who took 20 diabinese tablets 15 minutes ago
    d. A comatose 20-year-old who took 50 phenobarbital tablets 30 minutes ago
26. Which of the following organisms associated with food poisoning can produce central nervous system symptoms?
    a. *Clostridium botulinum*
    b. *Campylobacter* species
    c. *Salmonella* species
    d. *Shigella* species
27. Anesthesia, blindness, changes in color perception, and seizures are likely findings in a patient who has experienced a significant _____ inhalation:
    a. Ammonia
    b. Carbamate
    c. Cyanide
    d. Hydrocarbon
28. Which of the following drugs can produce a life-threatening reaction if the patient ingests a small amount of alcohol?
    a. Diazepam
    b. Diltiazem
    c. Diphenhydramine
    d. Disulfiram
29. The human immunodeficiency virus is present in all of the following body fluids, *except:*
    a. Blood
    b. Cervical secretions
    c. Semen
    d. Urine
30. Which of the following patients is *not* at increased risk of developing infectious diseases?
    a. 75-year-old woman
    b. 46-year-old alcoholic
    c. 50-year-old person with hypertension
    d. 20-year-old person with human immunodeficiency virus
31. Why might the patient suffering from heat exhaustion have decreased blood pressure?
    a. Cardiac depression
    b. Red blood cell loss
    c. Vasomotor failure
    d. Water loss
32. What is the most common dysrhythmia associated with moderate hypothermia?
    a. Atrial fibrillation
    b. Atrial flutter
    c. Ventricular tachycardia
    d. Ventricular fibrillation
33. Which of the following home medicines greatly increases the older person's risk of falling?
    a. Alprazolam
    b. Digoxin
    c. Hydrochlorothiazide
    d. Dipyridamole (Persantine)
34. Causes of dementia may include:
    a. Alzheimer's disease
    b. Epilepsy
    c. Hyperglycemia
    d. Pneumonia
35. Which of the following illnesses is likely to be seen in the neonatal period?
    a. Asthma
    b. Croup
    c. Febrile seizure
    d. Meningitis

36. *A 2-year-old child who has had a cold for 3 days awakens with a barking cough, stridor, and a temperature of 100.6° F (38.1° C). What illness do you suspect?*
  a. Bronchiolitis
  c. Epiglottitis
  b. Croup
  d. Pneumonia

37. What is the correct *initial* intravenous dose of epinephrine to be given to a child in cardiac arrest?
  a. 0.01 mg/kg
  c. 0.1 mg/kg
  b. 0.02 mg/kg
  d. 0.2 mg/kg

DIVISION FIVE
OB/GYN AND NEONATAL

CHAPTER 28
OBSTETRICAL AND NEONATAL EMERGENCIES

● **READING ASSIGNMENT**

Chapter 28, pp. 862-901, in *Mosby's Paramedic Textbook*

● **OBJECTIVES**

As a paramedic, you should be able to:
1. Label an anatomical diagram of the female reproductive system.
2. Outline the events in the normal menstrual cycle.
3. Outline fetal development from ovulation through birth.
4. Explain normal maternal physiological changes during pregnancy and how they influence prehospital patient care and transport.
5. Describe appropriate information to be elicited during the obstetrical patient history.
6. Describe specific techniques for assessing pregnant patients.
7. Discuss the implications of prehospital care based on the effects of trauma on the fetus and mother.
8. Describe the assessment and management of patients with preeclampsia and eclampsia.
9. Explain the pathophysiology, signs and symptoms, and management of the processes that cause vaginal bleeding in pregnancy.
10. Outline the role of the paramedic during normal labor and delivery.
11. Compute an Apgar score for a newborn.
12. Discuss the identification, implications, and prehospital management of complicated deliveries.
13. Describe the pathophysiology, assessment, and prehospital management of maternal pulmonary embolism.
14. Describe prehospital care of the normal neonate.
15. Outline steps in resuscitating a distressed neonate.

● **REVIEW QUESTIONS**

Match the types of abortion in Column 2 with their description in Column 1. Use each term only once.

Column 1	Column 2
_____ 1. Abortion before 12 weeks not externally induced	a. Complete abortion
_____ 2. Legal termination of pregnancy to preserve the mother's health	b. Incomplete abortion
	c. Induced abortion
_____ 3. All of the products of conception passed before 12 weeks	d. Missed abortion
	e. Spontaneous abortion
_____ 4. Symptoms of impending abortion with a closed cervix	f. Therapeutic abortion
	g. Threatened abortion

_____ 5. Failure to pass a fetus after
4 weeks of fetal death
_____ 6. Intentional termination of
pregnancy

Match the problems of pregnancy in Column 2 with their description in Column 1.

	Column 1	Column 2
_____	7. Painless bleeding in third trimester of pregnancy	a. Abortion
_____	8. Hypertension, proteinuria, and visual disturbance in the third trimester	b. Abruptio placentae
		c. Eclampsia
		d. Ectopic pregnancy
_____	9. Severe abdominal pain, shock, and easily palpable fetal parts	e. Placenta previa
		f. Preeclampsia
_____	10. Painful third-trimester bleeding	g. Uterine rupture
_____	11. Third-trimester seizure after a new onset of hypertension	
_____	12. Abdominal pain, scant vaginal bleeding, and shock in the first trimester	

13. Between what ages can pregnancy occur?

_____

14. In what lunar month do the following fetal development characteristics typically occur?
   a. Fetal movement:

_____

   b. Fetal heart beat:

_____

   c. Distinct fingers and toes:

_____

   d. Eyebrows and fingernails:

_____

   e. Possible viability if born:

_____

15. Why do the arteriovenous shunts close at birth?

_____

_____

16. What do the following pregnancy terms mean?
   a. A patient is gravida 6 para 5 (G6 P5).

_____

   b. She is a multipara.

_____

c. The patient has postpartum bleeding.

___

d. You are called to care for a nullipara who is term.

___

17. *A woman in her fortieth week of pregnancy complains of heartburn, dizziness, and frequency of urination. Her heart rate is 100; respirations are 20 and deep; and blood pressure is 90/60 mm Hg (she says her normal is 100/70 mm Hg). She has slight edema of the ankles and tortuous varicose veins.* Explain how the physiological alterations of pregnancy cause each of the signs or symptoms she is experiencing.
    a. Heartburn:

___

___

    b. Dizziness:

___

___

    c. Frequency of urination:

___

___

    d. Hypotension:

___

___

    e. Pedal edema and varicose veins:

___

___

18. Briefly explain why each of the following historical findings would cause concern if delivery is imminent in the field:
    a. No prenatal care:

___

___

    b. Diabetic mother:

___

___

    c. Vaginal bleeding:

___

___

d. Current heroin intoxication:

_____

_____

Questions 19 to 21 pertain to the following scenario: *A 28-year-old woman who is in her third trimester has no obvious external trauma but complains of abdominal pain after an automobile accident. She is pale, and her vital signs are blood pressure, 90/60 mm Hg; pulse, 134; and respirations, 28. Her abdomen is tender to palpation, and you note some vaginal bleeding.*

19. What other subjective information do you need from the mother?

_____

_____

20. How can you determine whether the infant is in distress?

_____

_____

21. Describe prehospital care and transport of this patient.

_____

_____

_____

Questions 22 to 26 pertain to the following scenario: *A 40-year-old primipara in the third trimester complains of headache, dizziness, and nausea. Vital signs are blood pressure, 160/100 mm Hg; pulse, 110; and respirations, 20. Her hands and feet are markedly swollen, and you note intermittent facial twitching. She says her doctor was worried about protein in her urine.*

22. What complication do you suspect?

_____

23. In what position should you transport this patient?

_____

24. List two drugs with appropriate doses that may be ordered by medical direction to stop seizure activity in these types of patients.

_____

25. Besides medications, what EMS actions will minimize the risk of seizures?

_____

26. What risks to the fetus exist with this condition?

_____

Questions 27 to 29 pertain to the following scenario: *A 30-year-old woman says she is 6 weeks pregnant and complains of severe cramping pain in the lower abdomen and vaginal bleeding. She states she has saturated 6 sanitary napkins and that she passed some "white stringy stuff" that her husband shows you in the toilet.*

27. What condition of pregnancy do you suspect?

_____

28. What actions should you take so that the physician can determine whether she has had a complete abortion?

_____

29. Estimate her blood loss if you feel the history was accurate.

_____

30. _An obstetrician calls you to his office to transport a 28-year-old woman who has an ectopic pregnancy (determined by ultrasound). She complains of severe abdominal pain and has frank signs of shock._
  a. What other signs or symptoms might she experience?

_____

  b. Describe interventions you will use on your 20-minute trip to the emergency department.

_____

_____

31. What general patient care measures should be taken for any patient who has third-trimester bleeding without shock?

_____

Questions 32 to 36 pertain to the following scenario: _You are called to a private residence 30 minutes from the nearest hospital to care for a woman in labor._
32. What information in the patient's past medical history will be important to help gauge how quickly labor will progress?

_____

33. What specific signs or symptoms lead you to believe delivery is imminent?

_____

34. As the baby's head delivers, what assessment and interventions should you perform?

_____

35. Describe the procedure to clamp the umbilical cord.

_____

36. When should the Apgar score be calculated?

_____

37. If needed, when should oxytocin be administered, and what is the proper dose and route?

---

38. *Labor fails to progress after a baby presenting in breech position is delivered to the level of the chest.* Describe the steps to be taken by a paramedic in this situation.

---

39. After the head of a baby with shoulder dystocia is delivered, what can the paramedic do to deliver the shoulders while minimizing fetal injury?

---

40. *A 35-year-old woman who is G6 P5 states that she is ready to deliver her baby at home. Her membranes have ruptured, her contractions are frequent, and she wants to push. When you examine her perineum, you see the umbilical cord protruding from the vagina.*

    a. What actions should you take immediately to prevent fetal hypoxia?

---

    b. Should you attempt to deliver this baby on the scene?

Questions 41 to 43 pertain to the following scenario: *A baby is born, his airway has been suctioned, and he has been properly positioned. Tactile stimulation has been provided; however, he is still not breathing.*

41. At what rate should you ventilate the neonate?

After ventilations are initiated, you detect a pulse of 70.

42. Where should you palpate the pulse on a neonate?

---

43. What steps should you take now?

---

44. Functions of the placenta include all of the following, *except:*
    a. Excretion of wastes
    c. Metabolism of drugs
    b. Hormone production
    d. Transfer of gases

45. The fetal structure that allows blood to bypass the liver and go directly into the inferior vena cava is the:
    a. Ductus arteriosus
    c. Foramen ovale
    b. Ductus venosus
    d. Umbilical vein

46. The primary role of amniotic fluid is:
    a. Excretion
    c. Nutrition
    b. Hydration
    d. Protection

47. The primary complication from administration of magnesium sulfate is:
    a. Increased hypertension
    c. Respiratory depression
    b. Precipitous delivery
    d. Ventricular dysrhythmias

48. *A minute after delivery, a baby has a weak cry, a pink body with blue extremities, and a pulse of 128; he actively moves about and sneezes when a catheter is introduced into his nose.* The Apgar score is:
    a. 6
    c. 8
    b. 7
    d. 9

49. What is a frequent complication of multiple gestation?
    a. Eclampsia
    c. Premature delivery
    b. Placenta previa
    d. Uterine rupture

50. Excessive traction on the umbilical cord during placental delivery may cause:
    a. Fetal distress
    c. Uterine inversion
    b. Placenta previa
    d. Uterine rupture

51. *A 30-year-old woman develops dyspnea and severe chest pain 24 hours after delivery of her third child. She is hypotensive and in acute distress.* Based on her history, you suspect:
    a. Eclampsia
    c. Pneumonia
    b. Myocardial infarction
    d. Pulmonary embolism

52. Priorities of care for neonatal resuscitation are:
    a. Prevent heat loss, administer intravenous fluids, and allow the infant to feed at the breast.
    b. Position the neonate and suction to clear the airway, minimize external stimulation, and initiate intravenous fluids.
    c. Prevent heat loss, position the neonate and suction to clear the airway, and provide stimulation.
    d. Position the infant and suction to clear the airway, administer intravenous fluids, and provide stimulation.

53. Deep suctioning of the posterior pharynx of the neonate may cause:
    a. Bradycardia
    b. Central nervous system depression
    c. Hypocarbia
    d. Tachypnea

54. Which of the following is an acceptable method of neonatal stimulation?
    a. Shouting loudly close to the baby's ear
    b. Holding the baby by the ankles and slapping her buttocks
    c. Slapping or flicking the soles of the feet or rubbing the back
    d. Vigorously shaking the baby by firmly grasping the shoulders

GYNECOLOGICAL EMERGENCIES

● **READING ASSIGNMENT**

Chapter 29, pp. 902-907, in *Mosby's Paramedic Textbook*

● **OBJECTIVES**

As a paramedic, you should be able to:

1. Describe the pathophysiology, assessment, and management of the following causes of abdominal pain in females: dysmenorrhea, mittelschmerz, pelvic inflammatory disease, and ruptured ovarian cyst.
2. Outline the assessment and physical and psychological management of the sexual assault victim.
3. Describe specific prehospital measures to preserve evidence in sexual assault cases.

● **REVIEW QUESTIONS**

Match the gynecological problems in Column 2 with their description in Column 1. Use each term only once.

Column 1	Column 2
_____ 1. Abdominal pain at ovulation	a. Dysmenorrhea
	b. Menarche
_____ 2. Infection of the female pelvic organs	c. Mittelschmerz
	d. Pelvic inflammatory disease
_____ 3. Menstrual cramps	
	e. Ruptured ovarian cyst
_____ 4. Fluid sac that ruptures	

5. Other than pain, list three signs or symptoms that a woman may experience during menses.
   a.
   b.
   c.

6. What measures can be taken in the prehospital environment to minimize the fear and stress experienced by a victim of sexual abuse?

_____

_____

7. Describe five guidelines for evidence preservation on a sexual abuse call.
   a.
   b.
   c.
   d.
   e.

8. Which of the following factors increases the incidence of dysmenorrhea?
   a. Increased age
   b. Frequent exercise
   c. Childbirth
   d. Infection
9. The most common cause of pelvic inflammatory disease is:
   a. Gonorrhea
   b. Herpes virus
   c. Human immunodeficiency virus
   d. Syphilis
10. A ruptured ovarian cyst may mimic all of the following, *except:*
    a. Appendicitis
    b. Cholecystitis
    c. Ectopic pregnancy
    d. Salpingitis
11. The most important role of the paramedic in caring for a victim of sexual abuse is to:
    a. Allow only a paramedic of the same sex to care for the patient.
    b. Provide a safe and secure environment for the patient.
    c. Preserve evidence exactly as outlined by protocol.
    d. Perform a complete history and head-to-toe examination.

DIVISION FIVE REVIEW TEST

1. A typical woman will have menstrual flow every _____ days.
   a. 14   c. 28
   b. 21   d. 35
2. In which of the following positions should the hypotensive pregnant patient more than 4 months gestation be transported?
   a. High Fowler's   c. Prone
   b. Left lateral recumbent d. Supine
3. How is eclampsia distinguished from preeclampsia?
   a. Edema   c. Hypertension
   b. Glucosuria   d. Seizures
4. Hemorrhage control in the postpartem period may include all of the following, *except:*
   a. Elevation of the mother's hips
   b. Delivery of oxytocin intravenously
   c. Having the baby breast-feed
   d. Vigorous uterine massage
5. Which of the following complications requires delivery by cesarean section?
   a. Breech presentation   c. Shoulder distocia
   b. Cephalopelvic disproportion d. Vaginal bleeding
6. The infant in fetal distress with thick meconium secretions should:
   a. Remain intubated until arrival at the emergency department
   b. Be vigorously suctioned with a bulb syringe and by endotracheal tube
   c. Not be suctioned because suctioning causes increased hypoxia
   d. Be given atropine for the bradycardia that will develop
7. *Immediately after birth, a newborn is breathing and has a pulse of 90.* You should:
   a. Administer oxygen by mask and observe.
   b. Initiate positive-pressure ventilation.
   c. Begin chest compressions and ventilations.
   d. Wrap the baby in a blanket and give her to the mother.
8. The correct dose of epinephrine (1:10,000) for a neonate is:
   a. 0.001 to 0.003 ml/kg   c. 0.1 to 0.3 ml/kg
   b. 0.01 to 0.03 ml/kg   d. 1.0 to 3.0 ml/kg
9. Which of the following gynecological problems may cause severe internal hemorrhage?
   a. Dysmennorhea   c. Salpingitis
   b. Mittelschmerz d. Ruptured ovarian cyst
10. Which of the following is *true* regarding preservation of evidence on a sexual abuse call?
    a. Ask the patient to shower.
    b. Thoroughly clean wounds.
    c. Place the clothing in a paper bag.
    d. Search the scene for evidence.

DIVISION SIX
BEHAVIORAL

BEHAVIORAL EMERGENCIES AND CRISIS INTERVENTION

● READING ASSIGNMENT

Chapter 30, pp. 910-921, in *Mosby's Paramedic Textbook*

● OBJECTIVES

As a paramedic, you should be able to:
1. List examples of interpersonal, situational, organic, and intrapsychic causes of behavioral emergencies.
2. List three critical principles in dealing with a patient having a behavioral emergency.
3. Describe effective interviewing techniques.
4. Distinguish among key symptoms and management techniques for selected behavioral (psychiatric) illnesses.
5. Identify factors that must be considered when assessing suicide risk.
6. Formulate appropriate patient interview questions to determine suicidal intent.
7. Explain management techniques for the patient who has attempted suicide.
8. Describe assessment of the potentially violent patient.
9. List situations when patient restraint can be used.
10. Outline steps in patient restraint.
11. Describe general safety measures to be taken when patient violence is anticipated.
12. Describe steps for self-protection when confronted with a violent patient.

● REVIEW QUESTIONS

Match the psychiatric conditions in Column 2 with their descriptions in Column 1. Use each condition only once.

Column 1	Column 2
_____ 1. Displays feelings of worthlessness and guilt	a. Conversion hysteria
_____ 2. Unfounded fear of situation or object	b. Depression
_____ 3. Individual loses touch with reality in this major mental disorder	c. Mania
_____ 4. Loss of sensory or motor function without organic cause	d. Neurosis
_____ 5. Excessive elation, irritability, talkativeness, and delusions	e. Panic attack
_____ 6. Logical, highly developed delusions	f. Paranoia
	g. Phobia
	h. Psychosis

7. *You pick up a 60-year-old man whose behavior is very erratic. He alternates among hysterical bursts of laughter, irritability, sitting quietly, and crying. You find chlorpropamide (Diabinese), hydralazine, and thyroxin in the medicine chest and note an ecchymotic area on the left temple. His skin is very warm and moist.* Based on this patient's history, what are some likely organic causes of his behavior that must be ruled out before assuming that this is a behavioral emergency?

_____

_____

_____

8. *You are called to a private residence by a woman who says her husband "beat her up." On arrival, you hear loud shouting coming from the house.*
   a. What measures should be taken before entering the home?

_____

   b. When you begin your examination, what measures should you take to enhance safety and allow for a better history and examination?

_____

9. Should a detailed secondary survey be performed on a patient with a behavioral emergency?

_____

10. *A patient with a phobia of heights must be rescued by ladder from a high bridge.* What measures can you take to prevent a panic attack?

_____

11. *A manic patient is being transported to the hospital for psychiatric evaluation.* Describe effective patient management techniques in this situation.

_____

12. *You are on the scene with a 25-year-old woman who was tackled just as she prepared to jump from a sixth-floor window. She is crying, "Let me go. Why didn't you let me do it?"*
   a. How can you best assess whether the patient intended to kill herself?

_____

   b. What are your goals in caring for this patient during transport?

_____

13. *Family members call you to the home of a 25-year-old man who they say has become increasingly out of touch with reality. He feels that aliens are trying to kidnap him so that they can remove his brain. He tells you that they are trying to control his thoughts. He states "They're here. Can't you hear them laughing?"*
   a. What behavioral illness does this presentation suggest?

_____

b. What patient approach will enable therapeutic communication with this person?

_____

_____

Questions 14 to 19 pertain to the following scenario: _A distraught family calls you to take their son to the hospital for psychiatric evaluation. They state that he has been breaking furniture for the past few hours and refuses to take his antipsychotic drugs. He is pacing, is verbally abusive, and is threatening injury to those who approach. He is not armed._

14. For what help should you call?

_____

15. When approaching the patient to prepare for restraint, what should you note about the physical environment?

_____

16. Assuming that he meets the criteria for involuntary detention in your state, how should the patient be restrained (including position and ways to secure extremities and torso)?

_____

_____

17. After restraints are applied, what should be monitored en route to the hospital?

_____

● STUDENT SELF-EVALUATION

18. The three general principles to use on all behavioral emergencies are:
   a. Restrain all patients, contain the crisis, and transport to the hospital.
   b. Show them that you are in charge, contain the crisis, and transport to the hospital.
   c. Restrain all patients, render emergency care, and show them that you are in charge.
   d. Contain the crisis, render emergency care, and transport to the hospital.

19. Which of the following questions would be most appropriate to elicit communication with a mentally ill patient?
   a. Did you start feeling this way today?
   b. Are you feeling bad now?
   c. How did this all begin?
   d. Are you OK?

20. _A middle-aged woman suddenly loses the ability to speak after catching her husband in an extramarital affair._ What behavioral illness may have caused her problem?
   a. Conversion hysteria   **c.** Panic attack
   b. Depression   **d.** Phobia

21. A panic attack may typically be characterized by any of the following, _except:_
   a. Chest pain and vertigo   **c.** Suicidal intent
   b. Hyperventilation   **d.** Trembling and sweating

22. The highest priority on a suicide call is:
   a. Ensuring safety of crew members
   b. Managing life threats
   c. Talking the person out of it
   d. Listening empathically

23. Which of the following statements regarding suicide is true?
   a. People who talk about killing themselves rarely do it.
   b. Men commit suicide more often than women.
   c. Suicide is an inherited tendency.
   d. When depression lifts, suicide risk disappears.

24. *You are transporting a person who clearly believes that he is Elvis Presley. His wife states that he quit his job, keeps calling her* Priscilla, *and is preparing to move to* Graceland. *You suspect that he is suffering from:*
   a. Delusions   **c.** Paranoia
   b. Neurosis   **d.** Phobia

25. When should a violent patient be released from physical restraints?
   a. Immediately after administration of haloperidol intramuscularly
   b. As soon as the patient assures you that he will cooperate
   c. When the police have adequate personnel to control him or her
   d. When an emergency department physician determines that he or she is no longer dangerous

EMERGENCY DRUG INDEX

1. List the actions, indications, and side effects of steroids.

_____

_____

_____

2. For each of the following two drugs, list the time of onset, duration, and dose.

   a. Methylprednisolone:

_____

   b. Dexamethasone:

_____

For each of the scenarios in Questions 3 through 26, complete the corresponding flashcard (flashcards begin opposite p. 332) with the appropriate drug information, including trade name, class, description, indications, contraindications, adverse reactions, onset, duration, dosage (adult and pediatric if appropriate), and special considerations. Verify your drug choice before completing the flashcard by looking at the generic drug name on the back.

3. *Your patient is experiencing urticaria and severe itching resulting from an allergic reaction. His vital signs are stable, and no wheezes are audible on auscultation of his lungs.* You will administer _____. (Complete Flashcard 23.)

4. *You are transporting a patient whose pulse is 30 and blood pressure is 80 by palpation. Administration of atropine, the use of the external pacemaker, and administration of dopamine and epinephrine have been unsuccessful.* The drug to increase the heart rate in this case will be_____. (Complete Flashcard 24.)

5. *Your crew is unable to initiate an intravenous line on an unconscious diabetic patient who is known to be hypoglycemic. Transport time is 45 minutes.* The drug of choice to increase the blood glucose level will be _____. (Complete Flashcard 25.)

6. *Lidocaine is unsuccessful in diminishing premature ventricular contractions for your 50-year-old patient whom you suspect is having a myocardial infarction. List two other drugs that may be appropriate to treat the ventricular ectopy in this situation.* (Complete Flashcards 26 and 27.)

7. *A 65-year-old female calls you complaining of shortness of breath and chest pain radiating down her left arm. Her blood pressure is 110/70 mm Hg.* The drug of choice to relieve her pain will be _____. (Complete Flashcard 28.)

8. *You place a 22-year-old patient with a pounding sensation in her chest on a monitor and discover ventricular tachycardia. The patient's blood pressure is normal, she has no chest pain, and the rest of the history and physical examination are unremarkable.* The appropriate drug to use to suppress ventricular dysrhythmia in this situation will be _____. (Complete Flashcard 29.)

9. *You are caring for a 72-year-old patient with chronic bronchitis who is in acute respiratory distress with mental status changes. His breath sounds are diminished, with inspiratory and expiratory wheezes audible throughout the chest. You have no inhaled bronchodilators available on your ambulance. He states that he has taken no home medicines in 3 days.* Which intravenous medication will you select? _____. (Complete Flashcard 30.)

10. *You are called to an outpatient surgery center to evaluate a nurse who is unconscious. Co-workers confide that they have suspected drug abuse for some time, and an empty meperidine (Demerol) tubex is found in her pocket. All other available medical history is negative. Pupils are pinpoints, and respirations are 12 and shallow.* What drug will you administer first if an overdose is suspected? _____. (Complete Flashcard 31.)

11. *Your 67-year-old patient is experiencing a severe headache and blurred vision resulting from his blood pressure, which is now 230/160 mm Hg. He is awake and cooperative.* What drug may improve this potentially disastrous situation by lowering the blood pressure? _____. (Complete Flashcard 32.)

12. *You are called to a nursing home to care for an 88-year-old woman who has fainted. The patient is extremely bradycardic (pulse, 40) and has a blood pressure of 80 systolic by palpation. Her only history is hypertension.* What emergency care drug is indicated initially to correct the bradycardia? _____. (Complete Flashcard 33.)

13. *Initial electrical countershocks do not successfully convert your cardiac arrest patient from ventricular fibrillation.* After the intravenous is initiated, the first drug of choice will be _____. (Complete Flashcard 34.)

14. *A 32-year-old patient fell while playing softball and has an apparent dislocation of the left shoulder, which is very painful. Medical direction wishes to administer a short-acting analgesic so that accurate emergency department evaluation will be possible.* What is an appropriate, self-administered analgesic agent in this situation? _____. (Complete Flashcard 35.)

15. *For 20 minutes you have been trying without success to resuscitate a 73-year-old woman who is in cardiac arrest. All appropriate airway, electrical, and fluid therapies have been used, but on arrival to emergency department, the blood gas levels reveal that the patient is extremely acidotic.* What drug may be considered at this point to increase the patient's pH? _____. (Complete Flashcard 36.)

16. *The police call you to evaluate an unconscious person. The patient is a known alcoholic, and friends say that he has not eaten for several days. Dextrostix analysis reveals a blood glucose level of 40 mg/dl (normal range 80 to 120 mg/dl). No drug use is suspected.* The two drugs indicated for this patient are _____ and _____. (Complete Flashcards 37 and 38.)

17. *A frantic husband calls you to evaluate his wife, who has been having seizures for 10 minutes. You find her to be experiencing repetitive grand mal seizures. The husband tells you that she is a known epileptic who has not taken any phenytoin (Dilantin) for 2 days.* What will your drug of choice be under these circumstances? _____. (Complete Flashcard 39.)

18. *Your 24-year-old patient is a known asthmatic who is experiencing an acute attack. Inspiratory and expiratory wheezes are audible throughout the chest, and the patient is tachypneic.* What drug would you initially administer by inhalation? _____. (Complete Flashcard 40.) What beta$_2$-selective drug will you initially administer via the parenteral route? _____. (Complete Flashcard 41.)

19. *You are called to treat a 32-year-old woman with a sudden onset of palpitations. The electrocardiogram reveals a rapid supraventricular tachycardia. The patient states that she has Wolff-Parkinson-White syndrome.* What will be the safest drug to use to convert this rhythm to sinus rhythm? _____. (Complete Flashcard 42)

20. *Airport authorities call you to care for a mechanic whose arm is trapped in the landing gear of a small aircraft. Extrication time will be lengthy, and the patient is in extreme distress because of pain. Vital signs are stable, and no other injuries are noted.* List two narcotic analgesics that may be administered to this patient. _____ and _____. (Complete Flashcards 43 and 44.)

21. *A frantic parent calls to report that her 16-year-old daughter reportedly ingested a large quantity of sleeping pills 10 minutes ago. The teenager is awake and alert, with stable vital signs.* What drug will you administer in an attempt to rid the body of these pills? _____. (Complete Flashcard 45.) When emesis is complete, what drug may be used to prevent absorption of any additional toxin that remains in the gastrointestinal tract? _____. (Complete Flashcard 46.)

22. *Your patient is 8 months pregnant and has been diagnosed with preeclampsia. Co-workers found her experiencing a grand mal seizure in the restroom. The patient appears to be in a postictal state. Blood pressure is 160/116 mm Hg.* What drug may be given to prevent a recurrence of seizure activity? _____. (Complete Flashcard 47.)

23. *You have a 30-minute estimated time of arrival to the hospital with an 86-year-old patient from a nursing home whose vital signs are blood pressure 80/50 mm Hg; pulse, 124; and respirations, 24. The urine in her Foley catheter bag is milky green and foul smelling. Cardiac history is negative, and there is no reason to suspect blood or fluid volume loss.* What will be the drug of choice to acutely correct her hypotension after fluid resuscitation in this situation? _____. (Complete Flashcard 48.)

24. *The 65-year-old patient you are called to evaluate has the following vital signs: blood pressure 130/90 mm Hg; pulse, 160; and respirations, 24. The electrocardiogram monitor shows atrial fibrillation with a rapid ventricular response. She has mild signs of congestive heart failure, but all other physical findings are negative.* What class IV antidysrhythmic drug will be indicated for this patient? _____. (Complete Flashcard 49.)

25. *Your 72-year-old patient is experiencing severe dyspnea that began suddenly during the night. She is in obvious distress, with cyanosis of the nail beds and lips. Lung sounds reveal rales and wheezes throughout, and she has a cough that produces frothy, pink sputum. History reveals two previous myocardial infarctions. Vital signs are blood pressure 170/108 mm Hg; pulse, 132; and respirations, 32.* Identify the diuretic that you will administer in an attempt to improve this patient's condition? _____. (Complete Flashcard 50.)

26. *You have just delivered a healthy baby boy, followed minutes later by a complete placenta. Despite vigorous massage, the patient's uterus is very soft, and she is experiencing profuse vaginal bleeding.* What pharmacological agent can you administer to help control this bleeding? _____. (Complete Flashcard 51.)

● STUDENT SELF-EVALUATION

27. When is the use of dopamine most clearly indicated?
    a. Cardiac arrest
    b. Cardiogenic shock
    c. Head injury
    d. Internal bleeding

28. Which of the following would be the appropriate drug to administer to a patient who was in a motor vehicle collision and is complaining of severe abdominal pain?
    a. Meperidine
    b. Morphine
    c. Nitrous oxide
    d. None of the above

29. Which of the following is an indication for administration of epinephrine 1:1000 subcutaneously?
    a. Anaphylaxis
    b. Asystole
    c. Electromechanical dissociation
    d. Ventricular fibrillation

30. Which of the following drugs is an anticonvulsant that may also be used for treatment of dysrhythmias in digoxin toxicity?
    a. Bretylium
    b. Lidocaine
    c. Phenytoin
    d. Procainamide

31. Which of the following is *not* true regarding use of atropine?
    a. It is indicated for management of bradycardia.
    b. The initial dose in bradycardia is 0.5 mg intravenously.
    c. It should be given in asystole.
    d. It is an antidote for verapamil.
32. Dopamine, when given at low doses (0.5 to 2.0 mcg/kg/min), will have what effect?
    a. Renal and mesenteric vessel dilation
    b. Profound arteriolar constriction
    c. Decreased cerebral edema
    d. Ventricular dysrhythmias
33. Which of the following should be the most appropriate drugs for the patient who has had a myocardial infarction and who is experiencing many premature ventricular complexes?
    a. Oxygen, verapamil, and lidocaine
    b. Oxygen, lidocaine, and procainamide
    c. Oxygen, adenosine, and procainamide
    d. Oxygen, phenobarbital, and lidocaine
34. Your patient is in ventricular fibrillation and has been shocked 3 times. An intravenous infusion has been started. Your *first* choice for drug therapy will be:
    a. Epinephrine   c. Morphine
    b. Hydralazine   d. Nifedipine
35. Drugs that cause bronchodilation include all of the following *except:*
    a. Albuterol   c. Diphenhydramine
    b. Epinephrine   d. Terbutaline
36. Verapamil is *contraindicated* if the patient is:
    a. Complaining of palpitations   c. Tachycardic
    b. Hypotensive   d. Under 45
37. Which drug is self-administered by mask for relief of pain?
    a. Albuterol   c. Nitroglycerin
    b. Morphine sulfate   d. Nitrous oxide:oxygen
38. A drug indicated for the management of hypertension is:
    a. Dobutamine   c. Phenytoin
    b. Hydralazine   d. Procainamide
39. Aminophylline should be administered with caution to patients with:
    a. Bradycardia   c. Drowsiness
    b. Bronchospasm   d. Tachycardia
40. Pharmacological management of the patient suffering from coma of unknown origin includes:
    a. Naloxone, glucagon, and D50W
    b. Butorphanol (Stadol), glucagon, and thiamine
    c. Naloxone, thiamine, and D50W
    d. Dexamethasone, glucagon, and D50W
41. When is mannitol indicated?
    a. Myocardial infarction   c. Digoxin toxicity
    b. Acute cerebral edema   d. Shock
42. Which pharmacological agent is useful in status epilepticus as an antianxiety agent, and as a skeletal muscle relaxant?
    a. Diazepam   c. Naloxone
    b. Morphine   d. Phenytoin
43. The drug indicated for management of postpartum bleeding is:
    a. Dopamine   c. Magnesium sulfate
    b. Insulin   d. Oxytocin
44. Diphenhydramine is contraindicated in:
    a. Anaphylactic shock   c. Allergic reactions
    b. An acute asthma attack   d. Patients over 35

45. Syrup of ipecac may be given to patients:
    a. Without a gag reflex
    b. Who have ingested prochlorperazine (Compazine)
    c. Who have ingested phenytoin (Dilantin)
    d. Who have ingested gasoline
46. Naloxone is an antagonist to all of the following, *except:*
    a. Propoxyphene   c. Meperidine
    b. Heroin   d. Phenobarbital
47. Which of the following medications may cause respiratory depression?
    a. Atropine   c. Magnesium sulfate
    b. Dexamethasone   d. Terbutaline
48. Administration of bretylium to a conscious patient may cause:
    a. Bradycardia   c. Sweating
    b. Nausea and vomiting   d. Tremors
49. What side effect may occur secondary to nitroglycerin ingestion?
    a. Headache   c. Burning under the tongue
    b. Hypotension   d. All of the above
50. Which of the following drugs will exert a positive chronotropic effect?
    a. Adenosine   c. Haloperidol
    b. Epinephrine   d. Propranolol
51. Furosemide is indicated in the management of:
    a. Angina   c. Hypotension
    b. Dysrhythmias   d. Pulmonary edema
52. A calcium channel blocker that slows conduction and is useful in management of paroxymal supraventricular tachycardia to slow the heart rate is:
    a. Adenosine   c. Dobutamine
    b. Albuterol   d. Verapamil
53. All of the following drugs are indicated to manage pulmonary edema that develops secondary to left-sided heart failure, *except:*
    a. Atropine   c. Morphine
    b. Furosemide   d. Nitroglycerin
54. When meperidine is given alone, what side effects should be anticipated?
    a. Increased heart rate   c. Vasoconstriction
    b. Nausea and vomiting   d. Hyperactivity
55. *Your patient is a 35-year-old man who is psychotic and violent. What is the drug of choice for his care?*
    a. Haloperidol   c. Meperidine
    b. Hydroxyzine   d. Nifedipine
56. Dexamethasone and methylprednisolone belong to what class of drugs?
    a. Analgesics   c. Sympathomimetics
    b. Inotropics   d. Steroids

PARAMEDIC CAREER OPPORTUNITIES

Since its inception in 1967, EMS has developed into a sophisticated profession, including various levels of care that result in improved care of the sick and injured. With the evolution of EMS has come career opportunities for EMTs, paramedics, nurses, and physicians. Although specific job opportunities depend on geographics, in general, opportunities for prehospital emergency responders have emerged from volunteer to paid career positions. For a certified EMT-Paramedic, many options are available.

Position	Description	Qualifications
Field parametic	Many paramedics enjoy the day-to-day operations of a field provider, administering emergency care to the sick and injured. Roles and responsibilities of paramedics will undoubtedly grow in the future as the emergency department extends into the community through advanced life support (ALS) personnel.	Usually requires current certification as an EMT-Paramedic (Some organizations also require National Registry certification.)
Paramedic supervisor	An ALS supervisor is usually an experienced paramedic with administrative or management skills. Responsibilities for this position generally include recruitment, scheduling, discipline, and supervision of emergency care personnel.	Usually requires substantial experience as a field provider and supervisory experience
Flight paramedic	A flight paramedic uses his or her knowledge and skills to care for victims who require air medical evacuation and rapid transport to hospitals. A flight crew is usually composed of a pilot, a flight medic, and a flight nurse.	Usually requires substantial experience as a field provider and the ability to work under pressure.

Interhospital transport medic	Some organizations hire paramedics to assist with the interhospital, intercontinental, or international transfer of patients requiring monitored transportation. Responsibilities for this position generally include monitoring patients during transport and initiating emergency care when necessary.	Usually requires certification as a paramedic.
EMS administrator	Experienced paramedics with backgrounds in management can act in administrative capacities within various organizations. Although advanced training is often necessary, it is possible to obtain administrative positions in hospitals, government emergency services organizations, and independent companies.	In addition to paramedic certification, often requires advanced degrees in EMS, business, or health care administration.
EMS educator	Many colleges and universities offer programs in emergency medical services, including paramedic certification programs, associate degrees, bachelor's degrees, and even master's degrees. Paramedics with experience in education can obtain positions as instructors for such programs.	Usually requires paramedic certification and experience as an instructor. Advanced-degree certification often desired for high-level training programs.

● OTHER AREAS OF INTEREST

Aside from traditional prehospital roles, some paramedics have taken on expanded duties. Although there has been much controversy regarding the use of paramedics within the emergency department, some hospitals in the United States use paramedics as orderlies, pathology assistants, intravenous team members, phlebotomists, and respiratory therapists.

Some hospitals have also extended emergency departments in which paramedics have a function. These facilities offer treatment for minor illnesses or injuries and perform physical examinations and health screenings. They are often located within industrial settings, universities, or a stand-alone building away from the hospital.

Finally, there are additional opportunities for paramedics with advanced educations. Many universities offer credits toward a bachelor's degree for anyone with a paramedic certification. For a field paramedic with experience, other advanced career opportunities might include training as a nurse or physician's assistant.

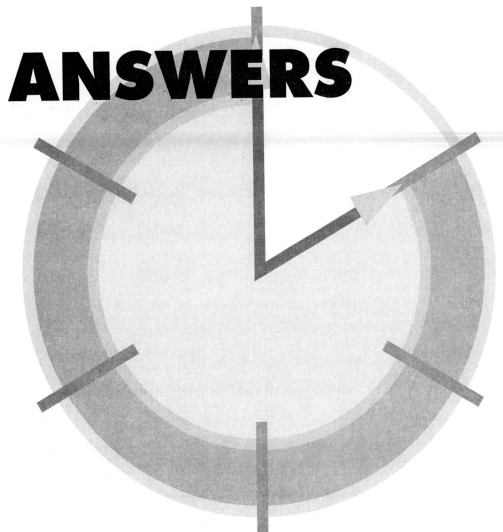

ANSWERS

CHAPTER 1
ROLES AND RESPONSIBILITIES

1. a (page 5)
2. d (page 6)
3. b (page 5)
4. c (page 5)
5. True (page 7)
6. Assessing the situation and the patient, assisting with extrication if necessary, calling for additional equipment if needed, and calming the patient; contacting medical control with the patient report; initiating necessary advanced life-support procedures and monitoring the patient's response to treatment; using protocols to provide care if communications fail; determining how and where the patient is to be transported; documenting the call; and restocking and replenishing supplies to prepare for the next call (p. 6)
7. Continuing education, refresher training, skill maintenance verification, and reexamination
8. To ensure the provision of quality care, learn new skills and treatments, and prevent decay of skills or knowledge (pp. 6-7)
9. Membership in professional associations; continuing education such as conferences and seminars, quality-improvement reviews, skill laboratories, certification and recertification programs, journal studies, videotaped presentations, and independent study; and involvement in community education, medical research, publication in EMS journals, and agency or community committee membership (p. 7)
10. In most situations a living will cannot be recognized without written documentation; in this situation the patient is comatose, so you have implied consent and a duty to treat. The decision may be ethical, depending on the paramedic's past experiences and religious and personal beliefs (p. 7).
11. Educational opportunities and participation in state or national issues relating to patient care and the EMS profession (p. 7)
12. d. Although this job may fall to the EMT-P in some systems, it is not an integral part of the role (p. 6).
13. a. Relicensure and recertification evaluate and enhance existing knowledge and do not reteach the curriculum (pp. 6-7).
14. e. All activities listed help ensure that the paramedic is familiar with current patient care management principles (p. 7).
15. a. Mass casualty training teaches us to give care to the most seriously injured patient. However, in a situation such as this, it may be difficult from a moral and ethical standpoint to turn to the perpetrator first for care. All other answers are clear-cut legal situations permitting care or enabling the paramedic to leave the scene without fear of increased patient injury (p. 7).

CHAPTER 2
THE EMS SYSTEM

1. True (p. 15)
2. False. Not all critically ill patients benefit from air medical transport. Factors that must be considered include ground transport times, road and weather conditions, and the expertise needed by the ground crew to care for the specific patient (p. 17).
3. Funding, first aid, and accessing the system (pp. 11-12)
4. a (p. 13)
5. The trauma patient typically needs rapid assessment, stabilization, and transportation to a medical facility where definitive care can often be provided only in the operating room. Advanced life-support procedures should usually be done en route to the hospital. The cardiac arrest patient may require extensive advanced life-support procedures in the prehospital setting, including defibrillation and drugs to resuscitate the patient before transport is initiated (pp. 13-14).
6. To train, evaluate skills, develop protocols, and monitor on-line medical control communications (p. 14)
7. To permit joint patient care decisions and ensure that hospital personnel are adequately prepared for the patient's arrival (p. 14)
8. They establish a standard of care, permit critical time-sensitive interventions to be initiated before physician contact, and provide guidelines for care if communications fail (p. 14)
9. Feedback regarding the effectiveness of prehospital care and a broader view of the long-term sequelae of the injury or illness can be gained (p. 15).
10. When the patient is physically delivered to the emergency department and the report is given to the receiving medical personnel (p. 15)
11. It provides an opportunity to learn from mistakes, vent hostilities, and prepare the crew for calls of a similar nature (p. 15).
12. KKK standards and the American College of Surgeons essential equipment list (p. 16)
13. Geographical area, topographical area, population, and traffic conditions (pp. 16-17)
14. a. Dispatcher; b. advanced life support; c. hospital delivery; d. patient rehabilitation and education (p. 12)
15. c. Other personnel should assume patient care and administrative and maintenance duties. The primary role of the EMS physician medical director is to ensure quality patient care (p. 14).
16. d. Although insurance reimbursement is necessary for the EMS system to operate, the insurance providers are not considered a part of the system (p. 12).
17. a. Although problems may surface in a critique, this should not be the focus of such a session. The

critiques should be conducted in a positive manner to decrease stress and to constructively review calls to improve future performance (p. 15).

18. c. Scene response time and availability of an ambulance to answer calls are the key elements in properly spacing EMS vehicles for maximal effectiveness (p. 16).

19. b. The patient with compromised circulation from a possible aneurysm needs rapid definitive care to prevent disability or death. Each of the other patients would appear not to need urgent hospital interventions (p. 17).

20. d. The on-line medical direction physician should be contacted to attempt to arbitrate the situation. If this is not possible, he or she may recommend police intervention (p. 14).

● CHAPTER 3
MEDICAL-LEGAL CONSIDERATIONS

1. c (p. 23)
2. h (p. 24)
3. e (p. 23)
4. d (p. 23)
5. f (pp. 23-24)
6. a (p. 23)
7. False. Violations of this nature can also be prosecuted in a criminal lawsuit, and offenders can be subject to fines, probation, or imprisonment (p. 23).
8. True (p. 27)
9. False. Group insurance policies offer the individual some protection from financial devastation if he or she is found guilty of negligence; however, they do not protect the EMS provider from litigation resulting from negligent acts (pp. 27-28).
10. Make regulations, license providers, revoke or suspend licensure, and enforce regulations under their jurisdiction (p. 21)
11. Training, competent patient care skills, and thorough documentation (p. 26)
12. Child or elder abuse, rape, animal bites, and gunshot or stab wounds (p. 24)
13. Duty to act, breach of duty, damage to the patient, and proximate cause (p. 22)
14. *Duty to act:* The unit was on duty and was called to care for this patient. *Breach of duty:* The standard of care would have indicated immobilizing and transporting this patient; the crew failed to act as the standard of care dictated. *Damage to the patient:* The patient lost movement, stopped breathing, and died after being abandoned by the paramedic crew. *Proximate cause:* The patient apparently died from spinal cord damage; the paramedic crew did not immobilize and protect the C-spine, which may have prevented death (pp. 22-23).
15. Informed, expressed, and implied (pp. 24-25)

16. Documentation of the incident, tracking of patient care skills, supplying of inventory, research, and billing (p. 26)

17. Document that the patient is awake and alert; explain to the patient the potential consequences of refusing care, including paralysis or death, and document same; have patient sign a refusal form; have witness sign a refusal form and document names of any additional witnesses; and give follow-up instructions and encourage the patient to call EMS if he elects to seek medical attention (p. 25).

18. d. Criminal law violations need not involve injury or criminal intent. Patients sue for damages in civil suits. A criminal law violation is based on proof that a statute has been violated (p. 22).

19. a. A patient who needs continuing advanced care should not be delivered to health care providers unable to provide that care (p. 23).

20. d. Buying malpractice insurance protects the paramedic's assets after a malpractice award has been made but does not protect the paramedic from a claim (pp. 27-28).

21. c. In all states but Louisiana, paramedics are permitted to discuss comments by patients in court. Professional transfer of information to receiving emergency department personnel is always permitted. Confidential release of patient information to quality-assurance committees is also protected (p. 24).

22. a. Implied consent permits a paramedic to render lifesaving care if the patient is unable to agree because of lack of mental competence. *Informed consent* means that the patient has been told the implications of the injury and illness, the treatment needed, and the potential complications. Referred consent does not exist (pp. 24-25).

23. d. The more thorough the narrative, the more useful it will be to health care professionals and the better it can be used as a means to protect against claims of negligence (p. 27).

● CHAPTER 4
EMS COMMUNICATIONS

1. c (p. 32)
2. i (p. 33)
3. a (p. 32)
4. j (p. 33)
5. b (p. 32)
6. e (p. 32)
7. k (p. 33)
8. h (p. 34)
9. False. The repeater increases transmission distance (p. 34).
10. True (p. 34)
11. Remote consoles (p. 34)

12. Decoder (p. 35)
13. Mountains, dense foliage, and tall buildings (p. 34)
14. Licensing and frequency allocation, establishing technical standards for radio equipment, and establishing and enforcing rules and regulations (pp. 35-38)
15. To receive calls for EMS assistance, dispatch and coordinate EMS resources, relay medical information, and coordinate with public safety agencies (pp. 40-41)
16. EMS response is initiated by bystanders through 9-1-1, emergency numbers or citizens band radios. The dispatcher obtains the necessary information and then dispatches appropriate emergency personnel and equipment. The EMS crew notifies dispatch while en route and obtains additional information. The EMS crew notifies the dispatcher on arrival to scene. The EMS crew contacts medical direction for orders and reports. The EMS crew re-contacts medical direction if necessary, updating patient information and the estimated time of arrival. The EMS crew notifies dispatch of arrival at the hospital. The EMS crew contacts dispatch for run times to document on the medical report. Finally, the EMS crew notifies dispatch when available for service (pp. 40-43).
17. Name and call-back number of individual who placed call; address of emergency and directions, including specific landmarks, because of the rural location; and the nature of the emergency (is the victim trapped, how seriously is he or she injured, and is he or she accessible to the EMS crew?) (p. 40)
18. Adjust squelch, listen for open channel, press transmit button for 1 second before speaking, speak 2 to 3 inches away from and across the microphone, speak slowly and clearly, and speak without emotion (pp. 41-42)
19. City Unit 7, paramedic Smith calling City Hospital. We are on the scene at an industrial site with a patient who fell approximately 20 feet onto a grassy area. Patient is a 30-year-old male weighing approximately 100 kg. Patient's chief complaint is back pain. Also complaining of bilateral heel pain. Patient states he got dizzy and fell. Past medical history of back pain for which he takes ibuprofen. Patient is awake, alert, and oriented x 3. Lungs are clear bilaterally; skin is warm and dry. Tenderness to palpation in lumbar region of back and bilaterally on heels. Soft tissue swelling present bilaterally at calcaneus. Distal pulse, sensation, and movement present in all extremities. V/S are BP 120/80, P 116, R 20. Patient placed on 100% oxygen by complete nonrebreather mask and immobilized on a backboard with cervical collar. Private physician is Dr. Jones. ETA will be 15 minutes. Standing by for any additional orders, over.

20. At 01:00 Unit 7 arrived on the scene of an industrial site. Found a 30-year-old, approximately 100-kg male lying on grassy area, where he landed after an approximately 20-foot fall. Patient is complaining of lumbar back pain and heel pain. Awake, alert, and oriented x 3. Lungs are clear. Pain on palpation of lumbar area and at calcaneus bilaterally. V/S at 01:00: BP 120/80, P 116, R 20. Patient states he got dizzy and fell. Patient states he takes ibuprofen for back pain. Placed on 100% oxygen by mask. Immobilized with cervical collar and backboard. At 01:20 Dr. Kane at City Hospital contacted for report. No further orders given. 01:25 BP 120/80, P 116, R 20. Patient status unchanged en route to City (p. 42).
21. c. A decibel is a unit of measurement for signal power levels. Frequency modulation is a deviation in carrier frequency resulting in less noise. A tone is a selective carrier wave used to selectively signal a receiver (p. 33).
22. b. Amplitude modulation is a radio frequency that fluctuates according to the applied audio. Range refers to the general perimeter of signal coverage. A watt measures power output (p. 32).
23. d. *Coverage* refers to the area where radio communication exists. A hot line is a dedicated line activated by merely lifting the receiver. Patching permits communication between different communication modes (p. 33).
24. c. All other equipment listed is part of a complex system (p. 31).
25. b. These tones can be set to *all call* for efficient disaster communication. Cellular telephones are used for ambulance-to-hospital contact in some areas. Satellite dishes and microwave transmitters extend transmission distance (p. 35).
26. d. This is the physician medical director's job (pp. 40-41).
27. b. "If it was not written, it was not done," is the common legal belief (p. 42).

● CHAPTER 5
RESCUE MANAGEMENT

1. True (p. 47)
2. False. Class ABC extinguishers are intended for use on ordinary combustible, flammable liquids and electrical equipment. Class D extinguishers are used for combustible metals (p. 48).
3. Impact-resistant helmet, safety goggles, turn-out coat, waterproof gloves, and rubber boots with steel insoles and toes (p. 46)
4. Hazardous materials, fuel supply hazards, fire, heat source hazards, gasoline spills, electrical hazards, unstable vehicles, and environmental hazards (pp. 48-49)
5. Response, other factors, and resources (pp. 50-51)

6. *Response:* Obtain en route any additional information regarding exact location (for example, what storefront or what parking lot locator). Determine whether the number of injured is known. *Other factors:* Determine whether extrication will be necessary. *Resources:* Determine what additional equipment, manpower, EMS crews, law enforcement officers, or rescue trucks you will need (pp. 50-51).

7. Immediately delegate several crowd members to move the crowd to a safe distance to allow for patient care and arrival of additonal equipment. Call for law enforcement officers to take charge of crowd control (p. 46).

8. Advanced life-support ambulance, rescue truck, pumper, and law enforcement officers (p. 50)

9. Begin initial patient assessment (p. 51).

10. Protect the patient with blankets, shields, or flame-retardant coverings (p. 51).

11. Securing an open airway, protecting the cervical spine, and assisting ventilations with high-concentration oxygen if necessary (p. 51)

12. *Disentanglement:* removal of the wreckage from the patient. Rescuers must protect the patient and maintain the airway, cervical spine immobilization, and breathing to the best of their ability. *Packaging and removal:* immobilization and removal of the patient from the scene to the emergency response vehicle. Rescuers must protect the patient's spine, splint, or bandage injuries if appropriate (based on how acute the patient's condition is), and ensure that the patient is adequately secured before removal begins. The paramedic should oversee safe transport of the patient by the rescue team to the ambulance or aircraft (pp. 51-52).

13. a. Contact utility workers to move downed wires or shut off power, keep bystanders away, and secure energized wires with a dry fire hose or other appropriate means. b. Advise occupants to stay in the car (p. 48).

14. Ropes, air tanks, pry bars, jacks, wedges, spreaders, and winches (pp. 48-51)

15. b. Initial efforts should ensure that the crew is uninjured so that their EMS functions can be maintained (pp. 45-46).

16. a. Although ear plugs are helpful on a response, they may impair communications on a rescue (p. 46).

17. b (p. 47)

18. d (p. 47)

19. d. In some cases, the battery may be left connected. The other measures would be unnecessary in the absence of flames (p. 47).

20. b (p. 48)

● **CHAPTER 6**
MAJOR INCIDENT RESPONSE

1. e (p. 57)
2. a (p. 57)
3. g (p. 57)
4. b (p. 57)
5. False. A major incident is any situation in which the resources available are inadequate to meet the needs at that time (p. 54).
6. Multiagency meetings, drills, a written plan (including mutual aid agreements and move-ups), and identification of special resources (p. 55)
7. Must be easily adapted to any emergency; must be part of standard operating procedures so that it is easily adapted to a major incident; must have common elements in organization, terminology, and procedures; must have implementation that minimizes disruption to existing systems; and must have minimum operational and maintenance costs (p. 56)
8. Air evacuation, aeronautical rescue, disaster services, hazardous materials emergency response, search and rescue, and heavy equipment (p. 55)
9. Four color tags are used: red—critically injured, yellow—less critically injured, green—non-life or non-limb threatening, black—dead or injuries that preclude the chance for survival (p. 62).
10. Immediate, delayed, or nonsalvageable or dead (p. 62)
11. Command is determined by the preplanned system of arriving emergency units. They must be familiar with ICS structure and the operating procedures of responding units (p. 57).
12. Assuming an effective command position that is away from any danger of the bleachers and that has a good vantage point, transmitting initial radio reports requesting additional equipment and alerting local hospitals, assessing the situation to determine special equipment and personnel needs, developing a strategy to move untrapped victims and begin safe extrication efforts, requesting additional resources (heavy equipment and local experts with knowledge of the structural design), assigning sectors, providing objectives for sectors, delegating authority (assigning a public sector commander), recording or having a delegated person record events of major incident so that more thorough documentation can be completed later, sending units no longer needed back into service and terminating command, and evaluating the effectiveness of operations (may be done retrospectively) (p. 57)
13. a. *Support:* procuring and distributing supplies (medical, food, water, protective gear) and resources (heavy equipment, special tools) (p. 60).

b. *Staging:* designating and staffing a safe helicopter landing zone and designating and staffing a staging area where all arriving apparatus will report and be assigned to areas where needed (p. 60). c. *Extrication:* triaging victims and moving them to designated treatment area, securing necessary experts to determine the safest extrication procedures for this structure, coordinating physical rescue operations (including direction of heavy equipment), and ensuring scene safety (p. 59). d. *Treatment:* selecting a site in close proximity but safely removed from actual collapse site, categorizing patients on arrival and designating them to the appropriate segment of treatment area or immediate or delayed zones, providing patient care and stabilization until transport can be provided, and communicating frequently with transportation sector so that appropriate patient transfers can be facilitated (p. 59). e. *Transportation:* coordinating patient transport with staging and treatment sectors, communicating with receiving hospitals so that appropriate resources can be selected, and assigning patients to ambulances or helicopters and directing them to the appropriate facilities (pp. 59-60).

14. Effective communications can be enhanced by using a common frequency for interdisciplinary communication when necessary; using the radio frequencies designated in the plan; using different frequencies for fire, EMS, and other support agencies; ensuring that common terminology is being used; ensuring clear, concise radio traffic; preparing messages before transmitting; and identifying the speaker only by sector (p. 61).

15. Air medical transport because of heavy traffic and heavy equipment to extricate victims from under bleachers (pp. 62-64)

16. *Site selection:* choosing a site that is 60 by 60 feet (day) and 100 by 100 feet (night); ensuring that there are few vertical structures around the site; choosing a flat area that is free of high grass or debris. *Site preparation:* placing bar lights around perimeter of zone at night; aiming white lights down; protecting the patient, informing the pilot of hazards and wind direction, and eliminating fire or explosion hazards (p. 64).

17. d. In most city EMS systems, this type of patient situation should not overwhelm the system and require a mass casualty plan (pp. 56-57).

18. a. This group initially developed the incident command system, which over time, was adopted nationally (p. 56).

19. c (p. 59)

20. a. As much verbal communication as possible should be done during the mass casualty incident to permit essential communication on the airwaves (p. 61).

21. d. Abnormal vital signs, obvious anatomical injury and other obvious preexisting illnesses and injuries should be considered when triaging patients (p. 62).

22. b. This patient has an obviously serious anatomical injury and abnormal physiological signs, indicating that urgent care is necessary (p. 62).

23. c. The minimum number of people necessary for patient transport should approach the aircraft from the front with long objects horizontal (p. 64).

● CHAPTER 7
HAZARDOUS MATERIALS

1. j, e (p. 76)
2. f, d (p. 76)
3. g (p. 76)
4. a (p. 76)
5. j, e (p. 76)
6. i (p. 76)
7. h, j, e (p. 76)
8. True (p. 67)
9. False. Hazardous materials are also found in transit by rail or truck, in the home, and in rural farm settings (pp. 67-68).
10. The Superfund Amendments and Reauthorization Act (SARA) of 1986 (p. 68)
11.

Category	Description
a. First responder awareness	May witness or discover hazardous materials release but does not have emergency response duties pertaining to hazardous material as part of the job duties (p. 68)
b. First responder operations	Responds to hazardous materials releases to protect nearby persons, property, or the environment without trying to stop the release (p. 68)
c. Hazardous materials technician	Responds to hazardous materials situations to stop the release (p. 69)
d. Hazardous materials specialist	Has a direct or specific knowledge of various hazardous substances and provides support to hazardous materials technicians (p. 69)
e. On-scene incident commander	Trained to assume control of a hazardous materials event (p. 69)

12. a. Placards on trucks, shipping papers, and Material Safety Data Sheets (p. 71). b. Visual indicators (vapor), container characteristics, company name on truck, and smell (p. 69).

13. Hazardous materials texts; poison control centers; Chemtrec; federal agencies; commercial agencies; regional, state, and local agencies (pp. 71-72)

14. a. Chemical splash protective clothing to protect the skin and eyes from direct chemical contact (p. 75). b. Structural firefighting clothing, including helmet, positive-pressure self-contained breathing apparatus, turnout coat and pants, gloves and boots, and a protective hood of fire-resistant material (p. 74). c. Vapor-protective clothing (suit with a self-contained breathing apparatus worn inside or outside the suit or an airline hose with emergency escape capabilities) (p. 75).

15. a. Irritants damage the upper and lower respiratory tracts and irritate the eyes (p. 76). b. Asphyxiants deprive the body tissues of oxygen (p. 76). c. Nerve gases, anesthetics, and narcotics act on the nervous system, causing disruption of cardiorespiratory function (p. 76). d Hepatotoxins destroy the liver's ability to function in a normal capacity (p. 76). e. Cardiotoxins may induce myocardial ischemia and cardiac dysrhythmias (p. 76). f. Neurotoxins may cause cerebral hypoxia or neurological or behavioral disruption (p. 76). g. Hemotoxins cause destruction of red blood cells, resulting in hemolytic anemia (pp. 76-77). h. Carcinogens are cancer-causing agents (p. 77).

16. Confusion, anxiety, dizziness, visual disturbances, changes in skin color, shortness of breath or burning of the upper airway, tingling or numbness of extremities, loss of coordination, seizures, nausea and vomiting, abdominal cramps, diarrhea, unconsciousness (p. 78)

17. Chemical burns and tissue damage (p. 78)

18. Apply protective gear, remove contact lenses, and flush with copious amounts of water, normal saline, or lactated Ringer's solution (p. 78).

19. a. Alpha particles are positively charged atoms with minimal penetrability; however, they are very dangerous when internal exposure occurs (p. 82). b. Beta particles are positively or negatively charged electrons that have more penetrating power than alpha particles and can permeate subcutaneous tissue (p. 83). c. Gamma particles have a much higher penetrating power than alpha or beta rays, requiring lead shielding to stop penetration (protective clothing does not stop these rays); exposure may produce local skin burns and extensive internal damage (p. 83).

20. a. Less than 100 rem usually causes no significant acute problems (p. 83). b. A total of 100 to 200 rem can cause symptoms such as nausea and vomiting but is not life threatening (p. 83). c. Greater than 450 rem exposure has a 50% mortality rate within 30 days (p. 83).

21. The rescuers and emergency vehicle should initially be positioned 200 to 300 feet upwind of the site. No eating, smoking, or drinking should be permitted at the site. The appropriate local authorities and medical control should be notified of the situation (p. 84).

22. Protective clothing should be worn if available. The victim should be approached quickly by trained rescue teams. Rescue personnel should trade off frequently until the victim can be stabilized sufficiently to remove him or her a safe distance from the contaminated area. If possible, the crew should position itself behind any protective barrier available (p. 84).

23. If ventilation is required for the radiation-contaminated victim, an airway adjunct should be used. The patient should be moved away from the radiation source as soon as possible, but lifesaving care should not be delayed if the patient cannot be moved immediately. Intravenous lines should be initiated only if absolutely necessary, and good aseptic technique should be used to minimize the risk of introducing contaminants into the patient's body (p. 84).

24. a. *Hot zone:* the area that includes the hazardous material and any associated wastes. Only specially trained and clothed personnel may enter this area (p. 79). b. *Warm zone:* the area that can become contaminated if the hot zone is unstable. Decontamination and patient care activities take place here (pp. 78-80). c. *Cold zone:* the area that encompasses the warm zone. Minimal protective clothing is required. The command post and other support agencies are located here (p. 80).

25. En route to the emergency scene, the EMS crew should attempt to identify the hazardous material, obtain preliminary information regarding the potential hazards and recommended safety equipment, initial first aid, and a safe distance factor for response to the area. Medical control should be notified so that appropriate measures can be taken at the hospital for potential victims. If a positive identification of the involved substance is made, the dispatching agency should contact the appropriate authorities and other experts such as Chemtrec to get additional information and support. The scene should be approached from uphill and upwind, and the EMS crew should call for additional help as needed. The arriving crew should be alert to any fire hazards and leakage of gas or liquid from the involved cars and remain clear of all vapors and spills (p. 78).

26. Nonambulatory patients should be removed from the hot zone by trained personnel who have adequate protective clothing. All patients in the hot

18. d. Mercury is an example of a hemotoxin (p. 77).
19. c. The brain would be affected by neurotoxins, nerve poisons, and narcotics. Kidney dysfunction occurs as a result of exposure to nephrotoxins. Irritants and asphyxiants interfere with normal lung function (p. 76).
20. b. Some dry chemicals produce an exothermic reaction when exposed to water, so it is desirable to brush away as much powder as possible (p. 77).
21. c (p. 80)
22. b. The blood pressure increases as the pulse rate increases, digestive rate decreases, and the pupils dilate (p. 89).
23. a. The family in crisis needs to be told what to do and when to do it and be helped to do it. Too many choices confuse the issue. It may be necessary to remove them from the scene if patient care is impaired; otherwise, observation from a safe distance is desirable (p. 91).
24. d. The five stages of death and dying are denial, anger, bargaining, depression, and acceptance (pp. 95-96).

● CHAPTER 9
MEDICAL TERMINOLOGY AND THE METRIC SYSTEM

1. d (pp. 102-103)
2. b (pp. 102-103)
3. c (pp. 102-103)
4. a (pp. 102-103)
5. g (pp. 102-103)
6. h (pp. 102-103)
7. f (pp. 102-103)
8. e (pp. 102-103)
9. a. *Adeno-*; b. *arthr-*; c. *gastroenter-*; d. *oto-*; e. *osteo-*; f. *nephro-*; g. *neuro-*; h. *hepat-* (pp. 102-103)
10. False. Medical terminology is important as a communications tool to understand and be understood in a consistent manner by other health care professionals (p. 100).
11. True (p. 101)
12. You are called to evaluate a patient who is *apneic* and has *bradycardia.* You note *cyanosis* of his skin. His family states that he had *dyspnea,* complained of *anesthesia* of his right arm, and became *aphasic* and then *syncopal.* His past medical history includes *cerebrovascular accident, cardiomegaly,* and *atherosclerosis.* Home medications include *antihypertensives, antidysrhythmics,* and *anticoagulants.* Physical examination reveals right *hemiplegia, hypertension,* and *unilateral* facial droop. There is no evidence of *otorrhea* or *rhinorrhea* (pp. 101-103).
13. The 78 yo pt was admitted stat to ICU to R/O MI. Her CC was dyspnea. VS were WNL except for BP of 200/100. In the ED she was given NTG 0.4 mg SL and MS 2 mg IV. Her past medical Hx (PMH)

included lung Ca, CAD, CVA, CHF and ETOH abuse (pp. 104-105).
14. c. The prefix precedes the root word and usually describes location or intensity (p. 101).
15. b. The root word for bladder is *cysto-*; for chest it is *thoraco-*, and for eye it is is *opthalmo-* (p. 103).
16. a (pp. 105-106)
17. d. Meters are the unit of measure for length (p. 106).
18. a. A zero should precede a decimal if a whole number does not. One space should be left between the number and the metric unit. Metric units should be noted in lowercase letters (p. 107).
19. c (pp. 105-106)

● CHAPTER 10
OVERVIEW OF HUMAN SYSTEMS

1. d (p. 114)
2. c (p. 114)
3. f (p. 114)
4. b (p. 114)
5. e (p. 114)
6. h (p. 114)
7. i (p. 114)
8. g (p. 114)
9. False. Some cells, such as those of the nervous system, divide only until birth (p. 115).
10. True (p. 123)
11. Person standing erect with palms and feet facing the examiner (p. 109)
12. a. Distal; b. lateral; c. superior; d. ventral (p. 111)
13. a. Limbs and extremities and their girdles; b. head, neck, thorax, and abdomen (p. 124)
14. Horizontally through the umbilicus and vertically from the xiphoid process through the symphysis pubis (p. 110)
15.

Subgroup	Type	Body Area	Function
Striated voluntary	Muscle	Skeletal muscle	Movement of bones (p. 117)
Bone	Connective	Bones of body	Support and protection (p. 116)
Epithelium	Epithelial	Skin, glands, lining of body cavities	Protection (p. 116)
Adipose	Connective	Subcutaneous tissue	Insulation, protection, storage of energy (p. 116)
Hemopoietic	Connective	Marrow cavities, spleen, tonsils	Formation of blood and lymph cells (p. 117)

Striated involuntary	Muscle	Cardiac muscle	Contraction of heart (p. 117)
Neurons	Nervous	Nervous system	Conduction of action potentials (p. 117)
Cartilage	Connective	Articulating surface of bones	Smooth movement (p. 116)
Areolar	Connective	Around organs, under skin	Cushioning and affixing (p. 116)
Nonstriated involuntary	Muscle	Smooth muscle of viscera	Vegetative muscle functions (p. 117)
Neuroglia	Nervous	Nervous system	Support cells Nourishment protection, insulation (p. 117)

16. Integumentary, skeletal, muscular, nervous, endocrine, circulatory, lymphatic, respiratory, digestive, urinary, and reproductive (p. 119)

17.

Structure	Function
Epidermis	Barrier against infection, protection, prevention of fluid loss (p. 119)
Dermis	sense organ containing sweat glands (p. 120)
Subcutaneous layer	Insulation, storage of energy, shock absorption (p. 120)

18. Lubrication to prevent drying, excretion of water and wastes, and temperature regulation (p. 120)

19. Decreased ability to perceive pain, decreased ability to regulate temperature, and decreased ability to preserve body fluids (pp. 119, 120)

20. a. Parietal; b. temporal; c. frontal; d. occipital; e. sphenoid; f. ethmoid; g. maxilla; h. mandible; i. zygomatic; j. nasal; k. lacrimal (p. 122)

21. a. Cervical (7); b. thoracic (12); c. lumbar (5); d. sacrum (1 fused); e. coccyx (1 fused) (p. 123)

22. Protects organs of the thorax and maintains lung inflation (p. 124)

23. a. Manubrium; b. body; c. sternum; d. xiphoid process; e. jugular notch; f. sternal angle (p. 124)

24. Injury to underlying organs and impaired ventilation (p. 124)

25. a. Scapula; b. clavicle; c. attach the upper extremity to the axial skeleton; d. sternoclavicular joint (p. 124)

26. a. Humerus; b. head; c. greater tubercule; d. radius; e. ulna; f. trochlea; g. medial epicondyle; h. lateral epicondyle; i. olecranon; j. styloid process; k. radial tuberosity; l. carpals; m. metacarpals (p. 125)

27. a. Obturator foramen; b. ilium; c. ischium; d. pubis; e. anterior superior iliac spine (p. 126)

28. Protection of the pelvic organs and point of attachment for the lower extremity to axial skeleton (p. 127)

29. a. Neck; b. head; c. shaft; d. greater trochanter; e. lesser trochanter; f. medial condyle; g. lateral condyle; h. medial epicondyle; i. lateral epicondyle; j. tibia; k. fibula; l. tibial tuberosity; m. head of fibula; n. lateral malleolus; o. tarsal bones; p. metatarsals; q. phalanges (pp. 126-127)

30. a. Fibrous, cartilaginous, synovial; b. little or no; c. skull; d. radius, ulna; e. teeth, mandible (or maxilla); f. sternum; g. sternal angle; h. symphysis pubis; i. intervertebral disks; j. synovial fluid; k. plane (or gliding); l. saddle joints; m. hinge; n. pivot; o. ball and socket; p. ellipsoid (pp. 128, 129)

31. a. Supinate (supination) or pronate (pronation); b. opposition; c. flexion and extension; d. rotation; e. abduction; f. adduction; g. inversion or eversion; h. excursion; i. depression (p. 131)

32. Movement, muscle tone, and heat production (p. 132)

33. a. Muscle fibers; b. myofilaments; c. actin, myosin; d. sarcomere; e. ATP (p. 132)

34. a. Isometric muscle contraction maintains constant length of the muscles in the body (p. 136). b. During an isotonic contraction, the amount of muscle tension is constant, but the length of the muscle changes, causing movement of a body part (p. 136). c. Muscle tone is the constant tension of muscles responsible for posture and balance (p. 136).

35. Excess energy from adenosine triphosphate in a muscle contraction is released as heat. If the body temperature falls below a certain level, muscles begin shivering, which can increase heat production up to 18 times the normal resting level (p. 137).

36. Regulation and coordination of the body to maintain homeostasis (p. 137)

37. a. Brain and spinal cord; b. nerves and ganglia (p. 137)

38. The somatic division transmits impulses from the central nervous system to skeletal muscle, and the autonomic division transmits impulses from the central nervous system to smooth muscle, cardiac muscle, and certain glands (pp. 137, 138).

39. a. Cerebral cortex; b. midbrain; c. pons; d. cerebellum; e. medulla; f. thalamus; g. hypothalamus (p. 138)

40. a. Is conduction pathway for ascending and descending nerve tracts; regulates heart rate, blood vessel diameter, breathing, swallowing, vomiting, coughing, and sneezing. b. Ascending and descending nerve tracts pass through, relays information from cerebrum to cerebellum, sleep and respiratory center. c. Involved in hearing and visual reflexes, regulates some automatic functions

such as muscle tone. d. Important for arousal and consciousness, sleep/wake cycle. e. Temperature regulation, water balance, sleep-cycle control, appetite, sexual arousal. f. Relays information from sense organs to cerebral cortex, influences mood (p. 137)

41. a. Frontal lobe: voluntary motor function; motivation, aggression, and mood. b. Temporal lobe: olfactory and auditory input; memory. c. Parietal lobe: reception and evaluation of sensory information (except smell, hearing, and vision). d. Occipital lobe: reception and integration of visual input (pp. 140, 141)

42. Coordination, balance, and smooth and flowing movement (pp. 140, 141)

43. Reflex center and transmits impulses to and from the brain and the rest of the body (p. 141)

44. a. Brain, spinal cord (p. 141); b. choroid plexus (p. 142)

45. Sensory, somatomotor and proprioception, and parasympathetic (p. 143)

46.

Affected Organ	Sympathetic	Parasympathetic
Heart	Increased rate and contractility	Decreased rate
Lungs	Bronchodilation	Bronchoconstriction
Pupils	Dilation	Constriction
Intestine	Decreased peristalsis	Increased peristalsis
Blood vessels	Constriction	No effect (p. 145)

47. Coordinates with the nervous system to regulate and control multiple body functions, including metabolic activities and body chemistry (pp. 145, 146)

48.

Hormone	Target Tissue	Action
Epinephrine	Heart, blood vessels, liver	Increased heart rate, contractility, increased blood to heart, release of glucose and fatty acids into blood
Aldosterone	Kidneys	Water retention
Antidiuretic	Kidney	Decreased urine output
Parathyroid	Bone, kidney	Increases bone breakdown, helps maintain Ca++ levels
Calcitonin	Bone	Decreased breakdown of bone, maintenance of blood calcium levels
Insulin	Liver	Promotes glucose entry into cells

Glucagon	Liver	Releases glucose into blood by glycogenolysis
Testosterone	Most cells	Male sex characteristics, behavior, spermatogenesis
Thymosin	Immune tissues	Development of immune system
Oxytocin	Uterus, mammary gland	Uterine contractions, milk expulsion from breasts.
Thyroid	Most cells	Increased metabolic rate (pp. 148, 149)

49. Hormones are secreted into blood and travel to all tissues of the body but only act on the target tissues (p. 146).

50. Transports nutrients, carries hormones, transports wastes, temperature regulation and fluid balance, and protection from bacteria (pp. 149, 150)

51. a. Erythrocytes; b. hemoglobin; c. oxygen; d. carbon dioxide; e. leukocytes; f. thrombocytes; g. defence; h. clots; i. plasma (pp. 149, 150).

52. a. Septum; b. right atrium; c. tricuspid valve; d. right ventricle; e. pulmonic valve; f. pulmonary arteries; g. pulmonary veins; h. left atrium; i. mitral or bicuspid valve; j. left ventricle; k. aortic valve; l. aorta (p. 154)

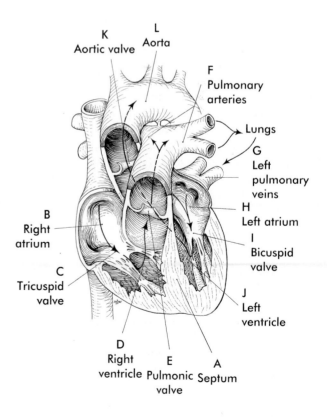

53. Aorta, smaller arteries, arterioles, capillaries, venules, veins, venae cavae, and right atrium (p. 154)

54. Blood vessels have smooth muscle walls that give them the ability to dilate, which increases their diameter, or to constrict, which decreases their diameter. This allows blood flow to be directed away from less vital organs to the heart and brain during emergencies (p. 155).

55. Some veins, especially in the lower extremities, have valves that prevent the backflow of blood in this low-pressure system (p. 156).

56. The arteriovenous shunt can selectively allow blood to bypass the capillaries. This is useful to help maintain body temperature (p. 156).

57. Maintains tissue fluid balance, absorbs fats and other substances from the digestive tract, and enhances the body's defense system (p. 158)

58. Lymph is gathered from the tissues by lymph capillaries that have one-way valves to prevent the backflow of lymph into tissues. It flows to larger lymph capillaries that resemble veins. Then it passes through the lymph nodes (in the groin, axilla, and neck), where microorganisms and foreign substances are removed. The lymph vessels meet to enter the right or left subclavian vein, where the lymph reenters the blood (p. 158).

59. a. Epiglottis: protection of lower airway; b. conchae and turbinates: warming and filtering of air; c. eustachian and auditory tube: joining of nasopharynx to ear; d. sinuses: production of sound and mucus; e. hard palate: separation of oropharynx from sinuses; f. soft palate: prevents food from entering nasal cavities (p. 159)

60. a. Epiglottis; b. thyroid cartilage or Adam's apple; c. cricoid cartilage; d. hyoid bone; e. vocal folds (p. 160)

61. a. Trachea; b. bronchi; c. alveoli; d. carina (p. 162)

62. Cartilage rings maintain patency of the airway. Goblet cells in the ciliated epithelium of the trachea sweep mucus, bacteria, and other small particles toward the larynx (p. 161).

63. The small bronchioles are surrounded by smooth muscle. Irritants cause constriction of that muscle, the airway size decreases, and a wheeze is produced as air is forced through a very tight airway (p. 162).

64. a. Alveoli are only one cell thick, which easily permits diffusion of gases from within them into the pulmonary capillaries (p. 162). b. Pulmonary surfactant decreases the surface tension within the alveoli, which inhibits collapse of the alveoli (p. 163).

65. The base of the lungs rests on the diaphragm; the apex extends to a point 2.5 cm superior to the clavicles (p. 163).

66. a. Three lobes further divided into 10 lobules; b. Two lobes further divided into 9 lobules (p. 163)

67. a. A potential space that forms a vacuum and causes the lung to adhere to the chest wall and re-

main expanded (p. 163). b. A lubricant that allows the pleural membranes to slide across one another and helps the visceral and parietal pleurae to adhere to one another (p. 163).

68. Provides the body with water, nutrients, and electrolytes (p. 164)

69.

Digestive Juice	Function
a. Salivary amylase	Begins digestion of carbohydrates
b. Hydrochloric acid, mucus, intrinsic factor, gastrin, pepsinogen	Produces chyme (a semisolid mixture)
c. Amylase, sodium bicarbonate	Neutralizes stomach acid, continues digestion
d. Bile	Dilutes stomach acid, emulsifies fat
e. Mucus	Aids movement of feces

70. Removes wastes from the body and helps maintain normal body fluid volume and composition (p. 166)

71. Control of red blood cell production and vitamin D metabolism (p. 166)

72. a. Nephron; b. filtration; c. reabsorption; d. secretion (p. 166)

73. a. Decreases; b. increases; c. increases; d. decreases (pp. 168-170)

74. a. Testis; b. epididymis; c. ductus deferens and vas deferens; d. urethra; e. seminal vesicles; f. prostate gland; g. bulbourethral glands; h. scrotum; i. penis (p. 170)

75. a. Ovary; b. fallopian tube; c. uterine body; d. fundus; e. cervix; f. vagina (p. 173)

76. a. Vagina; b. urethra; c. labia minora; d. labia majora; e. clitoris; f. clinical perineum; g. anus (p. 173)

77. a. Nasal; b. olfactory tract; c. thalamic; d. olfactory (p. 174)

78. a. Taste buds; b. tongue; c. palate, lips, throat; d. sweet, sour, bitter, salt (p. 175)

79. a. Optic (p. 175); b. oculomotor (p. 175); c. cornea (p. 176); d. iris (p. 176); e. rods (p. 176); f. cones (p. 176); g. aqueous (p. 177); h. vitreous (p. 177); i. intraocular pressure (p. 177)

80. a. Shade eyes from direct sun and prevent perspiration from entering eyes; b. protect against foreign objects; c. moistens the eye, lubricates the eyelids, and washes away foreign objects (p. 177)

81. a. Hearing; b. hearing, balance; c. vestibulocochlear; d. pinna; e. auditory; f. tympanic membrane; g. incus, stapes, malleus; h. organ of Corti; i. vestibule; j. semicircular canals (pp. 177, 178)

82. d. The anatomical position is standing erect with palms forward. A person lying in the lateral recumbent position is reclining on the right or left

side. The *prone position* refers to a patient who is lying on the stomach (p. 109).

83. d. The liver and gallbladder are located in the right upper quadrant, and the appendix is in the right lower quadrant (p. 112).

84. c. The thymus is located in the mediastinum, but the thyroid gland is found in the neck (p. 112).

85. b. Striated voluntary muscle is skeletal muscle, and nonstriated involuntary muscles are found in the viscera. Nonstriated muscles are always involuntary (p. 117).

86. c. A dendrite is a component of the neuron. Neuroglia are types of nerve cells that support the cells in the nervous system. Synapses are the gaps or spaces between nerve cells or effector tissues (p. 132).

87. c (p. 119)

88. a (p. 124)

89. b. The lateral malleolus is on the outside of the ankle, the olecranon is at the elbow, and the patella is over the knee (p. 127).

90. b. Actin and myosin are the actual myofilaments (thin, threadlike structures) that pull together to cause movement. A sarcomere is the contractile unit that contains actin and myosin (p. 132).

91. d. The other actions described are attributed to the occipital lobe (a), temporal lobe (b), and parietal lobe (c) (p. 140).

92. b (p. 141)

93. d. The layers from innermost to outermost are pia, arachnoid, and dura. The choroid plexus is where the cerebral spinal fluid is manufactured (p.141).

94. b (p. 146)

95. a. Immunoglobulins are antibodies, leukocytes are white blood cells, and platelets are cell fragments that aid in hemostasis (p. 149).

96. a. Pulmonary arteries carry deoxygenated blood from the heart to the lungs. Pulmonary veins carry oxygenated blood from the lungs to the heart, and the vena cava carries blood from the systemic circulation to the heart (p. 151).

97. d. Sinoatrial node impulses travel to the atrioventricular node, the bundle of His, and then to the Purkinje fibers (p.153).

98. d (p. 158)

99. a (p. 161)

100. a. The trachea and bronchus convey air to the alveoli. The capillary is not part of the respiratory system (p. 162).

101. d. Absorption occurs in the other areas of the small intestine (duodenum and ileum) and to a much lesser extent in the colon; however, the primary site of absorption is the jejunum (p. 164).

102. c (p. 165)

103. c. Roughly 180 L/day is filtered from the glomerulus; however, all but approximately 2 L/day is reabsorbed into the blood. Potassium and ammonia are secreted from the blood into the urine (p. 168).

104. a. Glucagon promotes conversion of glycogen stored in the liver back to glucose. Oxytocin is a female sex hormone that stimulates uterine contractions and plays a role in lactation. Testosterone is the male sex hormone responsible for male sexual characteristics (p. 169).

105. d. Final maturation but not production of the sperm occurs in the epididymis. The prostate and seminal vesicle produce seminal fluid (p. 171).

106. d (p. 174)

107. b. The organ of Corti lies within the cochlea. The semicircular canals and vestibule are involved in balance (p. 178).

● **CHAPTER 11**
GENERAL PATIENT ASSESSMENT

1. b (p. 195)

2. g (p. 196)

3. e (p. 200)

4. f (p. 201)

5. c (p. 195)

6. a (p. 195)

7. d (p. 200)

8. h (p. 200)

9. False. The purpose of the secondary survey is to find additional injuries or abnormal findings. Treatment is to be addressed while providing definitive care unless a life-threatening condition is found in the secondary survey. If this occurs, the paramedic returns to the primary survey for resuscitation (p. 187).

10. True (p. 187)

11. Perpetrators with firearms who may still be in the immediate area, hostile crowd, and risk of fire and smoke in area where victims are located (p. 181)

12. Do not enter until police can verify that firearms are confiscated, call for additional law enforcement officers for crowd control, call for fire and rescue assistance, and wear protective clothing (bullet-proof vests, turn-out gear, breathing apparatus) if indicated (p. 181).

13. Primary survey, resuscitation, secondary survey, history, definitive field management, and reevaluation (p. 182)

14. a. *Airway:* Inspect for foreign bodies, edema, teeth, emesis, and blood. Determine whether the patient can speak. Auscultate for stridor or gurgling. b. *Breathing:* Inspect for chest rise and fall, symmetry, open wounds, trauma to the chest, and accessory muscle use. Palpate briefly for structural integrity. Auscultate briefly for bilateral breath sounds if an abnormality is suspected. c. *Circulation:* Inspect the

skin for color and look from head to toe for obvious signs of uncontrolled external bleeding. Palpate the pulse for rate, quality, regularity, and location. Palpate the skin for temperature and moisture. Assess capillary refill by depressing the nail bed and observing for color return within 2 seconds. d. *Disability:* Assess whether the patient is alert, responds appropriately to verbal stimuli, responds to painful stimuli, or does not respond to any stimulus. e. *Expose:* Undress the patient as necessary to reveal abnormalities that may be concealed and to permit appropriate patient management and resuscitation. Maintain body warmth as patient is exposed (p. 182).

15.

Life Threat	Management
a. Tongue occludes	Head-tilt/chin-lift (if no trauma Jaw thrust
Occlusion by blood or other debris	Suction
Decreased level of consciousness	Manual airway maneuvers Airway adjuncts (nasal airway, oropharyngeal airway, endotracheal intubation)
Foreign body obstruction	Heimlich maneuver, abdominal thrusts, cricothyrotomy
b. Absent	Ventilation with 100% oxygen
Respiratory infection with hypoxia	Supplemental oxygen
Tension pneumothorax	Needle chest decompression
Open chest wound	Seal on three sides with occlusive dressing
Flail chest	Intubation, positive-pressure ventilation
Anaphylaxis, asthma	Medication, oxygen
c. Hemorrhagic shock	Intravenous fluids, rapid transport, pneumatic antishock garments (for approved situations)
Uncontrolled external bleeding	Direct pressure, elevation, pressure points, tourniquet (with medical direction)
Cardiac rhythm disturbance	Medication, electrical therapy

NOTE: For all airway management maneuvers, simultaneous cervical spine precautions should be used if a risk of traumatic injury exists (pp. 182-185).

16. Protect the cervical spine, sweep or suction the oral cavity, insert a nasal or oral airway, and assist ventilations with a bag-valve-mask, pocket mask, or demand valve and 100% oxygen (consider intubation). Apply pressure to the spurting wound and consider pneumatic antishock garment if protocol permits. Initiate a large-bore intravenous line for fluid resuscitation en route (pp. 182-186).

17. Assess patient's level of consciousness and expose the patient to reveal other life-threatening conditions. Continue resuscitation en route and perform secondary survey en route as time and circumstances permit (pp. 182-186).

18. A. *Medical patient:* oxygen, airway, intravenous line, blood samples, medications, pneumatic antishock garments, electrical therapy. b. *Trauma patient:* oxygen, airway, cervical spine control, intravenous line, medications, pneumatic antishock garments (p. 186).

19. a. *Inspection:* Observe the environment (scene), general patient appearance, and specific body regions to gather data (pp. 189, 190). b. *Palpation:* Use the palmar surface of the hands and fingers to feel for texture, mass, fluid, temperature, and crepitus in various body regions (p. 190). c. *Auscultation:* Use a stethoscope or the unaided ear to assess sounds generated by the movement of air or gases within the body (p. 190).

20. Vital signs assessment (blood pressure, pulse, respirations, and temperature if appropriate); skin; pupil response; and inspection, palpation, and auscultation of the head and neck, chest, abdomen, pelvis, extremities (musculoskeletal system), and back (p. 187)

21.

Abnormality	Cause
a. Dilated/unresponsive	Cardiac arrest, hypoxia, drug use or misuse
b. Constricted/unresponsive	Injury or disease of the central nervous system, narcotic drug use, use of eye medications
c. Unequal, one dilated and unresponsive	Cerebrovascular accident, accident, direct trauma to the eye, use of eye medications, use of an ocular prosthesis
d. Dull/lackluster	Shock or comatose states (p. 189)

22. Inspect for shape and symmetry of the skull and facial bones. Note bleeding, trauma, deformity, or drainage around the face or from the ears or nose. Inspect the mouth for bleeding and loose or missing teeth. Observe for pupil response to light and assess to see whether the patient's vision is intact. Palpate the scalp and face for deformities, swelling, inden tations, or bleeding, noting pain or tenderness. Be fore application of cervical collar while maintaining cervical immobilization, inspect to ensure that the trachea is midline and note

43. d. If the patient's physiological signs deteriorate, the rescuer should intervene (p. 238).

44. c (p. 238)

45. b. Because the tongue is the most frequent cause of airway obstruction, repositioning the airway may be the only maneuver necessary to permit air exchange (p. 238).

46. a. The mechanism of injury and signs are consistent with this life-threatening emergency, which will necessitate aggressive airway management (p. 240).

47. a. It is a frequently underused adjunct usually well tolerated by a semiconscious patient with a gag reflex (p. 245).

48. b. The tube should be in the esophagus of a patient more than 5 feet tall, and no sounds should be audible over the gastric area when the patient's lungs are ventilated (p. 247).

49. d. The tube is designed to function correctly in the trachea or the esophagus (p. 250).

50. a. Repeat attempts should be performed after hyperventilation (p. 248).

51. d. Percutaneous transtracheal ventilation is a short-term (less than 45 minutes) airway device used when other measures to secure the airway are unsuccessful. The demand valve does not provide sufficient pressure to ventilate by this method. It offers no protection from aspiration (p. 265).

52. c (p. 271)

53. b. Demand valves are not recommended for children or patients with chronic obstructive pulmonary disease. If the patient has apnea, the manual mode should be used (p. 272).

54. a. Suction should be applied for no longer than 10 seconds. A cough is stimulated frequently and may increase intracranial pressure. Suction should be set between 80 and 120 mm Hg (p. 274).

55. b (p. 278)

56. b. A patient with this mechanism and symptoms of hypoxia clearly needs the highest percentage of oxygen available (p. 279).

● **CHAPTER 13**
SHOCK

1. b (p. 286)

2. g (p. 287)

3. e (p. 287)

4. a (p. 286)

5. d (p. 286)

6. f (p. 286)

7. False. Shock is a clinical situation in which there is inadequate capillary perfusion. Alterations in the physical parameters of blood pressure and pulse alone are not sufficient to define this condition (p. 284).

8. False. A milliequivalent is one thousandth of an equivalent (the molecular weight divided by the charges on an ion) (p. 288).

9. a. An adequate amount of oxygen is available to red blood cells. There is a sufficient FiO_2, his airway is patent, and his lungs are clear. b. Red blood cells must be circulated to all tissue cells. Based on the history of significant blood loss and the physical findings that indicate decreased cerebral perfusion (anxiety and confusion) and decreased peripheral perfusion (pale, cyanotic lips and nailbeds), it is evident that red blood cell transport is inadequate. c. Red blood cells must be able to adequately off-load oxygen. It would appear that this is occurring in this situation, although acid-base abnormalities can impair this ability and there is insufficient information to accurately determine this (p. 285).

10. a. Muscle is lost; therefore contractility and stroke volume decrease, lowering the cardiac output. b. The additional fluid volume improves the preload, thereby increasing stroke volume and cardiac output. c. A sudden drop in the heart rate results in a decrease in cardiac output. d. Fear and anxiety cause the heart rate and stroke volume to accelerate, increasing cardiac output (p. 284).

11. All blood vessels larger than capillaries are surrounded by layers of connective tissue that counter the pressure of blood in the vascular system, have elastic properties to dampen pressure pulsations and minimize flow variations throughout the cardiac cycle, and have muscle fibers to control vessel diameter (pp. 284, 285).

12. a. Systemic; b. systolic; c. diastolic; d. pulse; e. heart, aorta; f. vena cava (pp. 284, 285)

13. a. Spinal cord injury results in a loss of sympathetic tone and therefore impairs the ability of the blood vessels to constrict below the level of the injury. This increases the container size, decreasing the effective circulating volume and preload. b. When blood loss occurs, a situation potentially exists in which the container is the same size but the volume has decreased, which reduces the preload. Body compensatory mechanisms attempt to decrease the size of the container by vasoconstriction in an effort to match the container to the volume (pp. 285, 286).

14. a. O positive, O negative, A positive, A negative; b. O negative; c. O positive, O negative, A positive, A negative, B positive, B negative, AB positive, AB negative; d. O negative, B negative (p. 232)

15. a. Extracellular; b. interstitial; c. intracellular (pp. 287, 288)

16. PO_4, phosphate, anion, intracellular; K^+, potassium, cation, intracellular; Na^+, sodium, cation, extracellular; HCO_3^-, bicarbonate, anion, extracellular; Mg^{++}, magnesium, cation, intracellular; Cl^-, chloride, anion, extracellular (p. 288)

17. a. The property of a cell membrane that freely permits the passage of water but selectively allows the passage of solute particles. This permits the cell to maintain a relatively constant internal environment (p. 289). b. A passive process that allows molecules or ions to move from an area of higher concentration to an area of lower concentration in an attempt to achieve a state of equilibrium (p. 291). c. A situation in which the solute concentration is greater at one point than another in a solvent. Solutes diffuse from the area of high concentration to the area of lower concentration until equilibrium is achieved (p. 291). d. The diffusion of water across a selectively permeable membrane from an area of higher water concentration to an area of lower water concentration (p. 289). e. A rapid, carrier-mediated process that can move a substance across a selectively permeable membrane from an area of low concentration to an area of high concentration. This process requires energy (p. 291). f. A carrier-mediated process (faster than diffusion) that can move a substance from an area of higher concentration to an area of lower concentration. This process does not require energy (p. 291).

18. D50W: hypertonic, into intravascular space; lactated Ringer's: isotonic, no net movement; normal saline: isotonic, no net movement; 0.45% normal saline: hypotonic, out of intravascular space; D5W: isotonic initially but rapidly hypotonic because of glucose metabolism, out of intravascular space (p. 290)

19. a. Overhydration: fluid restriction, intravenous normal saline to keep the vein open (p. 293). b. Hypokalemia: lactated Ringer's solution intravenously to keep the vein open, preparation to assist ventilations, and high-flow oxygen (p. 294). c. Hypocalcemia: possible calcium ions (calcium chloride) intravenously, airway management, seizure precautions, anticonvulsant therapy intravenously (p. 294). d. Isotonic dehydration: evaluation of the airway, breathing, and circulation; assessment for shock, possible intravenous therapy with lactated Ringer's solution 20 ml/kg as ordered by medical direction (p. 292). e. Hyponatremic dehydration: evaluation of the effectiveness of ventilations, high-flow oxygen, intravenous therapy with lactated Ringer's solution or normal saline, and evaluation of vital signs (p. 293). f. Hypermagnesemia: open airway, assistance with ventilations as necessary, high-flow oxygen, evaluation of vital signs, intravenous line with normal saline to keep the vein open, possible intravenous administration of calcium salts (p. 295).

20. a. Buffers produce an immediate response to changes in pH. They represent the body's ability to adjust the concentration of bicarbonate and carbon dioxide in the blood to maintain a relationship of 1 mEq of carbonic acid to 20 mEq of base bicarbonate. If this relationship can be maintained, hydrogen ion concentration will be within normal limits (p. 295). b. The respiratory system can increase alveolar ventilation within minutes in response to an increase in hydrogen ion concentration. Hydrogen ions combine with bicarbonate to form carbonic acid, which in turn breaks down into carbon dioxide and water. Therefore by increasing the amount of carbon dioxide that the body eliminates, the process can be accelerated and hydrogen ion concentration reduced (p. 296). c. The renal system takes hours to days to act. It restores normal pH by reabsorbing or excreting bicarbonate or hydrogen ions (p. 296).

21. a. Respiratory alkalosis: Treat cause of underlying hyperventilation (p. 297). b. Metabolic alkalosis: Initiate intravenous lactated Ringer's solution or normal saline (pp. 298, 299). c. Metabolic acidosis: Initiate intravenous administration of normal saline (p. 297). d. Respiratory acidosis. Assist ventilations (p. 296).

22. Abnormal, acidosis due to increased pCO_2: Increase ventilations. b. Abnormal: Increase amount of oxygen delivery to patient. c. Abnormal: Increase rate of ventilations (pp. 299, 300).

23. a. The vasoconstrictor center of the medulla is inhibited, and the vagal center is excited, resulting in peripheral vasodilation and a decrease in myocardial rate and the strength of contraction. This results in a decrease in blood pressure. b. Vagal stimulation is reduced, resulting in a sympathetic response that causes increased peripheral vasoconstriction, heart rate, and strength of contraction. This results in an increase in blood pressure (p. 305).

24. a. The low pressure results in a decrease in oxygen to the chemoreceptor cells, which in turn stimulates the vasomotor center of the medulla. This results in peripheral vasoconstriction. b. Chemoreceptors are also stimulated by an increase in P_{CO_2}, which causes vasoconstriction and increased blood flow to the lungs, enhancing their ability to eliminate carbon dioxide (p. 306).

25. The central nervous system ischemic response is initiated when the blood pressure drops below 50 mm Hg and causes intense vasoconstriction in an attempt to improve perfusion to the brain. If the ischemia lasts longer than 10 minutes, the vagal center may be activated, resulting in peripheral vasodilation and bradycardia (p. 306).

26. a. Increased sympathetic stimulation causes adrenal medulla to release epinephrine and norep-

inephrine, which results in increased heart rate, stroke volume, and vasoconstriction (p. 306). b. Low flow to the kidneys results in a release of renin, which by a series of chemical reactions causes plasma proteins to synthesize angiotensin II. Angiotensin II causes vasoconstriction and initiates the release of aldosterone. Aldosterone causes increased retention of sodium and water by the kidneys (p. 306). c. The hypothalamic neurons are stimulated by a drop in blood pressure or an increase in plasma solutes, and the secretion of antidiuretic hormone (vasopressin) is increased. This results in vasoconstriction and a decrease in the rate of urine production (pp. 306-309).

27. Nutrients diffuse across the capillary wall into the interstitial fluid and then into the cells. Wastes diffuse across the cell membrane into the interstitial fluid and then into the plasma. At the arterial end of the capillary, the forces pushing fluid from the capillary exceed those holding it in, resulting in a net movement of fluid out of the capillary and into the tissues. At the venous end, blood pressure is lower, and the forces attracting fluid into the capillaries exceed those pushing it out, so approximately nine tenths of the fluid that left the capillary at the arterial end reenters at the venous end. The remaining one tenth enters lymphatic capillaries and later returns to the general circulation (pp. 309, 310).

28. a. Acidosis resulting from anaerobic metabolism causes vasodilation. This opposes constriction of the precapillary sphincters, resulting in an increase in hydrostatic pressure. This pressure increase pushes fluid from the vascular space into the interstitial space. In addition, potassium is released into the extracellular space, which can lead to cellular damage (p. 303). b. Flow to capillaries is intermittent and is controlled by constriction and dilation of arterioles, metarterioles, and precapillary sphincters. A decrease in oxygen concentration causes the intermittent flow to the capillaries to increase, enhancing blood flow and oxygenation of the adjacent cells. Intermittent blood flow is much greater in active organs such as the heart and skeletal muscle (p. 303). c. Nervous control of circulation is regulated by the autonomic nervous system, as described in Questions 23 through 25 (p. 305).

29. a. Oxygen to cells in vasoconstricted areas decreases. Anaerobic metabolism occurs. Leaky capillary syndrome evolves. Pale, sweaty skin; rapid, thready pulse; elevation in blood glucose; dilation of coronary, cerebral,and skeletal muscle arterioles occur (pp. 309-310). b. Precapillary sphincters open. Blood pools, and vascular space is greatly expanded, resulting in increased container size. Decreased preload and congestion of the viscera

occur. Increased anaerobic metabolism results in increased respiratory rate. Rouleaux formation inhibits perfusion in visceral capillaries and impedes flow. Hypercoagulability develops (p. 310). c. Blood coagulates in microcirculation, clogging capillaries and causing congestion, pulmonary edema, and hemorrhage. Cell membrane function is lost, and anaerobic metabolism increases. Water and sodium leak into and potassium out of cells. Cells swell and die. Oxygen absorption and carbon dioxide elimination is impaired in the lungs, and acute respiratory distress syndrome may result (p. 310). d. After 1 to 2 hours, a dramatic decrease in blood pressure occurs. Cellular metabolism stops. Organ failure develops and may include liver, kidney, and heart failure; gastrointestinal bleeding; pancreatitis; and pulmonary thrombosis (pp. 310, 311).

30. a. Cardiogenic shock: Administer high-flow oxygen, continue assessment, initiate intravenous normal saline to keep the vein open, consider a fluid challenge of 100 to 200 ml of lactated Ringer's solution or normal saline, monitor lung sounds and patient response very carefully, and consider vasopressor drug therapy (p. 311). b. Neurogenic shock: Apply cervical spine immobilization, assess the need to assist ventilations, administer high-flow oxygen, initiate intravenous lactated Ringer's solution or normal saline (avoiding excessive amounts), monitor lung sounds frequently, apply and inflate pneumatic antishock garments if local protocol permits, continue assessment, and consider vaso pressor drug therapy (p. 311). c. Hypovolemic shock: Administer high-flow oxygen, place patient in modified Trendelenberg position, transport rapidly, initiate two large-bore (14- or 16-gauge) intravenous lines with lactated Ringer's solution or normal saline and infuse rapidly, and apply pneumatic antishock garments if local protocol permits and prepare to inflate if patient's condition deteriorates (p. 311). d. Anaphylactic shock: Ensure a patent airway, administer high-flow oxygen, initiate intravenous Ringer's lactate solution or normalsaline with a 14- or 16-gauge catheter, administer epinephrine, consider administration of diphenhydramine HCl (Benadryl) (p. 311). e. Septic shock: Administer high-flow oxygen, determine whether the patient has preexisting obstructive pulmonary disease, initiate intravenous therapy with a 14- or 16-gauge catheter, and obtain an accurate patient history (pp. 311, 312). f. Cardiogenic shock: Assess for a patent airway, administer high-flow oxygen, initiate a 16- or 18-gauge intravenous line with normal saline to keep the vein open, institute electrocardiographic monitoring, initiate maneuvers to decrease heart rate based on the electrocardiographic tracing and

patient symptoms (drugs, defibrillation), and apply dressing to head wound (p. 311).

31. a. Uncompensated shock: The compensatory mechanisms can no longer sustain a normal systolic blood pressure. The pulse pressure is narrowed. Blood oxygenation is decreased, as evidenced by cyanosis (p. 312). b. Compensated shock: Systolic blood pressure is adequate, but other signs of shock are evident (cool, pale skin and increased pulse and respiratory rate) (p. 311).

32. Irreversible shock may occur suddenly or 1 to 3 weeks after the event. Clinical signs include bradycardia; pale, cold, clammy skin; and cardiac arrest (p. 314).

33. Preexisting disease, medication, older or young age (p. 324)

34. a. Drug therapy: Neither pneumatic antishock garments nor rapid fluid infusion would be considered because this patient is already in failure. Therapy should be directed at improving the function of the heart with drugs (p. 324). b. Pneumatic antishock garments, rapid fluid replacement, blood transfusions, intraosseous infusion: The patient has a mechanism of injury for significant blood loss and is exhibiting signs of uncompensated shock. Pneumatic antishock garments may decrease the container size and maximize flow to the vital organs. Rapid fluid infusion may restore circulation volume. Blood transfusion may be necessary on arrival to emergency department to enhance oxygen-carrying capability and restore the vascular volume. Rapid peripheral intravenous therapy may be impossible in this situation, making intraosseous infusion the vascular access method of choice (p. 324). c. Drug therapy: The heart rate is very slow and is likely the reason that this person is exhibiting signs of shock. None of the other interventions increases heart rate (p. 324). d. Drug therapy, rapid fluid replacement: The primary cause of the shock state in this patient is probably histamine release. Drug therapy is the only intervention that can ar rest and reverse these symptoms. Rapid fluid replacement may also help restore circulating volume until drug therapy is effective (p. 324). e. Pneumatic antishock garments, rapid fluid replacement, blood transfusions: The primary cause of the shock symptoms acording to the patient history is loss of blood. Pneumatic antishock garments and rapid fluid replacement can restore cir-culating volume. At the emergency department, the blood transfusion helps restore oxygen-carrying capacity and circulating volume (p. 324). f. Rapid fluid replacement: At this time, the patient is maintaining a normal blood pressure. The pulse and respiratory rate are somewhat elevated, so as assessment continues, the effects of a rapid fluid bolus can be monitored

to determine whether the patient has lost a significant amount of blood. Other interventions may be necessary if the patient's condition deteriorates (p. 324).

35. a. Stabilize the vein by applying distal pressure and tension to the point of entry. b. With the bevel of the needle up, pass into the vein from the side or directly on top. c. Slide the catheter over the needle and into the vein and withdraw the needle while stabilizing the vein. d. Release the tourniquet and attach the intravenous tubing. e. Open the tubing clamp and allow fluid infusion to begin at the prescribed flow rate. Cover the puncture site with antimicrobial ointment and a dressing and secure the catheter with tape (p. 328).

36. a. Hematoma, cellulitis, thrombosis, phlebitis, sepsis, pulmonary thromboembolism, catheter embolism, fiber embolism, infiltration. b. All complications in (a), plus air embolism, hematoma, damage to arteries or nerves, pneumothorax, hemothorax, and infiltration of fluid into the pleural space or mediastinum. c. All complications in (a), plus hematoma, thrombosis extending to deep veins, phlebitis extending to deep veins, and an inability to use the saphenous vein (pp. 331, 332).

37. a. 30; b. 100; c. 50; d. 38; e. 23; f. 30; g. 83 (pp. 332, 333)

38. c. A systolic blood pressure less than 90 mm Hg may be normal in certain individuals. Loss of blood volume may lead to shock but does not define it. Shock leads to decreased myocardial blood flow (p. 284).

39. a. Peripheral vascular resistance influences blood pressure. Contractility and preload are reflected in the stroke volume (p. 284).

40. c. The Fick principle states that adequate oxygen must be available to red blood cells through the alveolar cells of the lungs. So that hemoglobin can be oxygenated, red blood cells must be circulated to the tissue cells, and red blood cells must be able to load oxygen at the lungs and unload oxygen at the peripheral cells (p. 285).

41. a. Vessel length and viscosity are relatively constant. Blood volume may influence pressure but not resistance (p. 285).

42. d. As peripheral vascular resistance decreases, vessel capacitance increases, and the container size increases. This makes the existing blood volume insufficient to maintain an adequate preload (p. 285).

43. a. Leukocytes, or white blood cells, aid in body defense. Plasma proteins maintain oncotic pressure, defend the body, and aid in clotting. Platelets help initiate blood clotting (p. 286).

44. d. Calcium, hydrogen, and magnesium carry positive charges and are cations. Phosphate carries a negative charge and therefore is an anion (p. 288).

45. c. All others are found chiefly in the extracellular fluid (p. 288).

46. a (p. 288)

47. d. Active transport involves movement of substances across a semipermeable membrane from an area of lower concentration to an area of higher concentration. This requires expenditure of energy. Diffusion is the movement of substances across a semipermeable membrane from an area of higher concentration to an area of lower concentration. Facilitated diffusion is a carrier-mediated process that moves substances into and out of cells from a higher to a lower concentration at a faster rate than diffusion (p. 289).

48. d. *Atonic* means without tone. A hypertonic solution has a greater solute concentration than the cells, whereas a hypotonic solution is less concentrated than the cells (p. 289).

49. c. D50W is hypertonic and draws fluid into the intravascular space. Lactated Ringer's solution and normal saline are isotonic and tend to remain in the intravascular space. 0.45% normal saline is hypotonic and rapidly moves out of the intravascular space (p. 290).

50. b. An isotonic fluid is desirable to replace fluid loss in dehydration. D5W rapidly converts to a hypotonic fluid, and 0.45% normal saline is hypotonic, so both rapidly leave the blood vessels. D50W is hypertonic and will not improve this patient's condition (p. 292).

51. b. The patient in renal failure is frequently hypocalcemic (p. 294).

52. d. It may be accompanied by hypocalcemia and cause hyperactive reflexes. Antacid abuse can cause hypermagnesemia (p. 295).

53. a (p. 294)

54. c. Tidal volume is frequently severely impaired in these patients. The resultant decrease in minute volume and thus ventilation inhibits the excretion of carbon dioxide from the lungs, causing increased carbonic acid levels and a decreased pH (pp. 296, 297).

55. b. Lactic acid decreases the peripheral response to catecholamines and can cause severe hypotension (p. 298).

56. a. A decreased pH and increased pCO_2 are signs of respiratory acidosis. An increased pH and decreased pCO_2 are signs of respiratory alkalosis. An increased pH and increased pCO_2 are signs of metabolic alkalosis (p. 297).

57. b. Arterioles give rise to capillaries or metarterioles, which in turn give rise to capillaries. Thoroughfare channels are a type of capillary arising from a metarteriole that connects arterioles and venules directly, bypassing the true capillary (p.300).

58. b. This fluid loss is due to the increased hydrostatic pressure created in this situation (p. 301).

59. c. Baroreceptors are stimulated by an increase in blood pressure. Therefore the body attempts to compensate by decreasing heart rate and contractility and causing vasodilation. Urine output would decrease only if the body was trying to increase blood pressure (p. 305).

60. d. Tachycardia and pupil dilation are sympathetic responses but are not secondary to vasoconstriction. The container size should decrease because of vasoconstriction (p. 305).

61. d. When blood flow to the vasomotor center of the medulla is reduced to the point of ischemia, this response initiates profound vasoconstriction (p. 306).

62. b. All other mechanisms decrease urinary output to conserve blood volume (p. 308).

63. d. The precapillary sphincter opens, whereas the postcapillary sphincter remains closed, increasing the pressure inside the capillary and forcing fluid out through the already compromised capillary walls (p. 310).

64. b. Cardiogenic shock results from pump failure (p. 311).

65. d. The compensatory mechanisms of vasoconstriction, increased heart rate, and increased contractility are no longer sufficient to maintain an adequate blood pressure (p. 312).

66. a. As peripheral vascular resistance increases, blood pressure increases (p. 313).

67. b. Use of pneumatic antishock garments is generally not recommended for any of the other situations (p. 318).

68. a (p. 321)

69. c (p. 322)

70. c. Packed red blood cells is the only fluid in this group that has oxygen-carrying capacity (p. 323).

71. d. Priorities of care always follow the ABCs; therefore oxygen should be first, and intravenous therapy should be initiated en route unless a transportation delay exists; in this case, definitive care may be expedited (pp. 323, 324).

72. b. The head-down position of the Trendelenberg position is thought to interfere with effective ventilation (p. 324).

73. d. Vasoactive drugs should be used only in patients who have hypovolemic shock after their fluid volumes have been restored (p. 324).

74. a. Increased lung congestion indicates that the failing heart cannot deal with the existing fluid volume. Jugular venous distention should increase with fluid overload. Peripheral edema would have a slow onset and is not an acute sign evident in the prehospital phase of care. A moderate decrease in heart rate indicates patient improvement (p. 324).

75. b. Epinephrine is the only treatment that rapidly improves all the life-threatening effects of anaphy-

laxis. Other adjunct therapy may be used after epinephrine has been given (p. 324).

76. a. The flow of fluid through a catheter is directly related to its diameter and inversely related to its length, so the shortest catheter with the largest diameter should be selected (p. 325).

77. a. This position should be maintained to keep air in the right side of the heart and away from the cardiac valves (p. 331).

78. b. Drops/min = (Volume to be infused × Drops/ml) ÷ Time (minutes) = (30 ml × 60 drops/ml) ÷ 60 min = 30 drops/min (p. 332)

79. c. Drops/min = (200 ml × 10 drops/ml) ÷ 20 min = 100 drops/min (p. 332)

● CHAPTER 14
GENERAL PHARMACOLOGY

1. h (p. 341)
2. b (p. 340)
3. j (p. 340)
4. i (p. 340)
5. k (p. 340)
6. l (p. 340)
7. a (p. 340)
8. c (p. 340)
9. g (p. 340)
10. True (p. 343)
11. True (p. 354)
12. Plants, animals, humans, mineral or mineral products, microorganisms, and synthetic chemical substances (p. 336)
13. a. Chemical; b. generic or nonproprietary; c. trade or proprietary; d. official (p. 337)
14. Protected the public from mislabeled drugs, prohibited the use of false and misleading claims for medications, and restricted sales of drugs with abuse potential. b. Prevented marketing of drugs until they were tested and required names of all ingredients and directions on labels. c. Controlled the sale of narcotics and established *narcotic* as a legal term (p. 338)
15. a. Federal Trade Commission; b. Food and Drug Administration; c. Drug Enforcement Administration; d. Public Health Service (p. 337)
16. a. For chronic control of bronchial asthma; b. contraindicated in the treatment of acute episodes of asthma or status asthmaticus or if a known hypersensitivity exists (*PDR*)
17. a. Idiosyncrasy; b. stimulant; c. drug allergy; d. antagonism; e. potentiation; f. side effect; g. syner-

gism; h. drug dependence; i. depressant; j. therapeutic action; k. contraindications; l. drug interaction; m. tolerance; n. cumulative action (p. 342)

18. The nature of the absorbing surface through which the drug must traverse, the blood flow to the site of administration, the solubility of the drug, the pH of the drug environment, the drug concentration, and the drug dosage form (pp. 344, 345)

19. Rectal (p. 346)
20. Subcutaneous (p. 346)
21. Intravenous (p. 346)
22. Nalaxone, atropine, epinephrine, and lidocaine (p. 347)
23. Intraosseous (p. 347)
24. Faster (p. 346)
25. Placenta and blood-brain barrier (p. 348)
26. *Subjective data:* Ask the patient if the pain has changed, and if so, try to quantify it. (For example, if the pain was a "10" before, what is it now? Does the patient appear more relaxed?) *Objective data:* Have the vital signs changed? Has the respiratory rate, pulse rate, or both, decreased as the pain lessened? Is the pulse regular now? Has the blood pressure decreased? Are the number of ventricular beats on the electrocardiogram diminishing? (Chapter 11)
27. a. 7 is the numerator, 8 is the denominator; b. 6 is the numerator, 13 is the denominator.
28. a. $1/4$; b. $3/4$; c. $1/2$; d. $1/6$; e. $1/5$; f. $1/4$; g. $1/5$; h. $9/25$; i. $1/10$; j. $2/5$; k. $17/23$; l. $2/3$
29. a. 15; b. 2; c. 3; d. $2\frac{1}{2}$
30. a. $43/8$; b. $7/4$; c. $37/12$; d. $47/3$
31. a. $18/24$; b. $48/60$; c. $79,000/100,000$
32. a. 45; b. 12; c. 24
33. a. Equal to; b. greater than; c. less than
34. a. $1\frac{3}{8}$; b. $3\frac{11}{12}$
35. a. 1; b. $1\frac{11}{12}$
36. a. $55/78$; b. $25\frac{1}{2}$; c. $13\frac{3}{4}$; d. $7/24$
37. a. $1\frac{1}{4}$; b. $3\frac{13}{14}$
38. a. 3.4; b. 5.35; c. 0.062
39. a. 0.25; b. 0.28; c. 0.02
40. a. $1/2$; b. $3\frac{6}{25}$; c. $6\frac{7}{1000}$
41. a. 0.47; b. 1.02
42. a. 29; b. 13.58
43. a. 0.0724; b. 1.08; c. 0.2175; d. 425.6; e. 29; f. 7052
44. a. 0.05; b. 2.58; c. 8; d. 4.0; e. 0.14237; f. 0.017
45. a. 7.6; b. 0.1; c. 0.9
46. a. 0.1; b. 5.63; c. 892.03
47. a. 5000:60 (5000 ml:60 seconds); b. 6000:60 (6000 ml:60 seconds); c. 100:30 (100 ml:30 minutes); d. 100:10 (100 mg:10 ml)
48. a. 83 ml/sec; b. 100 ml/sec; c. 3 ml/min; d. 10 mg/ml
49. a. True; b. not true; c. true
50. x = 3; b. x = 4; c. x = 10.5; d. x = 15; e. x = 27; f. x = 36; g. x = 28; h. x = 9

51. a. $x = \dfrac{10 \times 150}{50} = \dfrac{10 \times \overset{30}{\cancel{150}}}{\cancel{50}} = 30$

b. $x = \dfrac{25 \times 2}{50} = \dfrac{\overset{1}{\cancel{25}} \times \overset{1}{\cancel{2}}}{\cancel{50}_{1}} = 1$

c. $x = \dfrac{2500 \times 500}{20,000} = \dfrac{\cancel{2500} \times 500}{\cancel{20,000}} = \dfrac{125}{2} = 62.5$

d. $x = \dfrac{1\,g \times 1\,L}{1\,g} = \dfrac{\cancel{1\,g} \times 1\,L}{\cancel{1\,g}} = 1\,L$

e. $x = \dfrac{2\,mg \times 1\,cc}{10\,mg} = \dfrac{\overset{1}{\cancel{2}}\,mg \times 1\,cc}{\underset{5}{\cancel{10}}\,mg} = \dfrac{1\,cc}{5} = 0.2\,cc$

f. $x = \dfrac{10\,mg \times 10\,ml}{100\,mg} = \dfrac{\cancel{10\,mg} \times 10\,ml}{\cancel{100\,mg}} = 1\,ml$

52. a. 0.25; b. 1.1; c. 0.005
53. a. 34%; b. 229%; c. 7%
54. a. 68%; b. 20%; c. 43%
55.

Fraction	Ratio	Decimal	Percentage
a. $5/6$	5:6 or 5 to 6	0.83	83%
b. $1/20$	1:20 or 1 to 20	0.05	5%
c. $7/33$	7:33 or 7 to 33	0.21	21%

56. a. 11.25; b. 1.25
57. a. Liter; b. gram; c. meter
58. Kilogram (kg), gram (g), milligram (mg), and microgram (mcg)
59. 1000
60. Right
61. Left
62. a. 2000 g; b. 4000 mcg; c. 2000 mg; d. 0.6 kg; e. 0.4 mg; f. 0.35 g; g. 250 mcg; h. 12500 mg
63. a. 1; b. 10; c. 0.25; d. 330
64. Grain (gr)
65. Minim
66. 600 mg
67. a. 0.4 mg; b. 0.3 mg
68. a. 3; b. 16; c. 16; d. 4; e. 2; f. 8
69. a. 5; b. 15: c. 30; d. 960; e. 10; f. 50
70. a. 240; b. 960; c. 30; 480; d. 58; e. 5.2; f. 480; g. 0.9 and 900 (pp. 356, 106)
71. a. Magnesium sulfate; b. Aug. 1, 1995; c. 10 ml; d. 5g; e. 500 mg/ml (4mEq/ml)
72. a. 10; b. 1; c. 10; d. 1; e. 0.4; f. 25; g. 50
73. a. 40 mg/4 ml = 10 mg/ml; b. 1 mg/10 ml = 0.1 mg/ml; c. 25 g/50 ml = 25,000 mg/50 ml = 500 mg/ml; d. 50 mg/2 ml = 25 mg/ml; e. 1 g/250 ml = 1000 mg/250 ml = 4 mg/ml
74. a. 100; b. 350; c. 80; d. 250; e. 0.05 (don't forget to convert to kilograms); f. 80

75. a. $x = \dfrac{20\,mg \times 4\,ml}{40\,mg} = 2\,ml$

b. $x = \dfrac{3\,mg \times 1\,ml}{1\,mg} = 0.3\,ml$

c. $x = \dfrac{150\,mg \times 10\,ml}{250\,mg} = 6\,ml$

d. $x = \dfrac{2.5\,mg \times 2\,ml}{10\,mg} = 0.5\,ml$

e. $x = \dfrac{12.5\,mg \times 1\,ml}{50\,mg} = 0.25\,ml$

f. $x = \dfrac{0.3\,mg \times 1\,ml}{1\,mg} = 0.3\,ml$

g. $x = \dfrac{0.5\,mg \times 500\,ml}{400\,mg} = 0.6\,ml$

76. a. 6 mg:x: :6 mg:2 ml
$x \times 6\,mg = 6\,mg \times 2\,ml$
$\dfrac{x \times 6\,mg}{6\,mg} = \dfrac{6\,mg \times 2\,ml}{6\,mg}$
$x = 2\,ml$
b. 1 ml; c. 1 ml; d. 1 g:x: :20 g:100 ml, x = 5 ml
77. a. 7.5 ml; b. 12 ml; c. 0.5 ml; d. 7.7 ml; e. 350 ml; f. 6 ml; g. 0.625 ml and 38 gtt/min; h. 0.5 ml and 30 gtt/min; i. 0.5 ml and 30 gtt/min
78. a. 5; b. 0.3; c. 7; d. 4.0
79.

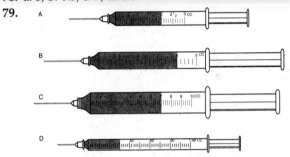

80. Avoid distractions; repeat orders to medical direction; verify that you are giving the right patient the right dose of the right drug at the right time by the right route; verify the correct drug on the label at least 3 times; verify the route of administration; ensure that the labeling information is correct for the drug you want to give; never give drugs from an unlabeled container; verify difficult calculations on paper, with a co-worker, or both; label the syringe immediately after withdrawing a drug that will not be completely administered immediately; do not give unlabeled drugs prepared by another person; do not give medications that are outdated or appear discolored, cloudy, or unusual; if the patient or a co-worker questions the drug or dose, double-check it; monitor the patient for adverse effects after administration; and document carefully (pp. 359, 360).
81. a. Upright (sitting) (p. 360); b. 4 to 8 ounces (p. 360); c. stomach (p. 360); d. tongue (p. 360); e. dissolve (p. 360); f. swallowed (p. 360); g., h., and i. infection, lipodystrophy, abscesses, necrosis, skin slough, nerve injuries, prolonged pain, and periostitis (p. 361); j. $1/2$ or $5/8$ (p. 361); k. 23 or 25 (p. 361); l. $1\frac{1}{2}$ to 2 (p. 361); m. 19 or 21 (p. 361); n. prohibited (p. 361); o. an appropriate sharp container (p. 362); p. air (p. 362); q. filter (p. 362); r. 45 (p. 362); s. upper arm, abdomen, thigh, and

back (p. 363); t. 90 (p. 363); u. deltoid muscle, dorsogluteal site, vastus lateralis muscle, rectus femoris muscle, and ventrogluteal muscle (p. 364); v. gloves (p. 367); w. 10 (p. 368); x. rapid onset and side effects (p. 368)

82. a. Less, more; b. decreased, more (p. 371)

83. a. Decreased renal function, altered nutrition habits, greater consumption of nonprescription drugs, reduced gastric acid, slowed gastric motility, decreased serum albumin, congestive heart failure, and decreased blood flow to the liver (p. 372)

84. Inability to pay for new drugs, forgetfulness or confusion, lack of symptoms (causing patient to become noncompliant), and other physical disabilities not mentioned (p. 373)

85. a. *Benzodiazepines:* alprazolam (Xanax), chlordiazepoxide (Librium), clorazepate (Tranxene), diazepam (Valium), flurazepam (Dalmane), lorazepam (Ativan), prazepam (Centrax), triazolam (Halcion) (p. 379). b. *Thrombolytic agents:* anisolated plasminogen streptokinase activator (Eminase), streptokinase (Streptase), urokinase (Abbokinase) (p. 389). c. *Antiemetics/antihistaminics:* diphenhydramine hydrochloride (Benadryl), hydroxyzine pamoate (Vistaril), meclizine hydrochloride (Antivert), promethazine hydrochloride (Phenergan) (p. 394). d. *Adrenergics:* dobutamine (Dubutrex), dopamine (Intropin), isoproterenol (Isuprel), norepinephrine (Levophed) (p. 382). e. *Antihypertensives (arteriolar dilator drugs):* diazoxide (Hyperstat), hydralazine (Apresoline) and *diuretics:* furosemide (Lasix), spironolactone (Aldactone) (p. 386). f. *Cardiac glycosides:* digitoxin (Crystodigin), digoxin (Lanoxin) (p. 384). g. *Anticonvulsants, barbiturate:* mephobarbital (Gemonil) (p. 379). h. *Narcotic analgesics, opioid analgesics-agonists:* codeine (Methylmorphine), meperidine (Demerol), methadone (Dolophine, Methadose), morphine sulfate (Astromorph and others), oxycodone (Percodan, Tylox, Percocet), propoxyphene (Darvon, Dolene) (p. 376). i. *Class IV antidysrhythmic:* verapamil (Isoptin) (p. 386). j. *Antiplatelet agents:* aspirin, sulfinpyrazone (Anturane) (p. 389). k. *Bronchodilators:* albuterol (Proventil, Ventolin), bitolterol (Tornalate), aminophylline (Amoline, Somophyllin, Aminophyllin), ephedrine (Ephed II), dyphylline (Dilor, Droxine, Lufyllin), epinephrine (Adrenalin, Asmolin, and others), epinephrine hydrochloride (Adrenalin Chloride 1:1000), epinephrine inhalation aerosol (Bronkaid Mist, Primatene Mist), epinephrine inhalation solution (Adrenalin), ethylnorepinephrine (Bronkephrine), epinephrine suspension (Sus-Phrine 1:200), isoproterenol hydrochloride inhalation aerosol (Isuprel Mistometer, Norisodrine Aerotrol), isoproterenol inhalation solution (Aerolone, Vapo-Iso, Isuprel),

racemic epinephrine inhalation solution (AsthmaNefrin, micro-Nephrin, and others), terbutaline sulfate (Brethine, Bricanyl), (p. 390). l. *Emetic:* syrup of ipecac (p. 393); m. *Anticoagulants:* heparin sodium (Liquaemin) (p. 389). n. *Opioidagonist-antagonist agents:* butorphanol tartrate (Stadol), nalbuphine hydrochloride (Nubain) (p. 378). o. *Other drugs used to treat respiratory emergencies:* dexamethasone sodium phosphate (Decadron Phosphate), glycopyrrolate (Robinul) (p. 392).

86. b. Antidote is a specific drug taken to minimize the adverse effects of an ingested drug or poison. *Parenteral* refers to a drug route. A vaccine is an injection of drug given to prevent disease (p. 366).

87. b (p. 339)

88. b. Only selected antibiotics pass through these barriers (p. 348).

89. d. LD 50 is the lethal dose for 50% of animals who took it. ED 50 is the effective dose for 50% of animals who took it. TI = LD 50/ED 50. Biological half-life is the time required to excrete half of the total amount of drug introduced into the body (p. 356).

90. d. Dose = 500 mg/kg × 100 kg = 50000 mg = 50 g
    Volume = $\frac{D}{H} \times Q = \frac{50 \text{ g} \times 100 \text{ ml}}{10 \text{ g}}$ = 500 ml (p. 358)

91. b (p. 368)

92. d. Then intramuscular, subcutaneous, and by mouth (p. 347)

93. b. All of the other routes listed give unpredictable, slow absorption because of poor perfusion in shock (p. 344).

94. b. Butorphanol tartrate and pentazocine are opioid agonist-antagonists, and oxycodone hydrochloride is an opioid analgesic-agonist (p. 378).

95. c. Nalbuphine is an opioid agonist-antagonist (p. 378).

96. c. Glucagon is a pancreatic hormone that increases blood glucose, lorazepam is a minor tranquilizer, and verapamil is an antidysrhythmic drug (p. 381).

97. a. Norepinephrine is the primary neurotransmittor for the sympathetic nervous system. Adrenalin is a trade name for epinephrine, and Aramine is the trade name for metaraminol (p. 382).

98. c (p. 382)

99. c (p. 382)

100. d. Increased chronotropic effect increases heart rate, increased dromotropic effect increases conduction velocity, and increased cholinergic effect slows heart rate (p. 385).

101. a. Influenza-like symptoms and a variety of dysrhythmias are associated with digoxin toxicity (p. 385).

102. d. Bretylium tosylate is a group III, lidocaine is a group IB, and procainamide is a group IA antidysrhythmic (p. 386).

103. d. Some also decrease heart rate and contractility; however, the majority achieve their effects by decreasing vascular resistance (p. 386).

104. d. All of the others prevent clot formation (p. 389).

105. a. Ephedrine and isoproterenol are nonspecific beta agonists, and aminophylline is a xanthine derivative (p. 391).

106. b. Antihistamines may worsen an acute asthma attack by thickening bronchial secretions (p. 392).

107. d. Insulin is continually secreted in amounts determined by the body's needs (p. 393).

108. b. Bretylium tosylate and meperidine frequently have the side effects of nausea and vomiting. Syrup of ipecac is an emetic (p. 394).

● DIVISION TWO REVIEW TEST

1. b. -asthenia means "weakness," -pathy means "disease," and -phasia means "speech" (p. 102).

2. b. cc stands for "cubic centimeter," c/o stands for "complains of," CHF stands for "congestive heart failure" (p. 104)

3. d (p. 106)

4. c. The pelvis is part of the appendicular skeleton (p. 120).

5. b. Lysosomes aid in cellular digestion, ribosomes synthesize protein, and the nucleus is the control center for the cell (p. 115).

6. a (pp. 116, 117)

7. b (p. 123)

8. b. The jugular notch is at the superior aspect of the sternum, and the xiphoid process is at the inferior end. The tragus is at the ear (p. 124).

9. d. A cartilaginous joint unites two bones by hyaline cartilage or fibrocartilage (symphyses). Fibrous joints have two bones united by fibrous tissue and have little or no movement (p. 129).

10. b. Abduction refers to movement away from the body. Pronation is rotation of the forearm so that the anterior surface is down, and supination is rotation of the forearm so that the anterior surface is up (p. 131).

11. a. The midbrain is involved in hearing, visual reflexes, coordination, and muscle tone. The pons contains ascending and descending nerve tracts and houses the sleep center and part of the respiratory center. The thalamus relays information from sense organs to the cerebral cortex and influences mood and general body movements (p. 139).

12. b. Afferent (sensory) pathways are carried on the dorsal roots of the spinal cord to the brain. Ganglia are a collection of neuron cell bodies (axons) (pp. 143-145).

13. c. The sympathetic (adrenergic) division of the autonomic nervous system is responsible for alarm or stress responses. B is not a division of the autonomic nervous sytem.

14. b. The aortic valve lies between the left ventricle and the aorta, the pulmonic valve between the right ventricle and pulmonary artery, and the tricuspid valve between the right atria and ventricle (p. 153).

15. d. The lymph system carries fluid only from tissue to blood, not in the opposite direction (p. 158).

16. c (p. 163)

17. b. The arytenoid and cuneiform cartilage are paired. The thyroid is the most superior unpaired cartilage in the larynx (p. 161).

18. d. Amylase and bicarbonate are excreted by the pancreas, and bile is excreted by the gallbladder (p. 164).

19. d (p. 166)

20. a. The fundus is the superior portion of the uterus. The ovaries and vagina are not part of the uterus (p. 172).

21. c. The sclera is the firm, white outer layer of the eye. The cornea is continuous with it and permits light to enter the eye. The iris is the colored smooth muscle that surrounds the pupil (p. 176).

22. b. Vital sign assessment is the first step in the secondary survey (p. 182).

23. d (p. 184)

24. a. Normocardia (not in text) indicates a rate within normal limits, whereas tachycardia indicates a rate faster than normal (greater than 100) (p. 184).

25. a. Simultaneous cervical spine and airway management take precedence over control of hemorrhage. Frequently, if enough help is on the scene, one paramedic takes control of the airway while another takes control of the bleeding (pp. 182-186).

26. d (p. 188)

27. d. Ataxic respirations are characterized by a series of inspirations and expirations and are usually associated with a lesion in the medulla. Biot's breathing consists of irregular respirations varying in depth and interrupted by periods of apnea. This does not repeat in a pattern like Cheyne-Stokes respirations and is frequently seen in patients with head injuries with increased intracranial pressure. Cheyne-Stokes respirations are a regular, periodic pattern of breathing with intervals of apnea followed by a crescendo/decrescendo sequence of respirations (p. 195).

28. d (p. 200)

29. d (p. 203)

30. c. First, one should observe for abnormalities, then listen, and finally palpate so that no bowel sounds are created by manipulation of the abdominal organs (pp. 202-204).

31. b. Bladder and blood vessel injury causing hemorrhage are frequently associated with pelvic fracture (p. 204).

32. b (p. 205)

33. b. All other questions invite only a "yes" or "no" answer (p. 208).

34. a (p. 209)

35. a. Many deaf people lip read, so the paramedic should speak slowly and clearly in full view of the patient (p. 215).

36. d. The diaphragm and thoracic muscles contract and result in an increase in anterior-posterior and superior-inferior chest dimensions. This causes a decrease in intrathoracic pressure, and air rushes into the lungs (p. 221).

37. d (p. 222)

38. c. Atmospheric pressure is 760 torr (mm Hg), and it contains 21% oxygen. $\frac{760 \text{ torr} \times 21}{100} = 159.6$ or 160 torr (p. 225).

39. b. Active transport frequently involves movement of molecules from an area of lower concentration to an area of higher concentration across a semipermeable membrane using energy. Osmosis is the movement of water from an area of lesser molecular concentration to an area of greater molecular concentration. Filtration is the passage of material through a material that prevents passage of certain materials (p. 228).

40. a. A pH of 7.0 is neutral, a pH less than 7.0 is acidic, and a pH greater than 7.0 is basic (pp. 229, 230).

41. b. When the metabolic rate decreases, carbon dioxide production decreases (p. 231).

42. b. The pons is also involved with respiratory control; however, it is primarily active only in labored breathing (p. 235).

43. b. Coughing and sneezing rid the airway of foreign particles. Periodic sighing expands collapsed alveoli (pp. 237, 238).

44. c. If the patient vomits, drainage will be facilitated in this position (p. 242).

45. d. After the airway is opened manually, adjuncts for airway and ventilation may be used when available (p. 243).

46. d. Because of the relatively straight line of the right mainstem, the tube will frequently pass into it if advanced too far (p. 255).

47. d (pp. 260, 261)

48. d. All other patients described should not be nasally intubated (p. 261).

49. a. The epiglottis is omega shaped, and the tongue is larger in proportion to the rest of the child's body. Because of the small airway size, right mainstem intubation is common (p. 252).

50. d. Increased thoracic rigidity and decreased alveolar surface area also occur. Although the pO_2 progressively decreases with age, the pCO_2 does not normally increase, except in patients with chronic obstructive pulmonary disease (p. 275).

51. c. Anaerobic metabolism occurs when oxygen is unavailable. It is less efficient than aerobic metabolism and produces lactic acid (p. 298).

52. d. As peripheral vascular resistance decreases, vessel capacitance increases, and the container size increases. This makes the existing blood volume insufficient to maintain an adequate preload (pp. 285, 286).

53. a. Leukocytes, or white blood cells, aid in body defense. Plasma proteins maintain oncotic pressure, defend the body, and aid in clotting. Platelets help initiate blood clotting (pp. 286, 287).

54. c. All others are found chiefly in the extracellular fluid (p. 288).

55. a (p. 288)

56. b. An isotonic fluid is desirable to replace fluid loss in dehydration (p. 292).

57. b. The patient in renal failure is frequently hypocalcemic (p. 294).

58. a (pp. 292-295)

59. a. Decreased pH and increased pCO_2 is respiratory acidosis. Increased pH and decreased pCO_2 is respiratory alkalosis. Increased pH and decreased pCO_2 is metabolic alkalosis (pp. 295-300).

60. d. Tachycardia and pupil dilation are sympathetic responses but are not secondary to vasoconstriction. The container size should decrease resulting from vasoconstriction (p. 310).

61. b. All other mechanisms decrease urinary output to conserve blood volume (p. 306).

62. d. The compensatory mechanisms of vasoconstriction, increased heart rate, and increased contractility are no longer sufficient to maintain an adequate blood pressure (p. 312).

63. a (p. 321)

64. c (p. 322)

65. d (pp. 315-316)

66. c. Drops/minute = $\frac{200 \text{ ml} \times 10 \text{ drops/ml}}{20 \text{ min}} = 100$ drops/min (p. 332).

67. d The generic name is *acetaminophen* (p. 337).

68. b. Antagonism is the inhibition of effects produced by other drugs or body functions. A side effect is an undesirable effect of a normal dose of a drug. An untoward effect is a harmful side effect (p. 342).

69. b (p. 356)

70. d (p. 356)

71. b (p. 358)

72. c. mcg/min = 10 mcg × 80 kg = 800 mcg/min
800 mcg = 0.8 mg
ml/min = D × Q = $\frac{0.8 \text{ mg} \times 250 \text{ ml}}{}$ = 0.5 ml
drops/min = 0.5 ml
× 60 gtt/ml\1 min = 30 gtts/min (p. 358)

73. c. Intramuscular injections should be given into the muscle at a 90-degree angle. Acceptable sites are in the deltoid, hip, and anterior and lateral thigh (pp. 364-365).

74. a (p. 379)

75. a. Naloxone is an opiate antagonist, propranolol is

a beta blocker, and succinylcholine is a neuromuscular blocking agent (p. 381).

76. a (p. 374)
77. c. The adrenergic or sympathetic receptors perform the alarm functions for the body (p. 377).
78. d. It may actually block bronchial dilation. It will not increase but may decrease blood pressure as it decreases heart rate and contractility (p. 383).
79. a. Captopril is an angiotensin-inhibiting enzyme (ACE) inhibitor, hydralazine is a vasodilator, and metoprolol is a sympathetic blocking agent (p. 387).
80. c. Bronchodilation is a desired effect, and central nervous system stimulation and muscle tremors will occur (p. 391).

● CHAPTER 15
TRAUMA

1. b (p. 401)
2. e (p. 401)
3. a (p. 401)
4. c (p. 401)
5. a (pp. 431, 432)
6. c (pp. 430, 431)
7. d (p. 432)
8. b (p. 432)
9. f and g (p. 476)
10. b, d, f, and g (p. 476)
11. b, d, f, and g (p. 476)
12. b, d, and f (p. 476)
13. b, d, and f (p. 476)
14. b and d (p. 478)
15. a, b, and d (p. 478)
16. c and e (p. 479)
17. c (p. 479)
18. c and h (p. 479)
19. c, b, and d (p. 479)
20. b and d (p. 479)
21. b (p. 481)
22. a (p. 481)
23. False. Injuries that may occur include abdominal trauma and thoracolumbar fractures and dislocations (p. 404).
24. True (p. 404)
25. False. The helmet should be removed to allow for proper assessment and to permit rapid airway-management techniques (p. 457).
26. True (p. 462)
27. True (p. 474)
28. a. Lacerations of the brain, brain stem, upper spinal cord, heart, aorta, or other large vessels; injury-prevention programs. b. Subdural or epidural hematoma, hemopneumothorax, ruptured spleen, lacerated liver, pelvic fracture, or multiple injuries associated with significant blood loss; time from injury to definitive care, which must be brief. c. Sepsis, infection, and/or multiple organ failure; early recognition and treatment of life-threatening injury in the field, with adequate fluid resuscitation and aseptic technique (p. 400).
29. a. The vehicle strikes the embankment, the passenger strikes the vehicle, and the internal organs pull forward rapidly and strike the bony structures inside the body (p. 401). b. Dislocated knees, patellar fractures, fractured femurs, posterior fracture or dislocation of the acetabulum, vascular injury, and hemorrhage (p. 402).
30. Whether the car struck remains stationary (injuries likely on the side of the impact) or moves away from the point of impact (injuries likely on the side opposite the impact) (p. 403)
31. b. The velocity that produces damage is determined by calculating the difference between the speed of the two vehicles. In example *a*, it would be 70 − 50 = 20, and in example *b*, it would be 40 − 5 = 35, which is greater (p. 403).
32. a. Intracerebral hemorrhage and cervical fracture; b. ruptured aorta; c. kidney, liver, and spleen lacerations (p. 405, 406)
33. a. Pneumothorax could be caused by displaced rib fractures that puncture a lung or a paper-bag injury, in which impact occurs after the patient has inhaled against a closed glottis (p. 407). b. Lacerated spleen, liver, or kidney and rupture of the bladder, diaphragm, gallbladder, duodenum, colon, stomach, or small bowel (p. 408).
34. a. Laying the bike down; b. head on (up and over the handle bars); c. angular (p. 408)
35. a. Fractures of lower legs, femur, pelvis, thorax, and spine; injuries to the intraabdominal or intrathoracic contents; and head and spinal injuries. b. Fractures of the femur and pelvis; abdomino-pelvic and thoracic trauma; and head and neck injuries (p. 409).
36. Energy forces involved, body part to which energy is transfered, speed of acceleration and deceleration, forces involved (compressive, twisting, hyperextension, hyperflexion), protective gear (p. 410)
37. a. Hearing loss, pulmonary hemorrhage, cerebral air embolism, thermal injuries, abdominal hemorrhage, and/or bowel perforation. b. Lacerations, contusions, fractures, and impaled objects. c. Fractures and abdominopelvic, thoracic, and head and spine injuries (p. 410).
38. a. Length and width of knives determine the depth and extent of the injury. With bullets, missile damage increases if the bullet is designed to rotate, flatten, or fragment during or after impact. b. Kinetic injury increases with increased speed, and tissue damage increases with increased energy applied.

c. As range increases, damage decreases because of decreased velocity. Close-range injuries have increased damage because of the direct injury of gases from combustion and the explosion of powder (p. 412).

39. a. Inspect and palpate head for lacerations, contusions, and deformities. Inspect face for asymmetry and soft tissue injury. Evaluate child's vision by holding up fingers and assessing pupil response. Inspect oral cavity for bleeding, soft tissue injury, and missing teeth. Palpate face for crepitus and question patient about tenderness. Ask child to open and close the mouth and move the lower jaw from side to side. Gently palpate for loose teeth. b. Immobilize the C-spine and secure the child to the backboard while frequently suctioning the oral cavity. Tilt the backboard to the side and secure it firmly with straps. Suction the oral cavity frequently and instruct the child to signal when he or she needs additional suctioning or if he or she has difficultly breathing (p. 420).

40. Observe for signs of external trauma, discoloration, injury to the lid, fluid or jelly extruding from the eye, bleeding, blood in the anterior chamber, and the presence of contact lens. Assess pupil response, extraocular movements, and visual acuity (p. 425).

41. a. Foreign body (or corneal abrasion). Irrigate with normal saline. b. Lid avulsion. Assess for underlying injury to the eye. Control bleeding with gentle pressure. For transport, cover with a dressing moistened with normal saline and an eye shield. c. Embedded foreign body. Patch uninjured eye. Stabilize hook and cover with cardboard cup secured with tape. d. Traumatic hyphema. Elevate head of ambulance cot 40 to 45 degrees. Instruct patient to avoid straining. e. Ruptured globe. Cover affected eye with damp, sterile dressings and an eye shield (p. 427).

42. a. Loss of consciousness (usually less than 5 minutes), retrograde or antegrade amnesia, vomiting, combativeness, transient visual disturbances, and problems with coordination. All symptoms should improve, not deteriorate (p. 433). b. Seizures, hemiparesis, aphasia, personality changes, and loss of consciousness (lasting hours, days, or longer) (p. 434). c. Headache, nausea, vomiting, decreasing level of consciousness, coma, abnormal posturing, paralysis, and bulging fontanelles in infants (p. 437). d. Transient loss of consciousness followed by a lucid interval (6-18 hours) and then a decreasing level of consciousness, headache, and contralateral hemiparesis (opposite the side of the bleeding) (50% are unconscious without improvement) (p. 436).

43. Headache, nausea, vomiting, altered level of consciousness, increased systolic blood pressure, widened pulse pressure, decreased pulse rate, abnormally slow respiratory pattern, unilateral dilated pupil, and abnormal posturing (p. 435)

44. Intubate tracheally (possibly nasally if basilar skull fracture is not suspected) using spinal precautions. Hyperventilate the lungs with 100% oxygen at a rate of 24 to 30/min. (Consider nasogastric tube if available.) Elevate the head of the backboard if possible (30 degrees). Maintain fluids to keep the vein open if fluid volume deficit is not suspected. Consider pharmacological agents such as mannitol, furosemide, and dexamethasone in consultation with medical direction. Notify medical direction and transport to closest appropriate trauma center (pp. 437-439).

45. Bleeding, shock, hematoma, pulse deficit, neurological deficit, dyspnea, hoarseness, stridor, subcutaneous emphysema, hemoptysis, dysphagia, and hematemesis (p. 441)

46. Secure airway and breathing. Maintain spine immobilization. Apply firm, direct pressure to the affected vessels and tamponade vessel with direct pressure with a gloved finger. If venous injury is suspected, keep the patient supine or in the Trendelenberg position to prevent an air embolism (p. 441).

47. Significant trauma with concurrent intoxication, seizures, unconsciousness with head injury, injury above the clavicle, fall greater than 3 times the patient's height, fall with bilateral heel fractures, injuries during a high-speed motor vehicle crash (pp. 444, 445)

48. a. Hyperflexion; b. hyperextension; c. ligamentous complex and joint capsule; d. dislocation (subluxation); e. whiplash; f. C5 to C7; g. C1 to C2; h. T12 to L2; i. compression (p. 446)

49. Absence of motor and sensory function below the nipple, relative bradycardia, hypotension, priapism, unstable body temperature, loss of bowel and bladder control, and decreased depth of respiration (loss of most intercostal muscles) (p. 446)

50. Increasing pain or neurological deficits during movement, resistance to movement, muscle spasm, airway compromise, and severe misalignment of head from midline (p. 448)

51. a. Rescuer 1 is positioned at the patient's head, providing in-line manual stabilization. Rescuers 2 and 3 are positioned at the patient's midthorax and knees. b. While maintaining immobilization, the rescuers, in one organzied move, slowly log-roll the patient onto his or her side perpendicular to the ground. c. Rescuer 4 positions the long spine board by placing the device flat on the ground or at a 30- to 40-degree angle against the patient's back. d. In one organized more, the rescuers slowly log-roll and center the patient onto the long spine board (pp. 450, 451).

52. Flail chest (p. 461)

53. The pulmonary contusion and injured segment of the chest will not expand; therefore insufficient negative pressure is generated in the chest to draw in a normal amount of air (p. 462).

54. Intubate if the Glasgow coma score is less than 8 or if the patient is hypoxic. Assist ventilations with positive pressure (demand valve, bag-valve) with 100% oxygen. Monitor vital signs, electrocardiogram, and oxygen saturation (pp. 461, 462).

55. Dyspnea, tachypnea, diminished breath sounds on the affected side, and chest pain on inspiration (p. 462)

56. a. During inspiration, some air will enter the wound instead of the trachea, which decreases air entering the lung for ventilation. b. Seal wound on three sides with occlusive dressing. Administer high-flow oxygen by nonrebreather mask (p. 463).

57. a. Cyanosis, tracheal deviation, tachycardia, hypotension, and distended neck veins (p. 464). b. Insert a 14-gauge catheter in the midclavicular line of the second intercostal space on the side of the pneumothorax. Listen for a rush of air, consider a flutter valve, reevaluate the patient, and repeat these steps en route if the needle clots (p. 465).

58. Hypoxia and hypovolemic shock (p. 465)

59. a. Traumatic asphyxia; b. maintenance of airway and ventilation and evaluation for associated injuries (p. 467)

60. a. Myocardial contusion; b. oxygen administration, electrocardiographic monitoring, and treatment of dysrhythmias per protocol (p. 467)

61. a. Pericardial tamponade; b. oxygen administration, fluid replacement, rapid transport, consideration of pericardiocentesis (p. 468)

62. Upper extremity or generalized hypertension, systolic murmur, paraplegia (rare), and severe shock (p. 469)

63. a. Spleen; b. referred pain caused by irritation of the diaphragm by a splenic hematoma or blood in the peritoneum (Kehr's sign) (p. 471)

64. Sepsis, infection, abscess formation, and peritonitis (due to leakage of the contents of hollow organs) (p. 471)

65. Compare with opposite extremity; palpate for crepitus and deformity; and assess for pain, pallor, pulselessness, paresthesias, and paralysis (p. 474).

66. Assess the injury, support the body part; remove jewelry or constrictive clothing; assess pulse, movement, and sensation distal to the injury; immobilize so that the joints above and below the injury are included in the splint; avoid excessive movement; leave fingers or toes exposed so that circulatory status can be evaluated; and reassess pulse, movement, and sensation after splinting (p. 475).

67. a. GCS = 12 and RTS = 11; b. GCS = 8 and RTS = 7 (pp. 417, 418)

68. a. The air bag will inflate and then rapidly deflate after the first frontal collision (p. 405).

69. b. Falls from greater than 3 times the height of the individual are likely to produce serious injury. Adults who fall from a height greater than 15 feet usually land on their feet (p. 411).

70. a (p. 413)

71. d. Pupil response should not be evaluated until the secondary survey (p. 423).

72. c (pp. 422, 423)

73. d (p. 430)

74. c. Loss of smell is associated with damage to cranial nerve I, blindness in one eye with damage to cranial nerve II, and facial paralysis with damage to cranial nerve VII (p. 433).

75. a. All other symptoms indicate increased intracranial pressure but may also point to another illness or injury (p. 434).

76. d. The patient in diabetic ketoacidosis has Kussmaul respirations in an attempt to correct acidosis (p. 435).

77. c. All other interventions are indicated (depending on medical control) to decrease intracranial pressure; however, hyperventilation is the fastest method with the least risk to the patient (p. 435).

78. d. $x = \dfrac{40\,g \times 100\,ml}{20\,g} = 200\,ml$ (p. 439)

79. c (p. 447)

80. d. Immobilize the torso first to prevent angulation of the cervical spine (p. 455).

81. d. Children have more elastic chests and are less likely to have rib fractures. The first rib is rarely fractured. The pancreas lies protected behind other abdominal organs and is unlikely to be affected by rib fractures (p. 461).

82. c (p. 462)

83. c (p. 470)

84. a (pp. 471, 472)

85. d (p. 471)

86. c. Followed by airway and oxygen, surgery may be necessary to stop the bleeding in this situation (p. 471).

87. a (p. 479)

88. d. A sprain is a partial tear of a ligament. Painful bruising secondary to minor bleeding may occur (p. 474).

● CHAPTER 16
SOFT TISSUE INJURIES AND BURNS

1. a (p. 512)

2. b (p. 512)

3. d (p. 512)

4. a (p. 513)

5. e (pp. 512-513)

6. a. Connective tissue, elastic fibers, blood vessels, lymphatic vessels, motor or sensory fibers, hair, nails, and glands (p. 486)

7. Protection and cushioning against injury, barrier against infection, temperature regulation, and preservation of body fluids (pp. 487, 119)
8. Release of platelet factors at injury site, formation of thrombin, and trapping of red blood cells in fibrin to form a clot (p. 487)
9. The warmth and redness is due to vasodilation and enhanced blood supply to the affected area. Swelling is caused by increased capillary permeability, which allows plasma, plasma proteins, and electrolytes to leak into extracellular space. Pain is secondary to chemicals and increased pressure resulting from fluid buildup (p. 488).
10. a. Apply direct pressure to the wound with a hand or bulky dressing and then secure it firmly (p. 489). b. Elevate affected anatomical area above the level of the heart (p. 489). c. Apply pressure-point control. Select the appropriate pressure point proximal to the wound and compress the artery against the underlying bone for at least 10 minutes (pp. 489-491). d. Immobilize by splinting. (Immobilization is used as an adjunct to other control devices.) Select the appropriate splint for the body area and apply it to minimize blood flow (p. 491). e. Use pneumatic pressure devices. (Devices such as air splints or pnematic antishock garments serve as adjuncts for pressure control after the bleeding is controlled by other methods.) (p. 491) f. Use a tourniquet only when other methods are unsuccessful in controlling bleeding and when preservation of life is selected over preservation of limb. Notify medical control, and select a site 2 inches proximal to the wound over the brachial or femoral artery. Place a tourniquet over the artery and a pad over the artery to be compressed. Place tourniquet twice around the extremity and tie it in a half knot over the pad. Place a windlass on the half knot and secure it with a square knot. Tighten the windlass until the hemorrhage stops and secure it. Note the time of application and TK on the patient's forehead and notify the receiving hospital (pp. 491, 492).
11. a. Compartment syndrome. Provide airway and ventilation support, administer oxygen, immobilize, replace fluid if needed, and rapidly transport patient to the appropriate medical facility (pp. 493, 494). b. Contusion or hematoma. Apply ice or cold packs and compression with manual pressure or compression bandage (pp. 492, 493). c. Crush syndrome. Provide airway and ventilation support, administer high-flow oxygen, maintain body temperature, rehydrate with expanding intravenous fluids, and administer pharmacological agents such as sodium bicarbonate, mannitol, furosemide, calcium chloride, and inhalation of beta agonists if ordered by medical direction (all controversial) (pp. 494, 495). d. Laceration.

Control hemorrhage and monitor for signs of hypovolemic shock (p. 495). e. Abrasions. Clean gross contaminants from injured surface and lightly cover with sterile dressing (p. 495). f. Dog bite. Ensure that animal is contained, control bleeding, rinse off gross contaminants, splint extremity, and obtain a medical history from the pet owner (p. 498). g. Penetrating or impaled object. Leave object in place, do not manipulate object unless it is necessary for patient extrication, control bleeding with direct pressure around the impaling object, stabilize the object with bulky dressings, and immobilize the patient. Treat shock if present (p. 496). h. Puncture wound. Evaluate wound, elevate affected extremity, immobilize, and transport (pp. 496). i. Avulsion. Control bleeding, retrieve the avulsed tissue, wrap tissue in gauze that is dry or moistened with lactated Ringer's or saline solution (per local protocol), seal in plastic bag, and place sealed bag on crushed ice (pp. 496, 497). j. Degloving. Control bleeding, evaluate for hypovolemia, elevate head of stretcher, and determine whether mechanisms for cervical spine injury are present (p. 497). k. Amputation. Control bleeding, retrieve amputated tissue, and treat as for avulsion (pp. 497, 498).
12. Time of injury (risk of infection increases with time), environment where injury occurred, mechanism of injury, previous medical history, and location of injury (p. 499)
13. Scene survey; primary survey; history: time and mechanism of injury, past medical history, current medications, tetanus immunizations, pain, and blood loss before your arrival; and physical: pain, movement, sensation and capillary refill distal to injury, and inspection for location, depth, associated injuries, foreign bodies, bleeding, tissue loss, deformity, and crepitus (p. 499)
14. Thermal, electrical, chemical, and radiation (p. 499)
15. a. Zone of coagulation: nonviable tissue. b. Zone of stasis: seriously injured but potentially viable. (Cells will die if no supportive measures are taken within 24 hours.) c. Zone of hyperemia: increased blood flow caused by inflammatory response (will recover in 7 to 10 days if no shock or infection develops) (p. 500).
16. Chemical mediators cause increased capillary permeability and a fluid shift from the intravascular space to burned tissues. Also, the sodium pump in cell walls is damaged, and sodium moves into injured cells and increases swelling (pp. 500, 501).
17. a. Decreased venous return, decreased cardiac output, increased vascular resistance except in zone of hyperemia, hemolysis, and rhabdomyolysis that

may lead to renal failure. b. Increased respiratory rate to meet increased metabolic demands. c. Adynamic ileus, vomiting, and stress ulcer. d. Decreased range of motion resulting from edema and immobilization and osteoporosis and demineralization later. e. Increased circulating levels of epinephrine, norepinephrine, and aldosterone. f. Increased basal metabolic rate. g. Increased susceptibility to infection and depressed inflammatory response. h. Pain, isolation, and fear of disfigurement (p. 501).

18.

Depth	Extent	Severity	Burn Center?
a. Second degree	36%	Major	Yes
b. Second degree	22.5%	Moderate	Yes
c. Third degree	9%	Major (involves feet)	Yes (pp. 501-505)

19. Jacket that created an enclosed space and loss of consciousness (p. 509)

20. Facial burns, singed nasal hair, and carbonaceous sputum (p. 510)

21. Increased dyspnea, decreased level of consciousness, hoarseness, and stridor (p. 510)

22. Above the glottis. Mechanism of injury does not suggest injury below glottis (p. 510).

23. a. Put out the fire and cool the burn; Perform ABCDE; monitor vital signs; assess burn depth (third degree), extent (82%), and severity (major); perform a head-to-toe survey; assess lung sounds; and assess distal pulse, movement, sensation, and capillary refill in all extremities. b. Cool burn with clean water, open airway, intubate as necessary, ventilate with 100% oxygen, remove remaining clothing and jewelry, cover patient to maintain warmth, initiate lactated Ringer's solution intravenously at 820 ml/hr (2 ml/kg/%BSA burned 24 hr [half of daily fluid to be given in first 8 hr]) − 1640 ml/hr (4 ml/kg/%BSA burned 24 hr) in an unburned extremity, rapidly transport patient (p. 508).

24. a. Realize that the burns may swell and be associated with airway problems. Raise head of stretcher 30 degrees if spinal injury is not suspected. If the ears are burned, do not use a pillow. b. Remove jewelry, assess neurovascular status frequently, and elevate extremities. c. Monitor distal pulse, movement, sensation, and respirations and rapidly transport patient to the nearest appropriate facility (pp. 509).

25. a. Rust removers, bathroom cleaners, and swimming pool acidifiers. b. Drain cleaners, fertilizers, heavy industrial cleaners, and cement and concrete. c. Phenols, creosote, and gasoline (p. 511).

26. a. What type, concentration, and volume of chemical was involved? How did the injury occur? When did the injury occur? Was there any first aid given? Is there any pain? b. With gloved hands and protective clothing, brush most of the powder off and then irrigate profusely (use a shower if available) (p. 511).

27. a. Amperage, voltage, resistance, type of current, current pathway, and duration of current flow (p. 513); b. flow (intensity); c. force (tension); d. 1000 volts; e. resistivity, size of object pathway, length of object pathway, and temperature; f. bone; g. alternating and direct; h. one; i. industry; j. direction; k. freeze; l. least resistance; m. shortest; n. increase (p. 513)

28. Direct contact, arc, and flash (pp. 513, 514)

29. a. Direct contact can cause large areas of coagulation necrosis. The entry wound is often a characteristic "bull's-eye" (dry and leathery), and the exit is ulcerated and explosive (p. 514). b. Dysrhythmias and damage to myocardium may occur. Cardiac arrest is the most common cause of death after electrical injury. Hypertension secondary to increased catecholamine levels is common (p. 514). c. Central nervous system injury may result in coma, seizures, peripheral nerve injury and may lead to sensory or motor deficits. Brain stem injury may cause respiratory depression or arrest or cerebral edema or hemorrhage, which can lead to death (pp. 514, 515). d. Blood vessel necrosis may cause immediate or delayed hemorrhage or thrombosis (p. 515). e. Muscle injury may result in release of myoglobin, which can cause renal failure (p. 515). f. Acute renal failure occurs in 10% of significant electrical injuries (pp. 515). g. Patient may have decreased ventilation or respiratory arrest secondary to central nervous sytem injury or chest wall dysfunction (p. 515). h. Fractures and dislocations can result from direct electrical injury or injury secondary to fall or electrocution (p. 515). i. Burns to conjunctiva or cornea and ruptured tympanic membrane are common (p. 515).

30. a. Electrical source must be safely removed from the patient, preferably by interruption of power by the electric company. b. Perform cervical spine immobilization and ABCDEs. Determine patient's chief complaint, source of electricity, duration of exposure, level of consciousness before and after injury, and past medical history. Perform head-to-toe survey, looking for entry and exit burn wounds or trauma associated with fall. Assess distal pulse, movement, sensation, and capillary refill in all extremities and document. Monitor electrocardiographic rhythm. c. Immobilize cervical spine, open airway, apply 100% oxygen, assess the need to assist ventilations, remove all jewelry, initiate lactated Ringer's solution intravenously at 20 to 40 ml/kg, monitor the electrocardiogram, and maintain body warmth (pp. 515, 516).

31. Linear, feathery, pinpoint appearance (p. 516)

32. a. Consciousness, confusion, amnesia, and stable

vital signs. b. Combative affect, comatose patient, associated injuries from lightning strike, first- and second-degree burns, tympanic membrane rupture (common), and possible internal injuries. c. Immediate brain damage, seizures, respiratory paralysis, and cardiac arrest (pp. 516).

33. b. The dermis provides the vascular supply to the epidermis. The sebaceous glands are in the dermis. The subcutaneous tissue lies under the dermis (p. 486).
34. b. Aldosterone aids in body fluid regulation (p. 487).
35. c. All others are late findings (pp. 493).
36. b. The most common sites are below the knee and above the elbow (p. 493).
37. b. All other interventions could cause further damage (pp. 497).
38. b. Men die more frequently than women secondary to burns. Three fourths of burn fatalities occur in the home. Deaths are also common in low-income homes (p. 499).
39. d (p. 499)
40. c. Evaporation of fluid from the injured area also accounts for significant fluid loss (p. 501).
41. d. The patient hyperventilates to adapt to the increased metabolic rate. The gastroinestinal tract slows and, with large burns, adynamic ileus is a frequent complication (p. 501).
42. c. The burn should be rapidly cooled, and then body temperature is maintained with sheets (p. 508).
43. d. Oxygen saturation levels may be normal because the hemoglobin is still saturated (with carbon monoxide, not oxygen), and the oximeter may not differentiate between the two. Intravenous fluid therapy is not helpful in these patients (p. 510).
44. c. Drying the chemical or delaying treatment only prolongs contact with the skin and increases the burn injury. Application of a chemical antidote is recommended only for a few chemicals (p. 511).
45. b (p. 512)
46. d. An arc occurs when electrical energy "jumps" from its source through the air to another conductive medium. Direct burns result when the current passes through a person. *Alternating* is a description of a type of electrical current (p. 514).
47. a. All of the other pathological conditions can occur secondary to lightning injury but cause death less frequently than cardiac or respiratory arrest (p. 516).

● **DIVISION THREE REVIEW TEST**

1. a. Kinetic energy = Mass × Velocity$_2$, so increased speed will cause the greatest increase in energy. By increasing the stopping distance, energy will decrease, and the force of the impact will be less (p. 401).

2. a. All other answers are a concern; in fact, bleeding and edema may be causes of airway obstruction. However, the airway is the primary concern (p. 420).
3. a. Larger impaled objects should not be removed, but sand and other small foreign objects that have not penetrated the globe should be irrigated (p. 428).
4. b. Mastoid ecchymosis (Battle's sign) and periorbital ecchymosis (raccoon eyes) are signs of basilar skull fracture; however, they typically take several hours to become evident (p. 432).
5. b. Concussion does not involve structural damage to the brain. Epidural hematoma needs surgical evacuation. Increased intracranial pressure is a secondary complication of another injury that requires treatment to correct (p. 434).
6. d. Chronic subdural hematomas have a slow onset, and an older patient with head trauma is at increased risk for this injury (p. 437).
7. d (p. 444)
8. d. A relative bradycardia is more common in high spinal cord injury (p. 446).
9. c (p. 450)
10. d. Although the other measures will help prevent some of the poor mechanics associated with this injury, only positive-pressure ventilation will substantially improve ventilation (p. 462).
11. b. The other measures may be appropriate if removal of the dressing fails; however, this is the fastest method to correct the problem (p. 465).
12. a. Although the mechanism of injury is appropriate for myocardial contusion, the diminished femoral pulses suggest vascular injury. Hypotension would be present in neurogenic shock and tension pneumothorax (p. 469).
13. c. Neither tracheal deviation nor hypertension is present in pericardial tamponade (p. 468).
14. c. Battle's sign is mastoid ecchymosis accompanying basilar skull fracture, Cullen's sign is periumbilical discoloration suggesting intraabdominal bleeding. Kernig's sign is pain during flexion of the knee and hip because of meningeal irritation (p. 471).
15. b. The kidneys are the only retroperitoneal organs listed (p. 472).
16. b. A traction splint should be used to treat this painful injury (p. 479).
17. b (p. 418)
18. c. The skin receives sensory input, and the central nervous system interprets it (p. 487).
19. d. There is vasodilation, increased vascular permeability, and accumulation of plasma in the interstitial space (p. 488).
20. c (p. 489)
21. a. Potassium is contraindicated, since potassium levels are typically high because of cellular disruption. Body temperature should be maintained at a normal level (p. 495).

22. a (p. 498)

23. d. The cells in this area are ischemic and will die if aggressive intervention is not provided. Cells in the zone of coagulation are already unsalvageable, and cells of the zone of hyperemia will likely heal spontaneously unless complicated by severe shock or infection (p. 500).

24. b. First-degree burns are dry and red, with good capillary refill. Third-degree burns are white or charred and leathery, without capillary refill (p. 502).

25. c. Each leg is worth 14% in children, according to the rule of nines (pp. 504).

26. c. 2 ml × 100 kg × 60(%) = 12,000 ml in first 24 hours. Give half of the total requirement in the first 8 hr = 12,000 ÷ 2 = 6000 (first 8 hours). Each hour in first 8 hours = 6000 ÷ 8 = 750 ml (p. 506).

27. a (p. 509)

28. c (pp. 511)

29. d. The most difficult tissue for electrical energy to traverse is bone (p. 514).

● CHAPTER 17
RESPIRATORY DISORDERS

1. c (p. 522)

2. a (p. 521)

3. e (p. 529)

4. j (p. 529)

5. b (p. 525)

6. g (p. 531)

7. i (p. 530)

8. f (p. 523)

9. h (p. 531)

10. a. Adult respiratory distress syndrome. b. Monitor the chest rising and falling to determine the effectiveness of ventilation; note any difficulty or increasing pressure necessary to ventilate patient; frequently assess vital signs, observing for increased heart rate; monitor electrocardiogram and oxygen saturation by pulse oximetry; and observe for cyanosis. Ventilate with high-flow oxygen, ventilate with positive end-expiratory pressure using Boehringer valve if trained and authorized by medical direction, and administer steroids and diuretics if ordered by medical direction (pp. 521, 522).

11. a. Pulmonary arteries become vasoconstricted secondary to changes of chronic obstructive pulmonary disease. The right ventricle must contract more forcefully to overcome the resulting increased pressure in the pulmonary arteries. Eventually, this increased work causes hypertrophy of the right ventricle and right ventricular failure. b. Hypertrophy and dilation of the right ventricle secondary to obstructive lung disease, restrictive lung disease, and vascular disease (p. 523).

12. a. "Blue bloater," chronic cough with production of large amount of sputum, hypercapnia, hypoxemia, cyanosis, pulmonary hypertension, and cor pulmonale. b. "Pink puffer," hyperexpansion of lungs, barrel chest, resistance to air flow (especially on expiration), pulsed lip breathing, and thinness (p. 523)

13. Oxygen should be administered initially at 2 L/min if the patient is not in respiratory failure. If continued deterioration occurs, the flow of oxygen may be increased while the paramedic carefully monitors the patient. If the patient's condition is critical, intubation and assisted ventilation may be necessary (p. 525).

14. Albuterol (Proventil) or aminophylline (p. 525).

15. Transport patient in a position of comfort, instruct patient to use pursed-lip breathing and minimize physical activity to conserve energy for breathing, calmly reassure and care for the patient, and provide a cool environment for transport (p. 525).

16. Albuterol 0.5 ml (2.5 mg) in 2.5 ml normal saline by nebulizer at 6 to 7 L/min O_2; epinephrine 0.3 to 0.5 ml (1:1000 solution) subcutaneously (pp. 923-924)

17. Ask the patient if his breathing is easier. Observe the patient for decreased anxiety, changes in level of consciousness, and ability to converse more easily. Note the degree of respiratory distress by observing patient position, use of accessory muscles, and respiratory rate. Monitor vital signs. (Pulse and respiratory rate should decrease, and pulsus paradoxis should decline to below 20 mm Hg. As the patient improves, first the inspiratory and then expiratory wheezes should disappear.) (p. 527)

18. Status asthmaticus (p. 528)

19. Ensure that oxygen is at 100% and is humidified, increase fluid rate to hydrate patient, administer other medications as ordered by medical direction, expedite transport, monitor patient closely for signs of respiratory failure, and prepare to intubate if necessary (p. 528).

20. Asthma, chronic obstructive pulmonary disease, heart failure, pulmonary edema, pulmonary embolism, bronchiolitis (infants), foreign body aspiration, toxic inhalation, and cystic fibrosis (p. 528)

21. Airway management, high-flow oxygen, bronchodilators as ordered by medical direction, and intravenous therapy (p. 529)

22. Extended travel; prolonged bed rest; obesity; older adulthood; burns; varicose veins; surgery of the thorax, abdomen, pelvis, and legs; pelvic or leg fractures; malignancy; use of birth control pills; pregnancy; chronic obstructive pulmonary disease; congestive heart failure; atrial fibrillation; myocardial infarction; previous pulmonary embolism; deep vein thrombosis; infection; diabetes mellitus; and multiple trauma (p. 530)

23. Cough, hemoptysis, pain, anxiety, syncope, hypotension, diaphoresis, increased respiratory rate, increased heart rate, fever, distended neck veins, chest splinting, pleuritic chest pain, pleural friction rub, crackles, and wheezes (localized) (p. 530)

24. Airway management, oxygen, preparation to assist ventilations if necessary, monitoring of vital signs, electrocardiogram, and pulse oximetry (p. 531)

25. Chronic obstructive lung disease, immune deficiency, malnourishment, older adulthood, infant, and exposure to infected persons (p. 531)

26. a. Inflammation; b. tuberculosis, lung tumor, pulmonary embolism, rib fractures, and pulmonary contusions; c. sharp (sudden, increases with respirations); d. chest wall or back; e. shoulder (pp. 531, 532)

27. a. Cough, fever, headache, myalgia, and mild sore throat; b. inhaled mucus droplets; c. bacterial pneumonia (p. 532)

28. a. Bacterial; b. water (natural and synthetic systems); c. bacterial pneumonia; d. renal failure, septicemia, and respiratory failure (p. 535)

29. Viral, bacterial, mycoplasma, and aspiration (pp. 532-534)

30. Shaking chills, tachypnea, tachycardia, cough with sputum (rust colored, hemoptysis, yellow, green, grey), malaise, anorexia, flank or back pain, vomiting, and fever (pp. 534-535)

31. Airway support, oxygen, ventilatory assistance if necessary, intravenous fluid administration, electrocardiographic monitoring, pulse oximetry, suctioning as necessary if the condition is aspiration pneumonia, and transport to hospital for definitive care (pp. 534, 535)

32. Homeless persons, migrants, persons with human immunodeficiency virus, and persons in correctional facilities (p. 535)

33. Fever, night sweats, malaise, weight loss, and cough with sputum (green-yellow). Advanced stages: dyspnea, hemoptysis, and respiratory failure (p. 536).

34. There is no classic symptom. The paramedic should wear personal protective measures when transporting *any* patient who has a respiratory illness of unknown cause (p. 536).

35. a. Right heart failure can develop secondary to pulmonary hypertension (cor pulmonale). The right side of the heart is increasingly forced to pump harder to overcome the excess pressure in the pulmonary arteries. Eventually, it cannot force the blood through, and fluid backs up to the venous side of the system (p. 523).

36. d (pp. 523)

37. c. The patient is more likely to be tachycardic than bradycardic. Capillary refill is an indicator of perfusion (flow), not oxygenation (p. 524).

38. c. This is an exocrine gland disease that causes excess production of thick mucus in the lungs and other organs (p. 529).

39. b. Both of these syndromes involve interference with normal nerve transmission that can lead to weakness or paralysis of the muscles of respiration and respiratory failure, respiratory arrest, or both (p. 531).

40. c. Atelectasis is collapse of the alveoli. Bronchitis is inflammation of the bronchi. Pneumonia is an inflammatory process of the respiratory bronchioles and alveolar spaces caused by infection (p. 531).

41. b. Immunization is the only intervention listed that can prevent influenza; however, there are often new strains of influenza, so the vaccine does not guarantee complete protection (p. 532).

42. b. Tuberculosis is most commonly found in the lung; however, it may also infect other organs. Hemoptysis is seen only in advanced stages of the disease. Symptoms may not appear for months or years (p. 535).

● CHAPTER 18
CARDIOVASCULAR EMERGENCIES

1. c (p. 544)
2. f (p. 543)
3. a (p. 544)
4. e (p. 543)
5. b (p. 544)
6. g (p. 544)
7. h (p. 543)
8. False. The strength of contractions can be indirectly measured in the field only by pulse quality and blood pressure (p. 557).
9.

	Sympathetic	Parasympathetic
a.	Increase	Decrease
b.	Increase	No effect
c.	Beta-bronchiolar dilation	Constriction
d.	Constriction	No effect (p. 545; also refer to Chapters 10 and 14)

10. a. Epinephrine: increased heart rate, contractility, bronchiolar dilation, and blood vessel constriction in skin, kidneys, gastrointestinal tract, and viscera. b. Norepinephrine: peripheral vasoconstriction (p. 545).

11. a. Magnetic; b. potential; c. permeable; d. potential; e. millivolts; f. negative; g. negatively; h. potential; i. negative; j. −90 mV; k. potassium; l. potassium; m. proteins; n. permeable; o. excitability; p. depolarization; q. threshold potential; r. action potential; s. depolarization; t. repolarization; u. positive; v. negative; w. depolarization; x. membrane potential (pp. 546, 547)

12. a. Sodium rushes into the cell through the fast sodium channels (p. 551). b. The membrane potential drops to approximately 0 (p. 551). c. The slow

calcium channels allow calcium to enter the cell while potassium continues to leave, maintaining the membrane potential of 0 (p. 552). d. The membrane potential returns to −90 mV (p. 552). e. The sodium pump allows the exchange of sodium and potassium to their proper compartments (p. 552). f. During phase 4, cardiac pacemaker cells slowly depolarize from their most negative membrane potential to a level at which threshold is reached and phase 0 begins. Cells other than pacemaker cells maintain a stable resting membrane potential and do not depolarize unless stimulated by a sufficiently strong stimulus (p. 552).

13. a. Action potentials; b. upward; c. automaticity; d. resting membrane potential (p. 557)

14. a. Sinoatrial node; b. intranodal pathways; c. Purkinje fibers; d. right bundle branch; e. left posterior bundle branch; f. common bundle of His; g. left anterior bundle branch; h. atrioventricular node (pp. 554, 555)

15. The next pacemaker (atrioventricular node) should take over and fire (p. 554).

16. a. Acceleration of phase 4 depolarization so that cells reach their threshold prematurely (may result from digoxin toxicity, increased catecholamine levels, hypoxia, hypercapnia, myocardial ischemia, infarction, increased venous return, hypokalemia, hypocalcemia, heating or cooling of the heart, or atropine administration). b. Reactivation of tissue by a returning impulse (p. 555).

17. (p. 558)

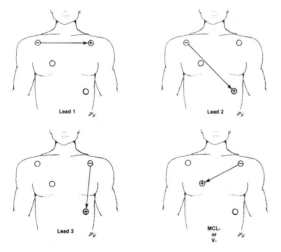

18. Excessive body hair: shave; diaphoresis: dry area and apply tincture of benzoin; poor electrode placement: reapply correctly; 60-cycle interference: run monitor on batteries; and poor cable connections: recheck all connections (p. 562).

19. a. 5 mm; b. 0.04 sec; c. 0.20 sec; d. 3 sec; e. 6 sec (p. 562)

20. a. P wave; b. QRS complex; c. T wave; d. PR interval; e. ST segment (pp. 563-566)

21. Muscle tremor, AC (60-cycle interference), loose electrodes, patient movement, loss of electrode contact, and external chest compression (p. 566)

22. Analyze the rate (p. 567); analyze the rhythm (p. 569); analyze the QRS complex (p. 572); analyze the P waves (p. 573); analyze the PR interval (p. 574).

23. a. Triplicate method (120/min): Find the R wave on the dark line, count 300-150-100-75 for each next dark line until the next R wave. The R wave falls between 100 and 150. Estimate rate to be 120/min (p. 567). b. R-R method: 300 ÷ Number of large boxes between R waves = 300 ÷ (almost) 3 = 100/min (p. 568). c. R-R method: 1500 ÷ Number of small boxes between R waves = 1500 ÷ 13 = 115/min (p. 568). d. 6-second method: 120/min number of R waves in a 6-second strip × 10 = 12 × 10 = 120/min (p. 559).

24. This reveals only the rate, not the perfusion status (p. 569).

25. a. R-R method (1500 ÷ Number of small boxes between the R waves) or triplicate method (but only if R waves both fall on dark lines). b. The 6-second method is the most accurate and quick estimate for irregular rhythm (p. 568).

26. The R-R distance should be equal when measured left to right across an ECG strip (can vary no greater than 0.16 sec) (p. 569).

27. a. Conduction through the ventricles is normal. b. Conduction through the ventricles is delayed and may follow an abnormal pathway (p. 572).

28. Are they regular? Is there a P wave in front of each QRS? Are they upright or inverted? Do they all look the same (p. 573)?

29. a. Electrical impulse progressed from the atria to the ventricles through pathways other than the atrioventricular node of the bundle of His. b. Normal conduction from the sinoatrial node through the atrioventricular node. c. Delay in conduction of impulse through the atrioventricular node or bundle of His (p. 574).

30. a. Rate: 75/min. (triplicate method). b. Rhythm: regular (R-R intervals =). c. QRS: 0.08 sec (normal is less than 0.12 sec). d. P waves: regular, one for each QRS complex, upright, all the same. e. PR interval 0.14 sec. Interpretation: normal sinus rhythm (p. 575).

31. Patient history, chief complaint, and physical findings (p. 576)

32. a. Parasympathetic stimulation; b. QRS less than 0.12 sec. (unless a conduction delay is present); c. P waves (regular, preceding each QRS, upright, similar); d. PRI 0.12 to 0.20 sec (p. 577).

33. a. Sinus node disease, increased parasympathetic vagal tone, hypothermia, hypoxia, and drug effects (digitalis, propranolol, verapamil). b. Exercise, fever, anxiety, ingestion of stimulants, smoking, hypovolemia, anemia, congestive heart failure, and excessive administration of atropine or vagolytic

or sympathomimetic drugs (cocaine, phencyclidine, epinephrine, isoproterenol) (p. 577)

34. Rate: 50/min. Rhythm: regular. QRS: 0.08 sec. P waves: present, upright, similar. PR interval: 0.16 sec. Interpretation: sinus bradycardia. Distinguishing features: all features of normal sinus rhythm except that rate is less than 60/min. Treatment: stable—monitor; unstable—atropine 0.5 to 1.0 mg every 5 min to a maximum dose of 0.04 mg/kg, transcutaneous pacing, dopamine 5 to 20 mcg/kg/min, epinephrine 2 to 10 mcg/min, AND isoproterenol 2 to 10 mcg/min (p. 577).

35. Rate: 110/min. Rhythm: regular. QRS: 0.06 sec. P waves: present, upright, similar. PR interval: 0.16 sec. Interpretation: sinus tachycardia. Distinguishing features: all features of normal sinus rhythm except that rate is greater than 100/min. Treatment: stable—none; unstable—seek and treat underlying cause (p. 579).

36. Rate: 70/min. Rhythm: irregular. QRS: 0.08 sec; P waves: present, upright, similar. PR interval: 0.12 sec. Interpretation: sinus dysrhythmia. Distinguishing features: All features of normal sinus rhythm but irregular rhythm that varies in cycles. Treatment: none (p. 581).

37. Rate: 50/min. Rhythm: irregular. QRS: 0.08 sec. P waves: normal, upright. PR interval: 0.16 sec. Interpretation: sinus arrest. Distinguishing features: Normal sinus rhythm until the sinoatrial node fails to fire. Treatment: stable—observe; unstable—atropine and transcutaneous pacing (p. 581).

38. a. Tissues; b. atria; c. internodal (p. 584)

39. a. QRS: normal; b. P waves (if present): different from normal sinus P waves; c. PR interval: abnormal, shortened or prolonged (p. 584)

40. Stress, overexertion, tobacco, caffeine, Wolff-Parkinson-White syndrome, digoxin toxicity, hypoxia, cor pulmonale, congestive heart failure, damage to sinoatrial node, rheumatic heart disease, and atherosclerotic heart disease (p. 584)

41. Rate: 75/min. Rhythm: Regular. QRS: 0.06 sec. P waves: changes from beat to beat. PR interval: variable. Interpretation: wandering atrial pacemaker. Distinguishing features: typically slightly irregular P-wave shapes and variable PR interval. Treatment: stable—monitor; unstable secondary to bradycardia—treat as bradycardia (p. 585).

42. Rate: 100/min. Rhythm: regular interrupted by premature beats. QRS: 0.06 sec. P waves: present, upright. PR interval: 0.10 sec (premature atrial contraction 0.16 sec). Interpretation: normal sinus rhythm with one premature atrial contraction. Distinguishing features: extra beat occurring earlier than next expected sinus beat; premature atrial contraction has features of sinus beat except that PR interval may be different. Treatment: none (p. 585).

43. Rate: 180/min. Rhythm: regular. QRS: 0.06 sec.

P waves: unable to determine, may be hidden in T wave. PR interval: unable to determine. Interpretation: supraventricular tachycardia. Distinguishing features: rate greater than 150/min, with complexes originating in atria, (QRS complex is narrow unless a conduction defect is present.) Treatment: stable—oxygen, intravenous line, consideration of vagal maneuvers, adenosine (6 mg, 12 mg, 12 mg at 1- to 2-minute intervals), verapamil (2.5 to 5.0 mg over 2 min [may repeat once at a dose of 5.0 to 10 mg in 15 to 30 min]), and consideration of digoxin, beta blockers, and diltiazem; unstable—sychronized cardioversion at 50, 100, 200, 300, and 360 joules (p. 587).

44. Rate: 100/min. Rhythm: regular. QRS: 0.06 sec. P waves: f-R waves. PR interval: none. FR interval: may vary. Interpretation: atrial flutter with 3:1 conduction. Distinguishing features: flutter waves. Treatment: stable—diltiazem, beta blockers, verapamil, digoxin, procainamide, and quinidine; unstable—synchronized cardioversion at 50, 100, 200, 300, and 360 J (p. 590).

45. Rate: 160/min. Rhythm: irregularly irregular. QRS: 0.06 sec. P waves: none. PR interval: none. Interpretation: atrial fibrillation. Distinguishing features: irregularly irregular, no P waves, fibrillation waves. Treatment: chronic—digitalis or calcium channel or beta blocker; acute but not seriously hemodynamically unstable—beta blockers and calcium channel blockers (verapamil, diltiazem); acute and associated with serious signs or symptoms—synchronized cardioversion at 100, 200, 300, and 360 joules (p. 592).

46. a. Junctional (nodal); b. QRS: normal; c. P waves: may occur before, during, or after QRS or may be absent; inverted in lead II. d. PR interval: often less than 0.12 sec (p. 594).

47. Increased vagal tone on sinoatrial node, pathological slowing of sinoatrial discharge, complete atrioventricular block, digitalis toxicity, damage to the atrioventricular junction, inferior-wall myocardial infarction, and rheumatic fever (p. 594)

48. Rate: 60/min. Rhythm: irregular. QRS: 0.08 sec. P waves: present, right, similar in underlying rhythm, absent in premature beats. PR interval: 0.16 sec (underlying rhythm), none in premature beats. Interpretation: sinus rhythm (borderline bradycardia) with two premature junctional contractions. Distinguishing features: premature beats occurring earlier than next expected sinus beat, lack of P waves, QRS complex within normal limits. Treatment: monitor patient and treat bradycardia if it is present and symptomatic (p. 594).

49. Rate: 40/min. Rhythm: regular. QRS: 0.08 sec. P waves: absent. PR interval: none. Interpretation: junctional escape rhythm. Distinguishing features: rate 40 to 60/min, inverted P waves if present

(may occur before, during [absent] or after QRS complex). Treatment: stable—monitor; unstable—atropine 0.5 to 1.0 mg every 5 min to max dose of 0.04 mg/kg, transcutaneous pacing, dopamine 5 to 20 mcg/kg/min, epinephrine 2 to 10 mcg/min, and isoproterenol 2 to 10 mcg/min (p. 595).

50. Rate: 80/min. Rhythm: regular. QRS: 0.08 sec. P waves: absent. PR interval: none. Interpretation: accelerated junctional rhythm. Distinguishing features: Rate 60 to 100/min, inverted P waves in lead II if present (may be absent or occur before, during, or after QRS complex). Treatment: monitor (p. 597).

51. a. 20 to 40; b. 100/min; c. 100/min (pp. 598, 599)

52. Failure of higher pacemakers, heart block, myocardial ischemia, hypoxia, acid-base or electrolyte imbalance, congestive heart failure, increased catecholamine levels, use of stimulants, medicine toxicity (digitalis, tricyclic antidepressant overdose), sympathomimetic drugs, cardiac trauma, and electrocution (p. 598)

53. Rate: 40/min. Rhythm: regular. QRS: 0.16 sec. P waves: absent. PR interval: none. Interpretation: ventricular escape rhythm. Distinguishing features: rate 20 to 40/min, absent P waves, QRS complex greater than 0.12 sec. Treatment: oxygen, atropine 0.5 to 1.0 mg every 5 min to a maximum dose of 0.04 mg/kg (class III recommendation in third-degree atrioventricular block), transcutaneous pacing, dopamine 5 to 20 mcg/kg/min, epinephrine 2 to 10 mcg/min, isoproterenol 2 to 10 mcg/min; if pulseless, treat as PEA (p. 600).

54. Rate: 75. Rhythm: regular interrupted by premature beats. QRS: underlying rhythm 0.10 sec. Premature beat: 0.16 sec. P wave: present, upright, except premature beat). PR interval: 0.16 (underlying rhythm). None: premaure beat. Interpretation: normal sinus rhythm with one premature ventricualr contraction. Distinguishing features: Ectopic beat occurs earlier than next expected sinus beat, wide bizarre QRS complex with T wave deflection opposite QRS complex, no P waves, compensatory pause. Treatment: In the absence of heart disease—no treatment; in presence of heart disease—oxygen, lidocaine 1.0 to 1.5 mg/kg repeated at 0.5- to 0.75-mg doses to a maximum of 3 mg/kg, procainamide 20 to 30 mg/min to maximum dose of 17 mg/kg (or until QRS widens by 50% or hypotension occurs), and bretylium 5 mg/kg intravenously over 8 to 10 min (p. 601).

55. Rate: 230/min. Rhythm: regular. QRS: 0.20 sec. P waves: absent. PR interval: none. Interpretation: ventricular tachycardia. Distinguishing features: rate greater than 100/min (usually greater than 150/min), regular, no p waves, QRS greater than 0.12 sec. Treatment: asymptomatic—oxygen, lidocaine, and procainamide; chest pain or dyspnea—

brief trial of lidocaine and synchronized cardioversion at 100, 200, 300, and 360 J; unconsciousness, hypotension, or pulmonary edema—unsynchronized cardioversion at 100, 200, 300, and 360 J; pulseless—treat as ventricular fibrillation (p. 606).

56. Rate: none. Rhythm: none, chaotic. QRS: none. P waves: none. PR interval: none. Interpretation: ventricular fibrillation. Distinguishing features: no organized rhythm, chaotic fibrillatory waves. Treatment: rapid defibrillation at 200, 300, and 360 J; cardiopulmonary resuscitation, intubation, epinephrine, lidocaine, bretylium, magnesium sulfate, and procainamide (p. 610).

57. Rate: none. Rhythm: none. QRS: none. P waves: none. PR interval: none. Interpretation: asystole. Distinguishing features: isoelectric rhythm. Treatment: cardiopulmonary resuscitation, transcutaneous pacing, epinephrine, atropine, and consideration of underlying cause (p. 611).

58. Rate: 80/min. Rhythm: regular. QRS: 0.16 sec. P waves: absent. PR interval: none. Interpretation: ventricular paced rhythm. Distinguishing features: pacemaker spike followed by wide- complex ventricular beat. Treatment: none (p. 614).

59. a. Heart blocks; b. conduction system (p. 616)

60. Myocardial ischemia, acute myocardial infarction, increased parasympathetic tone, drug toxicity (digitalis, propranolol, verapamil), and electrolyte imbalance (p. 616)

61. Rate: 60/min. Rhythm: regular. QRS: 0.06 sec. P waves: present, upright. PR interval: 0.32 sec. Interpretation: sinus rhythm with first-degree atrioventricular block. Distinguishing features: PR interval greater than 0.20 sec. Treatment: Monitor (p. 618).

62. Rate: 60/min. Rhythm: irregular. QRS: 0.08 sec. P waves: present, upright, more P waves than QRS complexes. PR interval: progressively longer until one is not conducted. Distinguishing features: more P waves than QRS complexes, progressively lengthens PR interval until a QRS complex is dropped. Interpretation: second-degree atrioventricular block (Mobitz type I or Wenckebach). Treatment: asymptomatic—observe; hemodynamic compromise—oxygen, atropine, transcutaneous pacing, dopamine, epinephrine, and isoproterenol (p. 618).

63. Rate: 50/min. Rhythm: irregular. QRS: 0.06 sec. P waves: present, upright, more P waves than QRS complexes. PR interval: 0.16 for conducted P waves. Interpretation: second-degree heart block (Mobitz type II). Treatment: stable—transport for transvenous pacemaker insertion; unstable—oxygen, transcutaneous pacing, atropine (class III recommendation for new-onset Mobitz type II with new onset with wide

QRS complexes), dopamine, epinephrine, and isoproterenol (p. 619).

64. Rate: 50/min. Rhythm: regular. QRS: 0.08 sec. P waves: present, upright. PR interval: no relationship between P waves and QRS complexes. Interpretation: third-degree (complete) heart block. Distinguishing features: R-R interval usually regular, more P waves than QRS complexes, no relationship between P waves and QRS complex. Treatment: stable—monitor and transport for transvenous pacemaker insertion; unstable—oxygen, transcutaneous pacing, atropine 0.5 to 1.0 mg (maximum dose 0.04 mg /kg [class III recommendation for new-onset third-degree atrioventricular block]), dopamine 5 to 20 mcg/kg/min, epinephrine 2 to 10 mcg/min, and isoproterenol 2 to 10 mcg/min (p. 622).

65. P—Is there anything that makes the pain better or worse? Q—What does the pain feel like? (Is it sharp, dull, crushing, squeezing?) R—Where is the pain? Does it go anywhere else? S—On a scale of 1 to 10, with 1 being no pain and 10 being the worst pain you have ever had, describe your pain. T—When did you first feel the pain (p. 633)?

66. Chest pain, dyspnea, syncope, or palpitations (p. 633)

67. How did you feel right before you passed out? What were you doing when you passed out? How long was the patient unconscious? Cardiac history, other significant medical history, current medicines, associated symptoms, and health over past several days (pp. 633, 634).

68. Pulse rate and regularity, ECG, vital signs, circumstances of occurrence, duration, associated symptoms, previous history of palpitations, past medical history, and daily medicines (pp. 633, 634)

69. Major medical illnesses, home medicines, and previous episodes like this (pp. 633, 634)

70. Atrial fibrillation with a slow ventricular response (p. 593)

71. Yes. Digoxin (Lanoxin) or calcium channel blocker (Cardizem) toxicity can cause this presentation. Digitalis toxicity is more likely in the patient who is also taking a diuretic (furosemide) (pp. 633, 634).

72. Neck: jugular venous distention. Chest: implanted pacemaker generator, median sternotomy scar, lung sounds (crackles), heart sounds (S3 gallop), and pulse deficit. Abdomen: generator for automatic implantable cardioverter defibrillator visible. Extremities: edema and ulceration. Back: sacral edema. Medical alert tags or medical information in wallet (p. 635).

73. a. Male gender, family history, and diabetes mellitus. b. Smoking, obesity, hypertension, and hypercholesterolemia (p. 636).

74. Unless 12-lead ECG interpretation is available, it will not be possible to distinguish between these two conditions in the field. Both patients should be managed as if they are having a myocardial infarction (excluding thrombolytic therapy) (p. 637).

75. Atherosclerotic plaque forms in coronary artery; thrombus forms on the plaque; as thrombus enlarges, it occludes the coronary artery. (Other causes are coronary vasospasm, coronary embolism, severe hypoxia, hemorrhage into diseased arterial wall, and shock.) (p. 638)

76. Lethal dysrhythmias, congestive heart failure, pulmonary edema, cardiogenic shock, and myocardial tissue rupture (p. 639)

77. Nausea; vomiting; diaphoresis; radiation of pain to the neck, jaw, arm, or back; palpitations; dyspnea; and a sense of impending doom (pp. 639, 640)

78. Normal sinus rhythm with multifocal premature ventricular contractions (pp. 603-605)

79. Administer oxygen via nasal cannula, minimize physical activity, monitor ECG and oxygen saturation (if pulse oximetry is available), assess vital signs frequently (including lung sounds for crackles), and establish an intravenous line to keep the vein open with normal saline or lactated Ringer's solution (pp. 640, 641).

80. Nitroglycerin 0.4 mg sublingually, repeated 3 times; morphine sulfate 2 to 5 mg intravenously titrated to relieve pain (pp. 641, 642)

81. 80 kg × 1.5 mg/kg = 120 mg
$$\frac{120 \text{ mg} \times 10 \text{ ml}}{100 \text{ mg}} = 12 \text{ ml (p. 358)}$$

82. 0.75 mg/kg (p. 582)

83. 6 ml (p. 358)

84. Infuse a maintenance lidocaine drip at 2 mg/min (p. 639-641).

85. a. Left ventricular failure leading to pulmonary edema and possible myocardial infarction (p. 643)

86. Pulmonary edema: orthopnea and frothy blood—tinged sputum. Myocardial infarction: chest pain, radiation of pain, nausea, and vomiting (p. 643)

87. Sinus tachycardia with frequent premature atrial contractions (pp. 642, 643)

88.

Drug	Dose	Desired Effect
Furosemide	20 to 80 mg intravenously	Venodilation and diuresis
Morphine	2 to 5 mg intravenously	Venodilation, decreased myocardial work, and decreased anxiety
Nitroglycerine	0.4 mg sublingually	Peripheral vasodilation and decreased preload and afterload
Nifedipine	10 mg sublingually (or have patient bite and) swallow	Peripheral vasodilation and decreased preload and afterload (p. 645)

89. 3.5 ml (p. 358)
90. a. Left heart failure, congestive heart failure, pulmonary embolism, right ventricle infarct, chronic hypertension, chronic obstructive pulmonary disease and valvular disease. b. Jugular venous distention, tachycardia, enlarged liver or spleen, peripheral and sacral edema, and ascites (p. 645).
91. Sinus bradycardia (pp. 577, 578)
92. Atropine 0.5 mg intravenously (p. 579)
93. Cardiogenic shock (p. 646)
94. High-flow oxygen by nonrebreather mask, supine position (if tolerated), intravenous therapy with normal saline to keep the vein open (consider fluid challenge of 250 to 500 ml in consultation with medical direction if no signs of pulmonary edema are present), dopamine infusion via intravenous piggyback 2.5 to 20 mcg/kg/min, and monitor ECG for dysrhythmias (pp. 646).
95. Expanding or ruptured abdominal aortic aneurysm (p. 648)
96. Palpation in this situation could cause a bulging aneurysm to rupture. If medical direction advises palpation, it should be done very gently (p. 648).
97. No. Increased intraabdominal pressure could cause rupture of the aneurysm (p. 648).
98. Administer oxygen, transport rapidly, apply pneumatic antishock garments (if indicated by protocol) but do not inflate unless the patient's condition deteriorates, initiate two large-bore intravenous lines en route and infuse normal saline or lactated Ringer's solution at a slow rate unless the patient's condition deteriorates (pp. 646-648).
99. Dissecting thoracic aortic aneurysm (pp. 648)
100. Unequal peripheral pulses, neurological deficit, or signs of pericardial tamponade (p. 649)
101. Minimize movement and anxiety, administer high-concentration oxygen, initiate a 14- or 16-gauge intravenous line in arm with good pulses (higher blood pressure) to keep the vein open, and monitor vital signs and the ECG frequently (pp. 648-650).
102.

	Embolic	Thrombotic
Causes	Clot breaks loose and travels to narrow area in blood vessel.	Clot develops at narrow spot in blood vessel.
Onset	Rapid	Gradual
Signs and symptoms	Pulseless extremity pain; decreased motor and sensory function; pallor; decreased skin temperature distal to the occlusion; decreased capillary refill; possible shock	Pain in hips, lower limbs, buttocks, leg, and abdomen (depends on affected artery); pain; decreased motor and sensory function; pallor; decreased skin temperature distal to the occlusion; decreased CR; possible shock (p. 650)

103. Control bleeding with direct pressure and elevation. The bleeding may be persistent and require hospital management (p. 653).
104. Pain, edema, warmth, erythema, tenderness, and a palpable cord (p. 654)
105. Hypertensive encephalopathy (p. 655)
106. Aphasia, hemiparesis, transient blindness, seizures, stupor, coma, and death (pp. 655)
107. Calm patient, apply oxygen and intravenous D5W to keep the vein open, monitor ECG, and transport rapidly (p. 655).
108. Nifedipine 10 mg: ask patient to bite and swallow or administer by rupturing capsule and administer sublingually (p. 655).
109. Determine unresponsiveness; go and call for help if no one else is available; look, listen, and feel for breathing; if there is none, deliver two rescue breaths; assess carotid pulse; if there is none, begin cardiopulmonary resuscitation until help arrives (pp. 656).
110. a. After intubation, intravenous therapy, and the first dose of epinephrine. b. Yes. Electric shock resulting in injury or death can occur (pp. 658).
111. Ventricular tachycardia (pp. 606, 607)
112. Defibrillate with 200 J (then 300 and 360 J if the rhythm is the same) and then reassess the rhythm and pulse (p. 609).
113. Amount of time patient has been in pulseless ventricular tachycardia (success decreases with time with bystander cardiopulmonary resuscitation), conductive gel applied to paddles, and proper paddle placement (p. 659)
114. Apply conductive gel on the patient's chest (or hands-off defibrillation patches); turn power on (on some monitors, there is a separate power source for the defibrillator and monitor); select correct energy level; charge the defibrillator; place paddles in an appropriate position on the patients chest; call "Clear" and visually check to ensure that no one is in contact with the patient or cot; lean firmly on paddles with 20 to 25 lb of pressure; discharge both paddle buttons simultaneously (or depress discharge button on monitor for hands-off defibrillator); and reassess pulse and rhythm (p. 660)
115. Unsynchronized cardioversion at 100, 200, 300, 360 joules; lidocaine 1.0 to 1.5 mg/kg; cardioversion at 360 joules; lidocaine 0.5 to 0.75 mg/kg, cardioversion at 360 joules, and repeat lidocaine to a maximum dose of 3 mg/kg (pp. 608, 582).
116. It is synchronized with the patient's heart beat, so there is less risk of firing on the relative refractory period and causing ventricular fibrillation (p. 662).
117. Depress the synchronize button before each

synchronized shock and hold the paddles firmly on the chest after activation until they discharge (pp. 662).

118. a. Third-degree atrioventricular block. b. Inform the patient that he may feel some discomfort; apply the pacing and monitoring pads; ensure adequate upright R wave on monitor; select pacing mode; select pacing rate (some sources say 20/min greater than patient's intrinsic rate, but commonly it is 70/min); set current (mA) at minimum and slowly increase until capture is observed; increase mA 10 milliamps above minimum energy required to cause capture; reassess patient's vital signs (use right arm for blood pressure); and document (pp. 663).

119. a. Pulseless electrical activity (the patient has a rhythm but no perfusing pulse). b. Cardiopulmonary resuscitation, intubation, intravenous therapy, epinephrine 1.0 mg every 3 to 5 min; consideration of causes (pulmonary embolus, acidosis, tension pneumothorax, cardiac tamponade, hypovolemia, hypoxemia, hypothermia, hyperkalemia, massive myocardial infarction, drug overdose) and treatment if causes are found; if rate is less than 60/min, administer atropine 1 mg every 5 min to a maximum dose of 0.04 mg/kg (p. 602).

120. a. Asystole; b. epinephrine 1.0 mg every 3 to 5 min and atropine 1 mg every 5 min until a maximum dose of 0.04 mg/kg is reached; c. transcutaneous pacing (p. 613)

121. a. Ventricular fibrillation; b. defibrillation; c. epinephrine 1.0 mg every 3 to 5 min, lidocaine 1.5 mg/kg repeated once, bretylium 5 mg/kg intravenously repeated in 5 min at 10 mg/kg, magnesium sulfate 1 to 2 g intravenously, and procainamide 30 mg/min to a maximum dose of 17 mg/kg (p. 609)

122. d. Adenosine is not indicated for atrial fibrillation, and verapamil is not indicated when a patient is hypotensive. The patient needs electrical cardioversion because her condition is unstable. Procainamide is indicated for ventricular dysrhythmias (p. 593).

123. c (p. 544)

124. b. Aortic valve separates the aorta and left ventricle, the pulmonic valve separates the pulmonary arteries and right ventricle, and the tricuspid valve separates the right atrium and right ventricle (pp. 542).

125. b (p. 635)

126. a. Hypotension secondary to pump failure and cardiac rupture can occur but are much less common than lethal dysrhythmias (pp. 639).

127. b. A small fluid challenge (250 ml) may be given to a cardiac patient who is hypotensive; however, in the normotensive patient, intravenous fluids should be infused to keep the vein open (p. 642).

128. a. Epinephrine will increase the work (and oxy-

gen demands) on the heart and may precipitate lethal dysrhythmias in this patient (p. 645).

129. d (p. 645)

130. b. Mortality is high in these patients and is often related to loss of functioning myocardium (p. 646).

131. a. Bretylium and lidocaine are used to treat ventricular dysrhythmias; calcium chloride is indicated only if there is a calcium channel blocker overdose, hyperkalemia, or hypocalcemia (p. 613).

132. a (p. 650)

133. a. It originates from tissue other than an intrinsic pacemaker (p. 587).

134. c. Isoproterenol is a beta stimulant, so it will increase the heart rate (p. 940).

135. c. In the conscious patient, it may also cause nausea and vomiting (p. 928).

136. a. Morphine will decrease the preload. It is contraindicated in the head-injured patient. It does not cause bronchodilation (p. 946).

137. a. It may cause bradycardia by slowing impulse conduction through the atrioventricular node. It should increase cardiac output by increasing the force of contractions (p. 931).

138. c (p. 655)

139. c. The correct dose is 2 to 10 mcg/min (p. 579).

140. c (p. 652)

141. b. The patient with diabetes is at higher risk for heart disease; however, hypertension does not precipitate diabetes (p. 654).

142. d. It may take a few milliseconds longer than unsynchronized cardioversion, but it is safer (p. 662).

143. b (p. 663)

144. b (pp. 618)

145. c (p. 614)

146. c (p. 604)

147. a (p. 618)

148. b (p. 590)

149. d (p. 579)

150. a (p. 597)

● CHAPTER 19
DIABETIC EMERGENCIES

1. a, b, d, e, f, i, j, k (p. 678)
2. b, f, h, i, j (p. 678)
3. b, c, g, h, i (p. 678)
4. a. Glucagon; b. insulin; c. somatostatin (p. 667)

5.

	Breakdown	
Food	Products	Storage
a. Carbohydrates	Glucose	Liver and muscles (excess converted to fat) (p. 670)
b. Proteins	Amino acids	Small amounts in cytoplasm of all cells (p. 671)
c. Fat	Fatty acids glycerol	Liver and fat and cells (p. 671)

6. a. As glycogen. b. As the blood sugar begins to drop, glucagon is released from the pancreas and stimulates the breakdown of glycogen to glucose (p. 670).

7. Breaks down glycogen, gluconeogenesis (formation of glucose from amino acids) (p. 671)

8. Glucose cannot be stored in the brain, so when blood sugar drops, there are no reserves. Also, the brain cannot use fats or proteins for energy (p. 670).

9. Blindness, neuropathy, kidney disease, heart disease, and stroke (p. 674)

10. Assess and protect the airway; place a nasal or oral airway and suction as necessary; evaluate breathing, assist if necessary, and apply oxygen; assess pulse; evaluate vital signs; determine blood glucose level; initiate an intravenous line (draw a blood sample) in the antecubital space; if the blood glucose level is less than 80 mg/dl, administer D50W 25 g intravenously; and reassess the patient (pp. 676, 677).

11. c (p. 667)

12. c. Insulin may be given only by the parenteral route (p. 674).

13. b. Although hyperosmolar hyperglycemic nonketotic coma can develop in these patients, life--threatening complications are more common in type I diabetics (p. 679).

14. d (p. 668)

15. b. The effects of glucagon are slow and unreliable (p. 679).

16. d. This will enhance the use of glucose by the brain and prevent Wernicke's encephalopathy (p. 678).

● CHAPTER 20
NERVOUS SYSTEM DISORDERS

1. a (p. 691)
2. e (p. 691)
3. d (p. 691)
4. b (p. 691)
5. d (p. 691)
6. f (p. 691)
7. (p. 691)
8. a. Neuroglia (p. 681); b. cell body (p. 681); c. dendrites (p. 681); d. axon (p. 681); e. white matter (p. 681); f. sensory (p. 683); g. motor (p. 683); h. inter (p. 683); i. negative (p. 683); j. positive (p. 683);
k. sodium (p. 683); l. depolarization (p. 683); m. nodes of Ranvier (p. 683); n. quickly (p. 683); o. synapse (p. 683); p. norepinephrine, epinephrine, and dopamine (p. 683)

9. Sensory receptor, sensory neuron, interneurons, motor neuron, and effector organ (p. 683)

10. Vertebral arteries and internal carotid arteries (p. 685)

11. a. Decrease; b. decrease; c. decrease; d. decrease (p. 688)

12. Assess pupils for shape, size, equality and response to light. Assess patient's extraocular movements by asking him or her to follow your finger movements with his or her eyes (to the extreme left, up and down, to the extreme right, and up and down) (p. 690).

13. a. Intracranial bleeding, head trauma, brain tumor, or another space-occupying lesion. b. Anoxia, hypoglycemia, diabetic ketoacidosis, thiamine deficiency, kidney and liver failure, and postictal phase of seizure. c. Barbiturates, narcotics, hallucinogenics, depressants, and alcohol; d. Hypertensive encephalopathy, shock, dysrhythmias, and stroke; e. Chronic obstructive pulmonary disease and toxic inhalation. f. Meningitis and sepsis (p. 691).

14. Assess for vigorous blinking or movement of the eyes (hysterical coma) and response to noxious (painful) stimuli. The patient who is hysterical generally responds to noxious stimuli (p. 691).

15. a. Structural; b. toxic-metabolic; c. structural (p. 692)

16. Secure the airway. Patient has no gag reflex, so she should be intubated. (Nasal intubation or manual in-line immobilization with oral intubation should be used if trauma is suspected.) Ventilate at 24 to 30 breaths/min using 100% oxgyen. Assess carotid and radial pulses. Assess vital signs, lung sounds, ECG, and pupil response. Scan body for obvious trauma. Draw a blood sample while initiating intravenous 0.9% normal saline. Assess blood glucose levels; if it is less than 80 mg/dl, administer thiamine 100 mg intravenously, reassess, administer 25 g of D50W, and reassess. If the blood glucose level is normal, administer Narcan 2 mg intravenously and reassess patient. Perform head-to-toe survey and transport (pp. 692-693).

17. Stroke, head trauma, toxins, hypoxia, hypoglycemia, infection, metabolic abnormalities, brain tumor, vascular disorders, eclampsia, and drug overdose (p. 693)

18. a. Simple sensory seizure (partial seizure) (p. 694); b. petit mal (generalized seizure) (p. 694); c. Jacksonian seizure (partial seizure) (p. 694); d. grand mal seizure (generalized seizure) (p. 694);

e. complex partial seizures (partial seizure) (p. 694)

19. Previous history of seizures, including frequency and medication compliance; description of seizure (length, features, incontinence, tongue-biting); history of head trauma; fever, headache, or nuchal rigidity before seizure; past medical history, including diabetes, cardiovascular disease, and stroke (p. 695).

20. There is no trauma to the tongue, there is no incontinence, there is no response to conventional therapy, and it may stop with a sharp command or sternal rub (p. 695).

21. a. Syncope; b. syncope; c. seizure; d. seizure (p. 696)

22. Lorazepam 1 to 2 mg intravenously and diazepam 5 to 10 mg intravenously every 15 min as necessary (p. 696)

23. Hypertension, diabetes mellitus, atherosclerosis, hyperlipidemia, polycythemia, and cardiac disease (p. 697)

24. Hemiparesis, hemiplegia on the side of the body opposite the lesion, numbness on the side of the body opposite the lesion, aphasia, confusion or coma, convulsions, incontinence, double vision, numbness of the face, dysarthria, headache, and dizziness or vertigo (pp. 697, 698)

25. Symptoms typically begin during stress or exertion. Abrupt onset of symptoms may include severe headache accompanied by nausea and vomiting, progressive deterioration in mental status from alert to lethargic to comatose, with hypertension and bradycardia; they may begin with an abrupt loss of consciousness or seizure progressing to coma (p. 698).

26. a. Intracranial pressure of less than 20 mm Hg typically does not interfere with blood flow. Intraocular fluid would not affect blood flow, and increased temperature would increase cerebral blood flow (p. 688).

27. d (p. 689)

28. a. Decorticate rigidity is due to the structural impairment of certain cortical regions of the brain. Flaccidity is due to brain stem or cord dysfunction. There is no such answer as c (p. 690).

29. c. Barbiturate overdose and medullary injury will more likely present with dilated pupils. Temporal herniation will cause a unilateral dilated pupil (p. 690).

30. d. Airway maintenance is critical and should be the top priority for this patient. Drug administration is not indicated unless the patient history indicates that the seizure was related to a correctable underlying cause or the patient's condition does not improve (p. 695).

31. b (pp. 698, 699)

● **CHAPTER 21**
ACUTE ABDOMINAL PAIN AND RENAL FAILURE

1. k (p. 705)
2. l (p. 703)
3. j (p. 705)
4. a (p. 703)
5. e (p. 707)
6. m (p. 706)
7. i (p. 707)
8. d (p. 706)
9. b (p. 707)
10. f (p. 706)
11. c (p. 703)
12. h (p. 703)
13. a. Urinary calculus (kidney stone) (p. 708); b. testicular torsion (p. 708); c. pyelonephritis (p. 708); d. Urinary tract infection (p. 707)
14. a. No. The pain of pancreatitis is located in the epigastric or right or left upper quadrant (p. 703). b. No. The pain of cholecystitis is located in the epigastric or right upper quadrant. It is more common in women younger than 50 (p. 703). c. Yes. It is common in older adults. Pain commonly occurs in the left lower quadrant (p. 706). d. No. It is common in men 30 to 50. Typically, there is flank pain that may radiate to the groin and testicle (p. 708). e. No. It is common in men younger than 30. Pain occurs in the epidydimis and scrotal sac (p. 708).
15. a. Somatic (p. 709); b. visceral (p. 709); c. referred (p. 710)
16. a. Does anything make the pain better or worse? What does the pain feel like (sharp, stabbing, cramping)? Can you point to the area where the pain is? Does the pain go anywhere else? On a scale of 1 to 10 with 1 being no pain and 10 being the worst pain you've ever had, rate the pain. When did the pain begin (p. 709)? *Associated signs and symptoms:* Do you or have you had any nausea or vomiting, diarrhea, constipation, unusual colored stools, chills, fever, shortness of breath (p. 709)? b. Myocardial infarction, abdominal aneurysm (p. 710).
17. a. Fever, chills, tachycardia, tachypnea, position (lying on side with knees flexed and pulled in toward the chest), reluctance to move, skin pallor, absent bowel sounds, generalized involuntary guarding, and rigidity of abdomen (p. 710). b. Oxygen by nonrebreather mask, intravenous 16-gauge catheter with normal saline or lactated Ringer's solution (rate at least 100 ml/hr, determined by patient's vital signs), electrocardiogram monitoring, and gentle transport in position of comfort (p. 712).
18. a. Trauma, shock, infection, urinary obstruction, and multisystem diseases; b. hypertension, dia-

betes, congenital condition, and pyelonephritis (p. 713)

19. a. Too much fluid taken off in dialysis and bleeding at fistula resulting from pseudoaneurysm (Any medical or traumatic cause for bleeding is significant because the patient is heparinized during dialysis.) (p. 714). b. Initiate large-bore intravenous line in the arm without the atrioventricular fistula, and infuse a small volume (200 to 300 ml), reevaluating the patient frequently for signs of fluid overload (crackles, engorged neck veins, pulmonary edema) (p. 715).

20. The patient has chronic anemia (resulting from lack of endogenous erythropoietin that is produced by the healthy kidneys and that is necessary for red blood cell production). Since there are fewer red blood cells to carry oxygen, the patient decompensates much more quickly when the body is stressed (p. 713).

21. High-flow oxygen by nonrebreather mask. Position patient on left side in Trendelenburg position. Initiate intravenous line with lactated Ringer's solution or normal saline in the arm without the atrioventricular fistula (p. 718).

22. b. Patient's age and gender and a description of patient history often yields more information about the cause of the abdominal illness than physical examination. However, the severity of the patient's present condition is determined by the physical examination (p. 709).

23. c. Melena (black or maroon stool) indicates the presence of bleeding. Tachycardia can be caused by bleeding, fever, pain, or other fluid loss (p. 706).

24. b. Appendicitis is more common in younger patients. Diverticulosis is most likely to cause rectal bleeding. Peptic ulcer symptoms do not typically include constipation (p. 705).

25. d. Administration of the pain medicines listed is contraindicated in the prehospital environment for the patient with undiagnosed abdominal pain (p. 712).

26. c. Loss of the testicle may occur if prompt treatment is not rendered. Pyelonephritis and urinary calculus also require urgent treatment but are not as time sensitive as testicular torsion (p. 708).

27. c. Infection at the site of catheter insertion is common and may lead to peritonitis (p. 714).

28. b. Atrioventricular fistula should never be accessed unless authorized by medical direction. (Some centers will not authorize access to this site under any circumstances.) The Port-a-cath should not be accessed unless the paramedic is trained in the use of a special Huber needle; if this needle is not used, the system may be punctured and ruined. The Tenckhoff catheter is used for peritoneal dialysis and is not a vascular access device (p. 716).

29. a. Peaked, tented T waves are associated with hyperkalemia, which is a common electrolyte imbalance in renal patients (p. 718).

30. b. Sodium bicarbonate may temporarily cause movement of potassium out of the vascular system and relieve the cardiac effects until definitive care (dialysis) can be given (p. 718).

● CHAPTER 22
ANAPHYLAXIS

1. f (p. 721)
2. h (p. 721)
3. e (p. 723)
4. g (p. 725)
5. c (p. 721)
6. a (pp. 721)
7. b (p. 721)
8. Collects microorganisms, cellular debris, and foreign material and delivers it to the lymph nodes, where it is disposed of by the immune response (pp. 721, 722)
9. a. Decreased blood pressure, increased gastrointestinal secretions, rhinorrhea, tearing, flushing, urticaria, and angioedema. b. Wheezing that may precipitate chest pain (resulting from coronary vasoconstriction) and enhance the hypotensive effects of histamine. c. Fever, chills, bronchospasm, and pulmonary vasoconstriction (pp. 725, 726).
10. a. Antibiotics (especially penicillin), local anesthetics, cephalosporins, chemotherapeutics, aspirin, nonsteroidal anti-inflammatory agents, opiates, muscle relaxants, anticancer agents, vaccines, and insulin. b. Wasps, bees, and fire ants. c. Peanuts, soybeans, cod, halibut, shellfish, egg white, strawberries, food additives, wheat and buckwheat, sesame and sunflower seeds, cotton seed, milk, and mango (pp. 725, 726).
11. a. Asthma, upper airway obstruction, pulmonary edema, drug overdose, and toxic inhalation (p. 726). b. Propranolol (Inderal) is a beta blocker and may interfere with epinephrine's ability to correct the symptoms. If the patient has already self-administered epinephrine (Epi-pen, Ana-pen), determine the time it was administered and whether symptoms have improved or worsened since administration (p. 728).
12. Foods such as crab, shrimp, nuts, and egg and some food additives are known to cause anaphylaxis in susceptible individuals (p. 725).
13. Epinephrine 0.3 to 0.5 mg (1:1000) subcutaneously and diphenhydramine (Benadryl) 25 to 50 mg intramuscularly or intravenously (p. 728)
14. Stridor, hoarseness, tachypnea, tachycardia, agitation, headache, seizures, decreasing level of consciousness, angioedema, tearing, swelling of the tongue, urticaria, pruritus, sneezing, coughing, tra-

cheal tugging, intercostal retractions, decreased breath sounds, dysrhythmias, chest tightness, nausea, vomiting, and diarrhea (pp. 726, 727)

15. Secure airway, ventilate with 100% oxygen, and intubate. Initiate intravenous therapy with large-bore catheter in antecubital space, infuse fluid rapidly, and administer epinephrine 0.1 to 0.2 mg (1:10,000) intravenously (if approved by medical direction). If patient's circulatory status improves but repeat doses of epinephrine are necessary, give epinephrine 0.3 to 0.5 mg subcutaneously; if necessary, administer diphenhydramine 25 to 50 mg intramuscularly or intravenously as a second-line drug (pp. 728, 729).

16. b. An antigen is a foreign protein that is introduced into the body and that activates the immune response. Lymphocytes are cells of the lymphatic system. Monocytes are a type of leukocyte that migrates out of the blood vessels to devour foreign material (p. 722).

17. b. IgA immunoglobulins are antibodies found in blood, secretions such as tears, and the respiratory system, IgG antibodies are the most common antibodies involved in the immune response, and production of IgM antibodies precede IgG production in acute infections (p. 723).

18. d. Chemotactic substances cause the attraction of phagocytic cells toward or away from the antigen, leukotactic substances attract leukocytes to the pathogenic agent, and opsonins bind phagocytes to the invading microorganism (p. 724).

19. b. All of the other choices are commonly associated with allergic reactions (p. 725).

20. a. The edema resulting from histamines and leukotrienes can rapidly occlude the airway and lead to death. All other choices can result in death but not as quickly (p. 727).

21. b. The skin will usually be erythematous (reddened) with urticaria because of the effects of histamine (pp. 726, 727).

22. b. It thickens bronchial secretions and may worsen the hypoxia secondary to bronchospasm, if that is the patient's primary problem. It does not increase the contractility of the heart (inotropic), and although it may produce drowsiness as a side effect, it is not a sedative hypnotic.

● CHAPTER 23
TOXICOLOGY, DRUG ABUSE, AND ALCOHOLISM

1. i (p. 738)
2. f (p. 739)
3. e (p. 740)

4. c (p. 745)
5. g (p. 736)
6. b (p. 736)
7. j (p. 749)
8. e (p. 766)
9. g (p. 767).
10. f (p. 768)
11. a (p. 769)
12. b (p. 766)
13. False. Some 25% of fatal tricyclic antidepressant overdose patients are awake and alert at the time of prehospital care (p. 767).
14. True (p. 776)
15. False. It may take several hours for the poison to reach the small intestine, where absorption occurs (p. 733).
16. False. Reports of toxic plant ingestions are second only to cleansing substance ingestions (p. 743).
17. True (p. 757)
18. Specific agent ingested, amount of agent ingested, time ingested, age, patient weight, medical condition, treatment rendered before arrival of EMS personnel (p. 732)
19. Coma, cardiac dysrhythmias, gastrointestinal disturbances, respiratory depression, and hypotension or hypertension (p. 733)
20. What was taken? Do you have the container? How much was in it and how much is left (may need to estimate based on date prescription issued, amount prescribed daily, and amount left in bottle)? When was the drug taken? Has the patient vomited or taken anything to induce vomiting since the drug was taken? Has any antidote been given to the patient? Ask the patient: Why did you do this? Were you trying to hurt or kill yourself (p. 733)?
21. A total of 30 ml of syrup of ipecac by mouth, followed by two to three 8-oz glasses of water (p. 734)
22. 30 to 100 g activated charcoal (p. 735)
23.

Poison/ Overdose	Ipecac?	Charcoal?	Other Interventions
a. Bleach	No	No	Dilution with milk or water (200 to 300 ml [adult] or 15 ml/kg [child]) (p. 736)
b. Ammonia	No	No	Dilution with milk or water as in a (p. 736)
c. Gasoline	No	No	Initiate intravenous line, monitor airway and electrocardiogram (p. 737)
d. Methanol	No	Controversial	Lavage, sodium bicarbonate intravenously (30 to 60 ml), and 80-proof ethanol by mouth (p. 738)

e. Ethylene glycol	No	Yes	Lavage, sodium bicarbonate intravenously (30 to 60 ml), 80-proof ethanol by mouth, and (rarely) furosemide, thiamine, and calcium gluconate (p. 739)
f. Isopropanol	No	Yes	Lavage (p. 740)
g. Cyanide	No	No	Amyl nitrite pearls, 3% sodium nitrite, and 25% sodium thiosulfate (p. 740)
h. Aspirin	Yes	Yes	D50W if patient is hypoglycemic
i. Acetaminophen	Usually not (varies by medical direction)	Usually not (varies by medical direction)	Mucomyst (p. 769)
j. Iron	Yes	No	Monitor airway, initiate intravenous line (p. 769)

24. a. Varies: chemical—1 to 2 hr, bacterial toxins—1 to 12 hr, viral or bacterial—12 to 48 hr (p. 742). b. Take personal protective measures, maintain airway and breathing, and initiate intravenous therapy with crystalloid solution to treat dehydration and fluid and electrolyte imbalance (p. 743).

25. a. Left lateral Trendelenberg (swimmer's) position. b. Endotracheal intubation before orogastric tube intubation if patient has a decreased level of consciousness with an absent gag reflex. c. After assessment for proper tube placement, normal saline (preferably warmed) should be infused into the orogastric tube in 200- to 300-ml boluses, and the tube should be allowed to drain after each bolus. This process is continued until the gastric drainage returns clear (pp. 734, 735).

26. a. Chemical asphyxiant: prevents oxygen from reaching tissues. b. Simple asphyxiant: displaces ambient oxygen and lowers inhaled oxygen concentration. c. Irritants and corrosives: damage cells of respiratory system and deter gas exchange (p. 745).

27. Ensure personal protection; open airway; administer high-flow oxygen; initiate a precautionary intravenous line to keep the vein open; and if pulmonary edema develops, consider administration of diuretics and bronchodilators (pp. 746, 747).

28. a. Carbamate and organophosphate (pp. 747, 748)

29. Pupil constriction, muscle fasciculation, headache, weakness, dizziness, hypotension, bronchoconstriction, anxiety, seizures, and convulsions (p. 748)

30. Sinus bradycardia (p. 578)

31. Don protective gear; suction oral secretions as necessary; prepare to intubate if patient's condition deteriorates; decontaminate as appropriate; initiate intravenous therapy with crystalloid to keep the vein open; administer atropine 2 mg intravenously every 5 to 15 min as necessary to induce relative tachycardia, flushing, and decreased secretions; monitor for dysrhythmias; administer pralidoxime 1 g intravenously over 15 to 30 min (adult) or 20 to 50 mg/kg intravenously over 15 to 30 min (pediatric); administer diazepam as necessary for seizures (pp. 747-749).

32. a. Assess for anaphylaxis; apply ice packs; and immobilize and elevate affected extremity. b. Scrape or brush off. (Do *not* squeeze because doing so will inject additional venom.) (p. 750).

33. *Lyme disease:* early—fever, lethargy, muscle pain, and general malaise; late—cardiac abnormalities, cranial nerve palsies, and arthritis. *Tick paralysis:* restlessness and paresthesia in hands and feet progressing to ascending symmetric flaccid paralysis (which may include respiratory muscles) (p. 754).

34. Apply gloves and grasp tick as close to skin surface as possible (may use tweezers or forceps if available), pull out with steady pressure (avoid squeezing tick), and cleanse wound and observe for any remnants of tick (p. 755).

35. a. Fang marks, pain and edema, weakness, diaphoresis, nausea, vomiting, and paraesthesias (p. 756). b. Ensure personal safety from another bite; monitor airway, breathing, and circulation; initiate intravenous therapy in unaffected extremity; immobilize affected extremity in dependent position; and keep patient at rest (p. 757).

36. a. Jellyfish, fire corals, and sea anemones. Rinse wound with seawater; apply vinegar, baking soda, isopropanol, ammonia, meat tenderizer (for 5 to 10 min only); remove visible tentacles with forceps; apply shaving cream, gently shave affected area or use knife or spatula to gently scrape remaining tentacles; and rinse again (pp. 757, 758). b. Sea urchins, star fish, and sea cucumbers. Remove embedded spines with forceps and immerse affected extremity (and unaffected extremity to prevent thermal injury) in hot water during transport (pp. 758, 759). c. Stingrays. Irrigate wound with salt or fresh water; remove venom apparatus if it is visible; and immerse the affected part in very hot water (p. 760).

37. a. Heroin, morphine, and methadone (p. 764). b. Barbiturates (secobarbital, phenobarbital), and benzodiazepines (diazepam, chlordiazepoxide) (p. 765). c. Amphetamines and cocaine (p. 765). d. LSD and phencyclidine (PCP) (p. 768).

38. a. He took fentanyl or heroin intravenously. b. She was smoking PCP and crack (cocaine) together. c. They were smoking purified crack cocaine. d. He injected morphine subcutaneously. e. She ingested PCP nasally (pp. 762, 763).

39. a. Respiratory depression (partial airway obstruction and decreased minute volume) (p. 764)

40. Naloxone (Narcan) 2.0 mg intravenously (pp. 764, 948)

41. Gooseflesh, tachycardia, diaphoresis, irritability, insomnia, abdominal cramps, tremors, nausea, vomiting, cold sweats and chills, fever, and diarrhea (pp. 764, 765)
42. Bilaterally dilated and slow to react to light (p. 765)
43. Flumazenil (Mazicon) (pp. 765, 935)
44. Tricyclic antidepressants (p. 765)
45. Cardiac dysrhythmias, seizures, or cerebrovascular accident (secondary to intracranial hemorrhage) (p. 766)
46. Personal safety (p. 767)
47. Quiet, calm approach and interview of the patient while minimizing external sensory stimuli (for example, bright lights, noise) (p. 767)
48. Euphoria, disorientation, seizures, hypertensive crisis, catatonia, unresponsiveness, bizarre and violent behavior (These patients are extremely difficult to manage and dangerous if found in or provoked into violent behavior.) (pp. 766, 767)
49. a. No. Patient is drowsy, and her level of consciousness could deteriorate further. Also, it has been more than 20 minutes since ingestion of the drug (pp. 734, 959).
50. Sinus tachycardia with delayed ventricular conduction (wide QRS complex) (p. 580)
51. Sodium bicarbonate 44 mEq intravenously (p. 767)
52. Delirium, depressed respirations, hypertension or hypotension, hyperthermia or hypothermia, seizures, coma, and dysrhythmias (p. 767)
53. No. Alcoholics frequently underestimate the number of drinks they have had (p. 770).
54. a. Short-term memory deficit, problems with coordination, and difficulty with concentration can mimic signs and symptoms of head injury. b. Nutritional deficiencies can cause muscle cramps, paresthesias, seizures, tremor or ataxia, and poor wound healing. c. Chronic dehydration may be difficult to distinguish from a new onset of fluid loss. (Patient will decompensate faster if there is acute fluid loss resulting from trauma.) d. Some $11/12$ of clotting factors are suppressed by alcohol. There is increased risk of bleeding, especially subdural hematoma, with minor trauma (pp. 771-774).
55. Protect airway (high risk of aspiration); ventilate as necessary; initiate intravenous therapy; draw blood samples per protocol; determine blood glucose levels, and if low, administer thiamine 100 mg intravenously and D50W 25 g intravenously; if opiate overdose is suspected or unknown, administer naloxone 2 mg intravenously; monitor airway, breathing, vital signs, and electrocardiogram (p. 775).
56. Manage as in Question 55 and protect from injury; administer valium 2.5 to 5.0 mg intravenously if additional seizures occur (p. 776).
57. Hyperactive motor, speech, and autonomic activity; confusion; disorientation; delusion; hallucina-tions; tremor; agitation; insomnia; tachycardia; fever; hypertension; dilated pupils; profuse diaphoresis; and in severe cases, cardiovascular collapse (p. 776).
58. a (p. 734)
59. b. Charcoal binds the drug by adsorption. It is often given with a cathartic that speeds the bound drug through the gastrointestinal tract (p. 735).
60. a. That is why emesis is usually contraindicated for these patients, unless the toxicity of the specific hydrocarbon is so great that the risks of absorption in the gastrointestinal tract outweigh the risks of aspiration (p. 737).
61. c. Methanol and ethylene glycol produce metabolic acidosis, so $NaHCO_3$ is indicated. In a tricyclic antidepressant overdose, it will decrease the toxic cardiac side effects. No metabolic acidosis is usually associated with isopropanol ingestion (p. 740).
62. a. Salivation and hypotension are likely to accompany the bradycardia. Symptoms vary according to the specific variety of mushroom ingested (p. 743).
63. a. All of the other chemicals are more likely to cause tachycardia (p. 748).
64. c. All other interventions are critical; however, rescuer safety should precede treatment because these poisons are readily absorbed through the skin, by ingestion, or by inhalation (p. 748).
65. d. $\dfrac{2 \text{ mg} \times 10 \text{ ml}}{1 \text{ mg}} = 20$ ml (p. 749)
66. d. Anaphylaxis would likely include respiratory distress and urticaria. His reaction was immediate and generalized and involved a large exposure to venom (p. 751).
67. a. The brown recluse produces a local reaction leading to delayed skin necrosis. Envenomation from most other spiders typically causes local versus systemic reactions (p. 751).
68. c. This description matches a coral snake, which is the only neurotoxic snake listed (p. 756).
69. a. Diazepam is not a narcotic; it is a benzodiazepine. Flumazenil (Mazicon) is a benzodiazepine antagonist (p. 765).
70. c. Oil of wintergreen contains a large amount of salicylate and has produced many fatal ingestions (p. 768).
71. c. Unless the patient volunteers information regarding an overdose of acetaminophen, he or she may be asymptomatic or complain of only mild influenza-like symptoms for the first 24 hours after ingestion (p. 769).
72. c. Ingestion of an overdose of iron is often lethal (p. 769).
73. d. This syndrome can lead to irreversible neurological problems and may be avoided by giving thiamine before administration of D50W (p. 777).

CHAPTER 24
INFECTIOUS DISEASES

1. c (p. 790)
2. g (p. 800)
3. i (p. 794)
4. e (p. 792)
5. h (p. 796)
6. f (p. 795)
7. b (p. 797)
8. j (p. 801)
9. False. These are all viral illnesses, and a virus cannot be controlled by antibiotic therapy (p. 785).
10. True (p. 787)
11. True (p. 795)
12. A pathological agent, a reservoir, a portal of exit from the reservoir, an environment conducive to transmission of the pathogenic agent, and susceptibility of the new host to the infectious disease (p. 779).
13. Burns, lacerations, abrasions, intravenous therapy, and urinary catheter (p. 681)
14. Human immunodeficiency virus, chemotherapy, and prolonged steroid therapy (p. 782)
15. a. Gloves, gown, mask, and eyewear. b. Gloves. c. Nothing is necessary according to the Centers for Disease Control; however, if bleeding is likely, gloves are indicated. d. Gloves, mask, and eyewear. e. Gloves, gown, mask, and eyewear. f. Gloves (p. 787).
16. a. Hepatitis A, B, or C (p. 790)
17. Take HBV vaccination and use strict universal precautions as warranted by each situation (p. 792).
18. Direct introduction of infected blood by needle or transfusion, introduction of serum or plasma through skin cuts, absorption of infected serum or plasma through mucosal surfaces, absorption of saliva or semen through mucosal surfaces, and transfer of infective serum or plasma via inanimate surfaces (p. 792)
19. Blood will be drawn, and if it is determined that you are not immune to the hepatitis B virus, an HBV vaccine will be given to protect against future exposures, and hepatitis B immune globulin will be given to provide temporary passive immunity to the hepatitis B virus (p. 792).
20. a. Fever, swollen lymph nodes, and sore throat; b. enlarged lymph nodes; c. bacterial pneumonia, oral lesions, shingles, and pulmonary tuberculosis; d. diarrhea, tumors, dementia, neurological symptoms, and opportunistic infections (p. 793)
21. a. None; b. just as you would after any patient (p. 794)
22. Annual skin test for purified protein derivative (of tuberculin) (and chest x-ray study if purified protein derivative [of tuberculin] text is positive) (p. 795)
23. a. Gloves and mask (respiratory spread); b. prophylactic antibiotic therapy (p. 795)

24. Paresis, wide gait, ataxia, psychosis, and signs of myocardial insufficiency (p. 796)
25. Gloves (p. 798)
26. a. Appearance like crabs or grey-blue spots and nits on abdomen, thighs, eyelashes, eyebrows, and axillary hair (p. 799). b. Elongated body with narrow head and three pair of legs and nits that look like dandruff and that cannot be brushed off (p. 799). c. Bites concentrated around webs of hands and feet, a child's face and scalp, a female's nipples, and a male's penis and vesicles and papules that become easily infected because of scratching (p. 800).
27. Yes (p. 791)
28. 13 to 17 days (p. 791)
29. Varicella can be transmitted 1 to 2 days before eruption of the rash until the lesions have all scabbed over (p. 802).
30. a. Acetaminophen has no antiinflammatory properties (p. 786).
31. c. The communicability period begins when the latent period ends and continues as long as the agent is present and can spread to others. The latent period begins with invasion of the body and ends when the agent can be shed or communicated. The disease period follows the incubation period and has variable lengths (p. 786).
32. b (p. 790)
33. d (p. 796)
34. d (p. 801)
35. b (p. 802)

CHAPTER 25
ENVIRONMENTAL EMERGENCIES

1. True. These findings occur in only 15% of freshwater drownings (p. 816).
2. True (p. 819)
3. a. Food metabolism; b. shivering; c. increased basal metabolic rate and vasoconstriction (pp. 806, 807)
4. a. Conduction, convection, and radiation; b. conduction and radiation; c. conduction, radiation, convection, and evaporation; d. conduction, radiation, convection, and evaporation (p. 807)
5. Skin vasodilation (becomes warm and flushed), sweating, decreased hormone secretion, and decreased muscle tone (p. 808)
6. Peripheral vasoconstriction (cool, pale skin), goose bumps, shivering, increased voluntary activity, increased hormone secretion, and increased appetite (p. 810)
7. a. Heat cramps. Remove patient from hot environment, replace sodium and water, and intravenously infuse saline solution if condition is severe (p. 806). b. Heat exhaustion. Remove patient from hot environment and intravenously infuse saline solution (p. 808). c. Heat stroke. Secure airway, as-

sess breathing, ventilate if indicated, administer high-flow oxygen, move patient to a cool environment, remove all clothing, wet the skin with cool fluid, fan the patient, initiate intravenous fluid therapy with normal saline, consult with medical direction regarding a fluid challenge, monitor for signs of fluid overload, if seizures recur administer diazepam, assess for hypoglycemia, and administer D50W if indicated (pp. 809, 810).

8. Increasing the metabolic rate increases the heart rate and contractility and increases the body's use of oxygen and other nutrients. The patient with preexisting trauma or illness will not tolerate these extra demands, and it may compromise organ response to illness or injury (p. 811).

9. a. Assess and secure the airway, assess breathing and assist with 100% oxygen (warmed and humidified if available) if indicated, assess circulation and begin cardiopulmonary resuscitation *only* after carefully verifying that no pulse is present, and move the patient to a warm environment and remove all clothing (pp. 812, 813).

10. a. Cardiopulmonary resuscitation; defibrillation at 200, 300, and 360 joules; intubation; ventilation with warm, humid oxygen; intravenous infusion of warm normal saline; and transport to the hospital. b. Cardiopulmonary resuscitation, defibrillation at 200, 300, and 360 joules; intubation; ventilation with warm, humid oxygen; intravenous infusion of warm normal saline; intravenous medications as indicated for ventricular fibrillation with a delay between doses; and another defibrillation as core temperature rises (pp. 812, 813).

11. When core temperature has reached 89.6° F (32° C) and resuscitation efforts are still unsuccessful (p. 812)

12. Move patient to warm area, remove any wet clothing, and wrap patient in warm blanket. If he is awake and alert, administer warm sugar-sweetened drinks (no alcohol, coffee, or tea). If necessary, apply hot packs wrapped in towels to the neck, armpits, and groin (p. 811).

13. a. Atrial fibrillation. b. Put the patient at rest and move to a warm environment after ensuring adequate airway, breathing, and circulation. Carefully remove all wet clothing and wrap patient in a blanket. Administer 100% oxygen (heated and humidified if possible) by nonrebreather mask. Initiate intravenous therapy of normal saline (initial fluid challenge of 250 to 500 ml may be ordered by medical direction [use warmed fluids if available]). Transport gently and monitor the patient carefully en route (p. 813).

14. In deep frostbite the underlying tissue is hard and not compressible, whereas in superficial frostbite the underlying tissue is compressible (p. 814).

15. Lack of protective clothing; preexisting illness or injury (diabetes or vascular insufficiency); fatigue; tobacco; tight, constrictive clothing; alcohol; and medications that cause vasodilation (some antihypertensives) (p. 814)

16. Elevate and protect the affected extremity, provide rapid transport to a medical facility, and assess for hypothermia (p. 815).

17. a. Temperature of water, length of submersion, cleanliness of water, and age of patient (p. 817)

18. Acute respiratory failure, dysrhythmias, decreased cardiac output, cerebral edema leading to central nervous system dysfunction, and renal dysfunction (rare) (p. 817)

19. Ensure scene safety, initiate cardiopulmonary resuscitation, secure the airway with an endotracheal tube and ventilate with 100% oxygen, assess cardiac rhythm and follow advanced life-support protocols to manage appropriately, assess for hypothermia, and transport to appropriate medical facility (pp. 817, 818).

20. Ears, sinuses, lungs and airways, gastrointestinal tract, thorax, and teeth (p. 819)

21. a. Focal paralysis or sensory changes, aphasia, confusion blindness or another visual disturbance, convulsion, loss of consciousness, dizziness, vertigo, abdominal pain, and cardiac arrest. b. If the patient's trachea is intubated, fill the balloon with normal saline instead of air; evaluate for POPS; and transport in the left lateral recumbent position with a 15-degree elevation of the thorax (p. 820).

22. a. Decompression sickness. b. Administer high-flow oxygen, initiate intravenous therapy, and rapidly transport for recompression (follow local protocol so that patient can reach hyperbaric chamber as quickly as possible) (p. 821).

23. a. Acute mountain sickness, high-altitude pulmonary edema, and high altitude cerebral edema; b. descent to a lower altitude (p. 821)

24. d. Vasoconstriction and vasodilation of the blood vessels in the skin are the major ways that the body releases or conserves heat (p. 805).

25. d (p. 809)

26. c. Damage to the body continues as long as the temperature remains elevated (p. 810).

27. b. Shivering should continue until the core temperature reaches 86° F (30° C). A tremendous amount of energy is needed for shivering, so glucose and glycogen must be available to fuel this increased muscle activity (p. 810).

28. b. Rapid rewarming in *warm* water is indicated only when sanctioned by medical direction if no chance of refreezing exists. Refreezing is very damaging to the tissues (p. 815).

29. c (p. 817)

30. a. Dalton's law states that the total pressure of a mixture of gases is equal to the sum of the partial pressures of the component gases. Henry's law states that the amount of gas dissolved in a given volume of fluid is proportional to the pressure of the gas with which it is in equilibrium. Newton's law says that a body at rest will remain at rest until acted on by an outside force, and a body in motion will remain in motion until acted on by an outside force (p. 818).

31. d. As trapped air in the lungs expands on rapid ascent, it ruptures alveoli and allows gas to leak into the subcutaneous tissues (p. 821).

32. b. The neurodepressant effects of nitrogen narcosis may lead to diving accidents resulting from impaired judgment and discrimination (p. 821).

33. a. Ataxia signals progression of the illness, and coma may ensue within 24 hours of its onset (p. 821).

● CHAPTER 26
GERIATRICS

1. a. Baseline pao_2 is lower, so there is less ability to compensate if chest trauma is sustained or if the patient is hypoxic resulting from trauma (for example, inhalation injury); the chest wall is less elastic and more susceptible to injury (p. 825). b. Myocardial contusion can cause pump failure resulting from poor cardiac reserve; decreased ability to increase heart rate can cause decreased ability to compensate for shock; and dysrhythmias can cause syncope and precipitate a fall (p. 826). c. Renal blood flow is decreased, so a sudden traumatic event that causes shock and hypoperfusion to the kidneys can precipitate the onset of renal failure; decreased renal function can make an older adult more susceptible to toxic drug effects, leading to central nervous system depression, disturbances in balance, hypotension, and dysrhythmias, all of which can increase the risk of falls (p. 826). d. Kyphosis may alter balance and predispose a person to falls, and osteoporosis increases the incidence of fractures after falls (p. 827). e. It can cause decreased ability for peripheral vasoconstriction, lowered metabolic rate, and poor peripheral circulation and can impair the body's ability to regulate temperature effectively, especially during time of stress such as traumatic injury; hypothermia may occur rapidly (p. 827).

2. a. His multiple illnesses and drugs will make it difficult to assess for new onset of signs or symptoms. *Diabetes:* It impairs pain perception and retards healing. *Heart attack and heart failure:* Cardiac output may be impaired from chronic conditions, and dysrhythmias may be chronic. *Lung disease:* Patient's baseline must be determined, and cyanosis, increased respiratory rate, and abnormal lung sounds may be chronic. *Lanoxin:* Therapeutic effects slow heart rate; patient may not become tachycardic in response to trauma; and toxic effects may cause dysrhythmias. *Insulin:* Excessive amounts may cause hypoglycemia and produce central nervous system impairment. *Dyazide:* Diuretics may cause an electrolyte imbalance that can affect muscle strength and may precipitate dysrhythmias that can cause syncope and falls. b. Dysrhythmias, visual impairment, neurological disabilities, arthritis, changes in gait, postural hypotension, syncope, cerebrovascular accident or transient ischemic attack, medications, slippery surfaces, loose rugs, objects on floors, poor lighting, pets, low beds or toilet seats, defective walking equipment, and lack of handrails on stairs (p. 830).

3. Cerebral atrophy inherent with aging allows for more blood to fill the cranial cavity before compression of the brain tissue (with associated symptoms) begins (p. 829).

4. His heart rate is slow relative to the rest of his clinical picture (everything else indicates impending shock or hypoxia) (p. 828).

5. He may have a pacemaker or be on medications (for example, digitalis or beta blockers) that prevent his heart from becoming tachycardic in response to a decrease in cardiac output (p. 828).

6. Abdominal injuries are frequently lethal in the older adult. His perception of pain may be impaired, and especially with signs of shock, this situation could deteriorate very quickly (p. 829).

7. Ensure a patent airway; deliver high-flow oxygen by nonrebreather mask; apply pneumatic antishock garments (if indicated by local protocol); en route to a trauma center, initiate two large-bore intravenous lines and administer small fluid challenges in consultation with medical direction; and frequently monitor vital signs and lung sounds (for increased rales [crackles]) to ensure that the patient is not developing a volume overload (pp. 822-823).

8. In the older adult, dyspnea and weakness may be the only presenting history for myocardial infarction. Carefully obtain a patient history, perform a physical examination, and treat with a high index of suspicion for myocardial infarction (p. 831).

9. Atrial fibrillation (p. 593)

10. Cerebrovascular accident and pulmonary embolism (p. 831)

11. Cholecystitis, colonic diverticular disease, appendicitis, aortic abdominal aneurysm, mesenteric artery occlusion, and mesenteric vein thrombosis (p. 832)

12. a. Rapid. b. Variable. It is usually self-limited and can be corrected quickly when the cause is identified. c. Electrolyte imbalance, hypoglycemia, hyper-

glycemia, acid-base imbalance, hypoxia, vital organ failure, and Wernicke's encephalopathy (p. 832).

13. Hypothyroidism, Cushing's syndrome, vitamin deficiencies, and hydrocephalus (p. 832)

14. a. Bleeding problems, increased hemorrhage from trauma, multiple contusions, and allergic reactions. b. Electrolyte abnormalities (sodium and potassium), and dehydration. c. Influenza-like symptoms, multiple dysrhythmias, and bradycardia. d. Dry mouth, tachycardia, ventricular dysrhythmias, seizures, and impaired level of consciousness. e. Impaired perception (increased risk of falls) and decreased level of consciousness with respiratory depression. f. Decreased heart rate (excessive) and bronchoconstriction. g. Tachycardia, dysrhythmias, and central nervous system stimulation. h. Dysrhythmias and clotting abnormalities (p. 834, Emergency Drug Index).

15. a. Follow local protocols and report to appropriate authority (local law enforcement, abuse hotline, medical direction) as indicated; report findings to receiving hospital; and document findings thoroughly on prehospital run report. b. Yes. Daughter lives with parent (p. 835).

16. a. Sinus bradycardia, rate 30/min (pp. 577, 578)

17. Atropine 0.5 mg intravenously (p. 579)

18. Acute myocardial infarction, drug toxicity, and vagal response (p. 831)

19. Sinus tachycardia (p. 580)

20. Bacterial pneumonia and pulmonary embolus (p. 831)

21. Must treat the patient and her underlying problem, not the rhythm (p. 581)

22. Administer high-flow oxygen via nonrebreather mask, initiate intravenous therapy and consider a small fluid challenge en route in consultation with medical direction, and monitor patient response and vital signs closely en route (p. 831).

23. a. Normal sinus rhythm with a premature atrial contraction and a premature ventricular contraction. b. Continue to monitor the patient and electrocardiogram rhythm (pp. 587, 606).

24. a. Junctional rhythm. b. Observe the patient for any signs of hemodynamic compromise related to the slow rhythm (monitor vital signs and electrocardiogram) (p. 579).

25. a. Delirium (sudden onset) (p. 832)

26. Normal sinus rhythm with a premature atrial contraction (p. 586)

27. No (pp. 586, 587)

28. Intoxication or poisoning, withdrawal from drugs, metabolic disturbances, infectious process, central nervous system trauma, and stroke (p. 832)

29. Second-degree heart block Mobitz type II (p. 620)

30. Below the left breast and inferior to the left scapula lateral to the spine (p. 664)

31. 70/min (p. 663)

32. Pacer spike followed by wide, bizarre QRS complex; a palpable pulse on the right side; and improved blood pressure (p. 663)

33. a. Atrial flutter with a rapid ventricular response; b. verapamil 2.5 to 5.0 mg intravenously over 2 min (pp. 591, 582)

34. d. The combination of elevated blood pressure, bradycardia, and irregular respirations is also a critical finding in head injury; however, each one by itself may indicate an underlying medical problem unrelated to the head injury (p. 829).

35. b. All other problems are possible; however, fractures account for the highest number of injuries secondary to falls (p. 830).

36. d. Many patients taking chemotherapy are immunosuppressed, and all efforts must be taken to minimize the risk of infection (p. 832).

37. b (p. 833)

38. c. Widowed women are at greater risk for abuse (p. 834).

● CHAPTER 27
PEDIATRICS

1. f (p. 856)

2. e (p. 856)

3. h (p. 856)

4. a (p. 856)

5. g (p. 856)

6. b (p. 927)

7. c (p. 856)

8. a. Neonate; b. infant, toddler, and preschooler; c. neonate; d. infant and toddler; e. infant, toddler, and school-age child; f. young infant, infant, toddler, school-age child, and adolescent (sexual abuse); g. preschooler and school-age child; h. adolescent (pp. 838-840)

9. Description of seizure activity, vomiting during seizure, history of epilepsy or another major medical illness, other current medicines, potential for toxic ingestion, recent head injury, and complaints of headache or stiff neck (p. 840)

10. Maintain airway and breathing; monitor vital signs; cool child with tepid water and fanning; monitor electrocardiogram and oxygen saturation (if available); depending on patient's vital signs and level of consciousness, initiate lactated Ringer's solution intravenously to keep the vein open and obtain blood sample; and assess blood sugar and treat if it is less than 60 mg/dL (p. 841).

11. Diazepam 0.2 to 0.3 mg/kg slow intravenous or intraosseous infusion (no faster than 1 mg/min); if intravenous or intraosseous infusion is not possible, administer medication rectally at higher dose (7 mg). Lorazepam 0.05 to 0.15 mg/kg intramus-

dia, hypertension, nausea, and vomiting. *Onset:* within 1 min. *Duration:* 9 to 17 min. *Dose:* Adult—0.5 to 1.0 mg intramuscularly, subcutaneously, or slow intravenous injection repeated in 20 min as necessary. Pediatric—0.03 to 0.1 mg/kg intramuscularly, subcutaneously, or intravenously repeated in 20 min as necessary. *Special considerations:* it is ineffective in chronic hypoglycemia, starvation, or adrenal insufficiency (p. 937).

6. a. Procainamide (Pronestyl). *Class:* antidysrhythmic (class 1-A). *Description:* reduces automaticity of ectopic pacemakers and suppresses reentry dysrhythmias by slowing intraventricular conduction. *Indications:* suppression of premature ventricular contractions refractory to lidocaine, suppression of ventricular tachycardia (with a pulse) refractory to lidocaine, suppression of ventricular fibrillation refractory to lidocaine if bretylium is not available, and paroxymal supraventricular tachycardia with wide-complex tachycardia of unknown origin (especially if Wolff-Parkinson-White syndrome is present). *Contraindications:* second- and third-degree atrioventricular block, digitalis toxicity, and torsades de pointes. *Adverse reactions:* hypotension, bradycardia, reflex tachycardia, atrioventricular block, widened QRS complex, prolonged PR or QT interval, premature ventricular contractions, ventricular tachycardia, ventricular fibrillation, asystole, central nervous system depression, confusion, and seizure. *Onset:* 10 to 30 min. *Duration:* 3 to 6 hr. *Dose:* Adult—20 mg/min to maximum dose 17 mg/kg, maintenance infusion after resuscitation or after initial bolus; mix 1 g in 250 ml of solution titrated to patient response (1 to 4 mg/min). Pediatric—3 to 5 mg/kg/dose slow intravenous injection; infusion: 20 to 80 mcg/kg/min. *Special considerations:* administration should be discontinued if dysrhythmia is suppressed, hypotension develops, the QRS complex widens by 50% of its original width, or a total of 1 g has been given. (b) Bretylium tosylate (Bretylol). *Class:* antidysrhythmic (class III). *Description:* increases ventricular fibrillation threshold. *Indications:* treatment of ventricular fibrillation and ventricular tachycardia refractory to lidocaine. *Contraindications:* none in the treatment of life-threatening dysrhythmias. *Adverse reactions:* vertigo, dizziness, vomiting, syncope, hypotension, bradycardia, increase in premature ventricular contractions, and angina pectoris. *Onset:* 2 to 15 min (antifibrillatory action) and 20 min (ventricular tachycardia and premature ventricular contractions). *Duration:* 2 to 6 hr. (ventricular fibrillation) and up to 24 hr (ventricular tachycardia). *Dose:* 5 mg/kg intravenous bolus repeated at 10 mg/kg (max dose 30 to 35 mg/kg) (ventricular fibrillation) and 5 to 10 mg/kg diluted in 50 ml administered over 8 to 10 min (ventricular tachycardia).

Special considerations: the patient should be kept supine to avoid postural hypotension (p. 954).

7. Nitroglycerin (Nitrostat). *Class:* vasodilator. *Description:* dilates peripheral venous and arteriolar blood vessels and reduces cardiac workload and oxygen demand. *Indications:* ischemic chest pain, hypertension, and congestive heart failure. *Contraindications:* hypersensitivity, hypotension, anemia, head injury, and cerebral hemorrhage. *Adverse reactions:* headache, postural syncope, reflex tachycardia, hypotension, nausea, vomiting, allergic reaction, muscle twitching, and diaphoresis. *Onset:* 1 to 3 min. *Duration:* 10 to 30 min. *Dose:* Tablet—0.3 to 0.4 mg sublingually that may be repeated in 3 to 5 min 3 times. Metered dose inhaler—0.4/spray, 1 to 2 inhalations that may be repeated in 5 min 2 times. *Special considerations:* it must be kept in airtight container protected from light; older adults have an increased risk of hypotension (p. 948).

8. Lidocaine (Xylocaine). *Class:* antidysrhythmic (class 1-B). *Description:* suppresses premature ventricular contractions and raises ventricular fibrillation threshold. *Indications:* acute ventricular dysrhythmias. *Contraindications:* hypersensitivity, Stokes-Adams syndrome, and second- or third-degree heart block in the absence of an artificial pacemaker. *Adverse reactions:* lightheadedness, confusion, blurred vision, hypotension, cardiovascular collapse, bradycardia, and central nervous system depression (including seizures) with high doses. *Onset:* 30 to 90 sec. *Duration:* 2 to 4 hr. *Dose:* Adult—given intravenously or via endotracheal bolus followed by a continuous infusion: for ventricular fibrillation, 1.5 mg/kg repeated in 3 to 5 min to a total loading dose of 3 mg/kg; for ventricular ectopy or stable ventricular tachycardia: 1 to 1.5 mg/kg intravenously repeated in 5 to 10 min at 0.5 to 0.75 mg/kg to a total dose of 3 mg/kg; given via infusion: dilution of 1 g of lidocaine in 250 ml of D5W and infusion at 1 to 4 mg/min. Pediatric—1 mg/kg/dose; infusion: 20 to 50 mcg/kg/min. *Special considerations:* it has a short half-life; if bradycardia is seen with premature ventricular contractions, the bradycardia is treated first with atropine; high doses can result in coma or death (p. 941).

9. Aminophylline (Amoline, Somophyllin, Aminophyllin). *Class:* xanthine bronchodilator (theophylline derivative). *Description:* causes bronchodilation, is a respiratory stimulant, has mild diuretic properties, and causes positive inotropic and chronotropic effects at high doses. *Indications:* bronchospasm associated with asthma, chronic bronchitis, and emphysema. *Contraindications:* allergy to xanthine compounds (such as caffeine), hypersensitivity, and cardiac dysrhythmias. *Ad-*

verse reactions: tachycardia, palpitations, premature ventricular contractions, angina pectoris, dizziness, anxiety, headache, seizure, nausea, vomiting, and abdominal cramps. Onset: less than 15 min intravenously. Duration: 4.5 hr. Dose: Loading dose—adult: 5 to 6 mg/kg in 50 to 100 ml of diluent over 30 min (not to exceed 20 mg/min) (should be lower in patients who have been receiving theophylline preparations); pediatric: 5 to 6 mg/kg in 50 to 100 ml intravenous infusion (not to exceed 20 mg/min). Maintenance infusion for first 12 hours—pediatric: 1 mg/kg/hr; young adult smokers: 1 mg/kg/hr; young adult nonsmokers: 0.7 mg/kg/hr; older adult: 0.6 mg/kg/hr; patients with heart failure or liver disease: 0.5 mg/kg/hr. Special considerations: beta blockers may oppose effects; barbiturates, phenytoin, and smoking may decrease theophylline levels; it should be used with caution in patients with cardiovascular disease, hypertension, and hepatic or renal insufficiency; if the patient has had a theophylline preparation in past 6 to 24 hr, the dose is reduced by half; rapid administration may cause hypotension; the therapeutic to toxic ratio is small (p. 924).

10. Naloxone (Narcan). Class: synthetic opioid antagonist. Description: is a competitive narcotic antagonist used to manage and reverse overdoses caused by narcotics and synthetic narcotic agents. Indications: complete or partial reversal of narcotic depression and ventilatory depression resulting from opioids, including narcotics (morphine sulfate, hydromorphone [Dilaudid], methadone, meperidine [Demerol], paregoric, fentanyl [Sublimaze], oxycodone [Percodan], and codeine), synthetic narcotics (butorphanol tartrate [Stadol], pentazocine [Talwin], propoxyphene [Darvon], and nalbuphine [Nubain]; decreased level of consciousness, coma of unknown origin, and circulatory support in refractory shock (investigational). Contraindications: hypersensitivity and caution with narcotic-dependent patients, who may experience withdrawal syndrome. Adverse reactions: tachycardia, hypertension, dysrhythmias, nausea, vomiting, and diaphoresis. Onset: within 2 min. Duration: 30 to 60 min. Dose: Adult—0.4 to 2.0 mg intravenously, intramuscularly, or subcutaneously or via endotracheal administration (diluted) that may be repeated in 5-min intervals to a maximum of 10 mg. Infusion—mix 2 mg in 500 ml of D5W (4 mcg/ml) and infuse at 0.4 mg/hr (100 ml/hr). Pediatrics—0.1 mg/kg/dose intravenously, intramuscularly, or subcutaneously or via endotracheal administration (diluted), maximum dose of 0.8 mg; if no response in 10 min, administer additional 0.1 mg/kg/dose. Special considerations: seizures have been reported; it may not reverse hypotension (p. 947).

11. Nifedipine (Procardia). Class: calcium channel blocker. Description: inhibits movement of calcium ions across cell membranes and depresses smooth muscle contraction, dilates coronary arteries and arterioles in normal and ischemic tissue, prevents coronary artery spasm, dilates peripheral vessels, and decreases total peripheral resistance. Indications: angina pectoris, hypertensive crisis, and pulmonary edema. Contraindications: hypersensitivity, compensatory hypertension, and hypertension. Adverse reactions: dizziness, headache, palpitations, hypotension, edema in extremities, muscle cramps, myocardial infarction, nausea, allergic reaction, and facial flushing. Onset: 15 to 30 min. Duration: 6 to 8 hr. Dose: Adult: 10 mg sublingually or buccally repeated in 30 min as necessary (have the patient bite and swallow). Pediatric: not recommended. Special considerations: beta blockers may potentiate its effects; antihypertensives may potentiate hypotensive effects; the effects of theophylline may be increased (p. 948).

12. Atropine sulfate (Atropine and others). Class: anticholinergic agent. Description: inhibits action of acetylcholine at postganglionic parasympathetic neuroeffector sites and blocks vagus and causes positive chronotropy and positive dromotropy. Indications: hemodynamically significant bradycardia, asystole, organophosphate poisoning, and pulmonary disorders. Contraindications: tachycardia, hypersensitivity, unstable cardiovascular status in acute hemorrhage and myocardial ischemia, and narrow-angle glaucoma. Adverse reactions: tachycardia; paradoxical bradycardia when pushed slowly or when used at doses less than 0.5 mg; palpitations; dysrhythmias; headache; dizziness; anticholinergic effects (dry mouth, photophobia, blurred vision, urine retention); nausea; vomiting; flushed, hot, dry skin; and allergic reactions. Onset: rapid. Duration: 2 to 6 hr. Dose: Brady-dysrhythmias—adult: 0.5 to 1.0 mg intravenously every 3 to 5 min as needed (maximum 0.4 mg/kg); pediatric: 0.02 mg/kg/dose intravenously (minimum dose 0.1 mg, maximum single dose 0.5 mg for a child and 1.0 mg for an adolescent). Anticholinesterase poisoning—adult: 2 mg intravenously every 5 to 15 min until signs of atropine poisoning appear, repeated as needed; pediatric: 0.05 mg/kg/dose (usual dose 1 to 5 mg) intravenously, repeated as needed every 15 min. Special considerations: potential adverse effects when given with digitalis, cholinergics, and neostigmine; the effects of atropine may be enhanced by antihistamines, procainamide, quinidine, antipsychotics, antidepressants, and benzodiazepines (p. 927).

13. Epinephrine (Adrenalin). *Class:* sympathomimetic. *Description:* stimulates alpha and beta receptors; causes bronchodilation and, when given via rapid intravenous injection, causes rapid increases in systolic pressure, ventricular contractility, and heart rate; causes vasoconstriction of the arterioles of the skin, mucosa, and splanchnic areas; and antagonizes the effects of histamine. *Indications:* bronchial asthma, acute allergic reactions, asystole, PEA, and ventricular fibrillation. *Contraindications:* hypersensitivity, nonanaphylactic shock, coronary insufficiency, and hypertension. *Adverse reactions:* headache, restlessness, weakness, dysrhythmias, hypertension, and precipitation of angina pectoris. *Onset:* 5 to 10 min (subcutaneously) 1 to 2 min (intravenously). *Duration:* 5 to 10 min. *Dose:* Asystole, PEA, or ventricular fibrillation—adult: initial, 1 mg intravenous push repeated every 3 to 5 min; intermediate, 2 to 5 mg intravenous push every 3 to 5 min; escalating, 1 mg–3 mg–5 mg intravenously (3 min apart); high, 0.1 mg/kg intravenous push every 3 to 5 min. Pediatric: first dose: standard (0.1 ml/kg 1:10,000) intravenously or intraosseously, high (0.1 ml/kg 1:1000) via endotracheal administration; second and subsequent doses: high (0.1 ml/kg 1:1000) intravenously or intraosseously, high (0.1 ml/kg 1:1000) via endotracheal administration. Bradycardia refractory to other interventions—adult: 2 to 10 mcg/min (1 mg 1:1000 in 500 ml of normal saline or D5W); pediatric: standard, 0.1 ml/kg 1:10,000 intravenously or intraosseously, high, 0.1 ml/kg 1:1000 via endotracheal administration. Anaphylactic reaction or bronchoconstriction—adult: mild: 0.3 ml (1:1000 subcutaneously, moderate to severe: 0.1 to 0.2 mg (1:10,000) slow intravenous injection. *Special considerations:* monoamine oxidase inhibitors and bretylium may potentiate effects of epinephrine; beta adrenergic agonists may blunt inotropic response; sympathomimetics and phosphodiesterase may exacerbate dysrhythmias; it may be deactivated by alkaline solutions (NaHCO$_3$ and furosemide); syncope has been reported after administration in children; it may increase myocardial oxygen demand (p. 934).

14. Nitrous oxide:oxygen (50:50) (Nitronox). *Class:* gaseous analgesic and anesthetic. *Description:* depresses the central nervous system and causes anesthesia. *Indications:* moderate to severe pain. *Contraindications:* impaired level of consciousness, head injury, chest trauma, inability to comply with instructions, decompression sickness, undiagnosed abdominal pain, bowel obstruction, hypotension, shock, and dizziness. *Adverse reactions:* drowsiness, dizziness, COPD, apnea, cyanosis, nausea, vomiting, malignant hyperthermia, and expansion of gas-filled pockets. *Onset:* 2 to 5 min. *Duration:* 2 to 5 min. *Dose:* adult—invert cylinder several times before use and instruct the patient to inhale deeply through the demand valve and mask or mouthpiece, which the patient must hold. Pediatric—same. *Special considerations:* it increases the incidence of spontaneous abortion; it will diffuse into gas-filled pockets trapped in the patient (e.g., pneumothorax, intestinal obstruction) and may cause rupture; nitrous oxide is a nonexplosive gas (p. 950).

15. Sodium bicarbonate. *Class:* buffer. *Description:* reacts with hydrogen ions to form water and carbon dioxide to buffer acidosis. *Indications:* metabolic acidosis, tricyclic antidepressant overdose, and alkalinization for treatment of specific intoxications. *Contraindications:* patients with chloride loss from vomiting or gastrointestinal suction, metabolic and respiratory alkalosis, hypokalemia, and hypocalcemia. *Adverse reactions:* metabolic alkalosis, hypoxia, rise in intracellular P_{CO_2} and increased tissue acidosis, electrolyte imbalance (tetany), seizures, and tissue sloughing at injection site. *Onset:* 2 to 10 min. *Duration:* 30 to 60 min. *Dose:* Urgent forms of metabolic acidosis—adult: 1 mEq/kg intravenously repeated in 5 min with 0.5 mEq/kg every 10 min; pediatric: same. *Special considerations:* it may precipitate in calcium solutions; vasopressors may be deactivated; if possible, arterial blood gas analysis should govern administration of this drug; it may increase edematous or sodium-retaining states; it may initially worsen cellular acidosis; it may worsen congestive heart failure (p. 956).

16. a. Thiamine (Betaxin). *Class:* vitamin (B$_1$). *Description:* is necessary for carbohydrate metabolism. *Indications:* coma of unknown origin (before administration of dextrose 50% or naloxone), delirium tremens, beriberi, and Wernicke's encephalopathy. *Contraindications:* none significant. *Adverse reactions:* hypotension (from rapid injection or a large dose), diaphoresis, nausea, vomiting, and allergic reaction (rare). *Onset:* rapid. *Duration:* depends on degree of deficiency. *Dose:* adult—100 mg slow intravenous or intramuscular injection; pediatric: 10 to 25 mg slow intravenous or intramuscular injection. *Special considerations:* large IV doses may cause respiratory difficulties; anaphylactic reactions have been reported (p. 960). Dextrose 50%. *Class:* carbohydrate and hypertonic solution. *Description:* is the principal carbohydrate used in the body for fuel. *Indications:* hypoglycemia, altered level of consciousness, coma of unknown etiology, seizure of unknown etiology, and refractory cardiac arrest (controversial). *Contraindications:* none for emergency care. *Adverse re-*

321

actions: warmth, pain, burning from medication infusion, thrombophlebitis, and rhabdomyositis. *Onset:* less than 1 min. *Duration:* depends on degree of hypoglycemia. *Dose:* adult—12.5 to 25 g slow intravenous injection (may repeat once); pediatric—0.5 to 1 g/kg/dose slow intravenous injection (may repeat once). *Special considerations:* blood sample should be taken before administration if possible; blood glucose analysis should be performed before administration if possible; extravasation may cause tissue necrosis; it may sometimes precipitate severe neurological symptoms (Wernicke's encephalopathy) in patients with thiamine depletion such as alcoholics; high-risk groups should receive thiamine before D50 (p. 930).

17. Diazepam (Valium and others). *Class:* benzodiazepine sedative-hypnotic and anticonvulsant. *Description:* raises the seizure threshold in the cerebral cortex and acts on the limbic, thalamic, and hypothalamic regions of the brain to potentiate the effects of inhibitory neurotransmitters. *Indications:* acute anxiety states, acute alcohol withdrawal, muscle relaxation, seizure activity, and preoperative sedation. *Contraindications:* hypersensitivity, substance abuse, coma, and shock. *Adverse reactions:* hypotension, reflex tachycardia, respiratory depression, ataxia, psychomotor impairment, confusion, and nausea. *Onset: 1 to 5 min* (intravenously), 15 to 30 min (intramuscularly). *Duration: 15 min to 1 hr* (intravenously), 15 min to 1 hr (intramuscularly). *Dose:* Seizure activity—adult: 5 to 10 mg intravenously every 10 to 15 min as necessary (maximum dose 30 mg); pediatric: 0.2 to 0.3 mg/kg/dose intravenously (less than 1 mg/min) every 2 to 5 min as necessary (maximum total dose 10 mg). Amnesia for cardioversion—adult: 5 to 15 mg intravenously 5 to 10 min before procedure. *Special considerations:* it may precipitate central nervous system depression and psychomotor impairment when the patient is taking central nervous system depressant drugs; it should not be administered with other drugs because it may precipitate; it may cause local venous irritation; dose should be reduced by 50% in older adults; resuscitation equipment should be readily available (p. 930).

18. a. Albuterol (Proventil, Ventolin). *Class:* sympathomimetic and bronchodilator. *Description:* is a beta$_2$-specific sympathomimetic stimulant that relaxes bronchiolar smooth muscle and peripheral vasculature. *Indications:* relief of bronchospasm in patients with reversible obstructive airway disease and prevention of exercise-induced bronchospasm. *Contraindications:* hypersensitivity, cardiac dysrhythmias associated with tachycardia, and tachycardia caused by digitalis intoxication. *Adverse reactions:* restlessness, apprehension, dizzi-

ness, palpitations, increased blood pressure, and dysrhythmias. *Onset:* 5 to 15 min via inhalation, 30 min by mouth. *Duration:* 3 to 4 hr via inhalation, 4 to 6 hr by mouth. *Dose:* Bronchial asthma—adults: via metered dose inhaler, 1 to 2 inhalations (90 to 180 mcg) every 4 to 6 hr (wait 5 min between inhalations); via inhalation: 2.5 mg (0.5 ml of 0.5% solution) diluted to 3 ml with 0.9% NaCl administered over 5 to 15 min. Pediatric: via solution, 0.01 to 0.03 ml (0.05 to 0.15 mg)/kg/dose to a maximum of 0.5 ml/dose diluted in 2 ml of 0.9% normal saline (may be repeated every 20 min 3 times). *Special considerations:* sympathomimetics may exacerbate adverse cardiac effects; antidepressants may potentiate effects on the vasculature; beta blockers may antagonize effects; diuretics may potentiate hypokalemia; it may precipitate angina pectoris and dysrhythmias; it should be used with caution with patients with diabetes mellitus, hyperthyroidism, prostatic hypertrophy, or seizure disorder; it should be administered only by inhalation in prehospital care. b. Terbutaline (Brethine). *Class:* sympathomimetic and bronchodilator. *Description:* is a beta$_2$ adrenergic receptor stimulant that causes relaxation of bronchiolar smooth muscles and bronchodilation. *Indications:* bronchial asthma, reversible bronchospasm associated with exercise, chronic bronchitis, and emphysema. *Contraindications:* hypersensitivity, tachydysrhythmias, and digitalis-induced tachycardia. *Adverse reactions:* (usually transient and dose related): restlessness, apprehension, palpitations, tachycardia, chest pain, coughing, bronchospasm, nausea, and facial flushing. *Onset: 15 to 30 min* (subcutaneously), 5 to 30 min (metered dose inhaler). *Duration:* 1.5 to 4 hr (subcutaneously), 3 to 6 hr (metered dose inhaler). *Dose:* adult—0.25 mg subcutaneously, may repeat in 15 to 30 min (max dose 0.5 mg/4 hr); pediatric: not recommended for children under 12, 0.01 mg/kg/dose subcutaneously every 15 to 20 min as necessary, (maximum dose 0.25 mg). *Special considerations:* sympathomimetics may exacerbate adverse cardiovascular effects; monoamine oxidase inhibitors may potentiate hypotension; beta blockers may antagonize terbutaline; vital signs should be carefully monitored; it should be used with caution in patients with cardiovascular disease or hypertension (p. 859).

19. Adenosine (Adenocard). *Class:* endogenous nucleotide. *Description:* slows tachycardia associated with the atrioventricular node via modulation of the autonomic nervous system without causing negative inotropic effects and acts directly on sinus pacemaker cells and vagal nerve terminals to decrease chronotropic and dromotropic activity. *Indications:* conversion of paroxysmal supraventricular tachycardia to sinus rhythm. *Contraindica-*

tions: second- or third-degree atrioventricular block, sick sinus syndrome, atrial flutter, atrial fibrillation, ventricular tachycardia, and hypersensitivity to adenosine. *Adverse reactions:* facial flushing, lightheadedness, paresthesia, headache, diaphoresis, palpitations, chest pain, hypotension, dyspnea, nausea, and metallic taste. *Onset:* 30 seconds. *Duration:* 10 seconds. *Dose:* Adult—Initial, 6 mg over 1 to 3 sec repeated; if there is no response in 1 to 2 min, administer 12 mg over 1 to 3 seconds, repeat 12 mg dose once as necessary. Pediatric: 0.1 to 0.2 mg/kg rapid intravenous injection (maximum single dose 12 mg). *Special considerations:* methylxanthines antagonize the action of adenosine; dipyridamole potentiates the effect of adenosine; carbamazepine may potentiate the atrioventricular-nodal blocking effect of adenosine; it may produce bronchoconstriction in patients with asthma or bronchopulmonary disease (p. 922)

20. Morphine sulfate (Astramorph/PF and others). *Class:* Opioid analgesic. *Description:* increases peripheral venous capacitance and decreases venous return. It promotes analgesia, euphoria, and respiratory and physical depression; decreases myocardial oxygen demand; and is a schedule II drug. *Indications:* chest pain associated with myocardial infarction, moderate to severe acute or chronic pain, and pulmonary edema with or without pain. *Contraindications:* hypersensitivity to narcotics, diarrhea caused by poisoning, hypovolemia, hypotension, head injury or undiagnosed abdominal pain, and patients who have taken monoamine oxidase inhibitors within 14 days. *Adverse reactions:* hypotension, tachycardia, bradycardia, palpitations, syncope, facial flushing, respiratory depression, euphoria, bronchospasm, dry mouth, and allergic reaction. *Onset:* immediate. *Duration:* 2 to 7 hr. *Dose:* adult—1 to 3 mg intravenously every 5 min titrated to relief of pain; pediatric—0.1 to 2.0 mg/kg/dose intravenously (maximum 15 mg dose). *Special considerations:* central nervous system depressants may potentiate effects of morphine; chlorpromazine may potentiate analgesia; monoamine oxidase inhibitors may cause paradoxical excitation; narcotics rapidly cross the placenta; it should be used with caution with older adults, patients with asthma, and patients susceptible to central nervous system depression; naloxone should be readily available. b. Meperidine (Demerol). *Class:* opioid analgesic. *Description:* is an opioid agonist that produces analgesia, euphoria, and respiratory and physical depression. *Indications:* moderate to severe pain. *Contraindications:* hypersensitivity to narcotics, diarrhea resulting from poisoning, concurrent use of monoamine oxidase inhibitors, labor or delivery of a premature infant, undiagnosed abdominal pain, and head injury. *Adverse reactions:* respiratory depression, euphoria, delirium, agitation, hallucination, seizures, headache, visual disturbances, coma, facial flushing, circulatory collapse, dysrhythmias, allergic reaction, nausea, and vomiting. *Onset:* 10 to 45 min (intramuscularly), less than 1 min (intravenously). *Duration:* 2 to 4 hr. *Dose:* adult—50 to 100 mg (intramuscularly), 10 to 25 mg (intravenously); pediatric—1 to 2 mg/kg/dose (intramuscularly or intravenously). *Special considerations:* it should be used with caution in patients with asthma and chronic obstructive pulmonary disease and may aggravate seizures in patients with convulsive disorders; nalaxone should be readily available (pp. 946, 944).

21. Syrup of ipecac. *Class:* emetic. *Description:* acts locally as an irritant on gastric mucosa and on emetic centers of brain, causing vomiting. *Indications:* acute oral drug or toxin overdose in alert patients. *Contraindications:* caustics, corrosives, petroleum distillates, unprotected airway, absent gag reflex, unknown ingestion, rapidly acting CNS depressants, and children younger than 6 months. *Adverse reactions:* prolonged vomiting, muscle aching, weakness, cardiac conduction disturbances or dysrhythmias, chest pain, and hypotension. *Onset:* 15 to 20 min. *Duration:* 80 min. *Dose:* Adult—30 ml by mouth followed by 1 to 2 glasses of water (may repeat once in 25 to 30 min if ineffective). Pediatric—1 to 12 years: 15 ml by mouth followed by water (4 ml/kg), 6 to 12 months: 5 to 10 ml by mouth followed by several swallows of water repeated once if ineffective. *Special considerations:* active charcoal adsorbs ipecac; airway should be carefully monitored; sample of emesis should be saved; patient should be kept awake; it should be administered with caution in tricyclic antidepressant overdose because rapid central nervous system depression may occur with this type of overdose (do not give unless the overdose was witnessed). b. Activated charcoal (Charcoaide). *Class:* adsorbant. *Description:* binds and adsorbs ingested toxins that may still be present in gastrointestinal tract after emesis. *Indications:* many oral poisonings and medication overdoses. *Contraindications:* corrosives, caustics, and petroleum distillates. *Adverse reactions:* nausea (indirectly), vomiting, and constipation. *Onset:* immediate. *Duration:* continual in gastrointestinal tract. *Dose:* Adult—0.5 to 1.0 g/kg diluted to a 500-ml aqueous slurry solution administered by mouth or by nasogastric tube. Pediatric: 0.6 to 2.0 g/kg diluted with 8 ounces of water in a slurry solution administered by mouth or nasogastric tube. *Special considerations:* it does not adsorb all drugs and toxic substances (e.g., cyanide, lithium, iron, lead and arsenic) (p. 922).

22. Magnesium sulfate. *Class:* central nervous system depressant. *Description:* reduces striated muscle

contractions and blocks peripheral neuromuscular transmission by reducing acetylcholine release at the myoneural junction. *Indications:* seizures resulting from eclampsia, torsades de pointes, and refractory ventricular fibrillation. *Contraindications:* heart block. *Adverse reactions:* diaphoresis, facial flushing, hypotension, depressed reflexes, hypothermia, reduced heart rate, circulatory collapse, and respiratory depression. *Onset:* immediate. *Duration:* 3 to 4 hr. *Dose:* seizures associated with pregnancy—1 to 4 g (8 to 32 mEq), maximum dose of 1.5 ml/min. Ventricular fibrillation unresponsive to therapy or torsades de pointes—1 to 2 g in 100 ml of D5W infused over 1 to 2 min. *Special considerations:* other central nervous system depressants may enhance central nervous system depressant effects; it should not be administered in the 2 hours before delivery; calcium gluconate or calcium chloride should be available as antidotes; it may be needed for up to 48 hours after delivery (p. 943)

23. Dopamine (Intropin). *Class:* sympathomimetic. *Description:* acts on alpha$_1$- and beta-adrenergic receptors, increasing systemic vascular resistance and exerting a positive inotropic effect on the heart, and dilates renal and splanchnic vasculature at low doses, maintaining blood flow. *Indications:* hypotension and low cardiac output states. *Contraindications:* tachydysrhythmias, ventricular fibrillation, and patients with pheochromocytoma. *Adverse reactions:* dose-related tachycardias, hypertension, and increased myocardial oxygen demand. *Onset:* 2 to 4 min. *Duration:* 10 to 15 min. *Dose:* Adult—place 200 mg in 250 ml of D5W and infuse at 2.5 to 20 mcg/kg/min (titrated to patient response); dopaminergic response: 2 to 4 mcg/kg/min; beta adrenergic response: 5 to 10 mcg/kg/min; alpha adrenergic response: 10 to 20 mcg/kg/min. Pediatric: 2 to 10 mcg/kg/min (titrated to patient response). *Special considerations:* it should be infused through a large common stable vein to avoide extravasation injury; patient should be monitored for signs of compromised circulation (p. 934).

24. Verapamil (Isoptin). *Class:* calcium channel blocker (class IV antidysrhythmic). *Description:* inhibits the movement of calcium ions across cell membranes, decreases atrial automaticity, reduces atrioventricular conduction velocity, prolongs the atrioventricular nodal refractory period, decreases myocardial contractility, reduces vascular smooth muscle tone, and dilates coronary arteries and arterioles. *Indications:* paroxymyl supraventricular tachycardia, atrial flutter with rapid ventricular response, and atrial fibrillation with a rapid ventricular response. *Contraindications:* hypersensitivity, sick sinus syndrome (unless the patient has a pacemaker), second- or third-degree heart block, hypotension, cardiogenic shock, severe congestive heart failure, Wolff-Parkinson-White syndrome with atrial fibrillation or flutter, patients receiving intravenous beta blockers, wide-complex tachycardias. *Adverse reactions:* dizziness, headache, nausea, vomiting, hypotension, bradycardia, complete atrioventricular block, and peripheral edema. *Onset:* 2 to 5 min. *Duration:* 30 to 60 min. *Dose:* Adult—2.5 to 5.0 mg intravenous bolus over 2 min, repeat with 5 to 10 mg in 15 to 30 min as necessary (maximum of 20 mg). *Special considerations:* It increases the serum concentration of digoxin; beta adrenergic blockers may have additive negative inotropic and chronotropic effects; antihypertensives may potentiate the hypotensive effects; vital signs should be closely monitored; the paramedic should be prepared to resuscitate the patient; atrioventricular block or asystole may occur because of slowed atrioventricular conduction (p. 961).

25. Furosemide (Lasix). *Class:* diuretic. *Description:* inhibits reabsorption of sodium and chloride in the proximal tubule and loop of Henle. *Indications:* pulmonary edema and congestive heart failure. *Contraindications:* anuria, hypersensitivity, and states of severe electrolyte depletion. *Adverse reactions:* hypotension, electrocardiogram changes, chest pain, dry mouth, hypochloremia, hypokalemia, hyponatremia, and hyperglycemia. *Onset:* within 5 min intravenously. *Duration:* 4 to 6 hr. *Dose:* adult—0.5 to 1.0 mg/kg slow intravenous injection; pediatric: 1 mg/kg/dose every 12 hr. *Special considerations:* it may potentiate digitalis toxicity because of potassium depletion; it may potentiate lithium toxicity resulting from sodium depletion; it has been known to cause fetal abnormalities; it should be protected from light (p. 936).

26. Oxytocin (Pitocin). *Class:* hormone. *Description:* indirectly stimulates uterine smooth muscle contractions, which stimulates contractions and transiently reduces uterine blood flow, and stimulates the mammary gland to increase lactation. *Indications:* postpartum hemorrhage after infant and placental delivery. *Contraindications:* presence of a second fetus. *Adverse reactions:* hypotension, tachycardia, hypertension, dysrhythmias, angina pectoris, anxiety, seizure, nausea, vomiting, allergic reaction, and uterine rupture (excessive dose). *Onset:* intravenous—immediate, intramuscular—3 to 5 min. *Duration:* intravenous—20 min, intramuscular—30 to 60 min. *Dose:* intramuscularly—3 to 10 units after delivery of the placenta; intravenously—mix 5 to 20 units in 500 ml D5W, normal saline, or lactated Ringer's solution and infuse at 20 to 40 milliunits/min titrated to the severity of bleeding and uterine response. *Special considerations:* vasopressors may potentiate hypertension;

vital signs and uterine tone should be closely monitored (p. 951).

27. b. To increase stroke volume (p. 934)

28. d. Narcotic analgesics and nitrous oxide are contraindicated in undiagnosed abdominal pain because they may mask symptoms (pp. 943-950).

29. a. Epinephrine 1:10,000 intravenously is indicated for all other conditions listed (p. 934).

30. c (p. 953)

31. d (p. 927)

32. a. It will cause vasoconstriction at high doses (p. 934).

33. b (pp. 941, 951, 954)

34. a (p. 934)

35. c. All others are beta agonists (p. 932).

36. b. Verapamil vasodilates and further decreases blood pressure (p. 961).

37. d (p. 950)

38. b. It will dilate blood vessels and decrease peripheral vascular resistance and blood pressure (p. 938).

39. d. Aminophylline causes tachycardia and may exacerbate a preexisting tachycardia (p. 924).

40. c. Naloxone is given to reverse potential narcotic intoxication. Thiamine promotes uptake of glucose in the brain and prevents the development of Wernicke's encephalopathy when glucose is given. D50W will correct underlying hypoglycemia (pp. 930, 947, 960).

41. b. It is an osmotic diuretic and pulls excess fluid from the brain, temporarily decreasing intracranial pressure (p. 943).

42. a (p. 930)

43. d. Oxytocin should be given only after delivery of all the babies (p. 951).

44. b. Benadryl causes thickening of the bronchial secretions and exacerbates an asthma attack (p. 932).

45. c. Syrup of ipecac is contraindicated in patients with no gag reflex because aspiration may occur. Compazine is an antiemetic and decreases the effect of the ipecac. Hydrocarbons such as gasoline pose a large risk of aspiration, so ipecac is not indicated (p. 958).

46. d. It is not effective against barbiturates (p. 947).

47. c. It may also cause hypotension (p. 942).

48. b. Bretylium may also cause hypotension, so it should be infused slowly over 8 to 10 minutes in the patient with a pulse (p. 927).

49. d (p. 948)

50. b (p. 934)

51. d. Furosemide decreases intravascular volume and causes vasodilation, which causes decreased preload and therefore less fluid to back up in the lungs (p. 936).

52. d. Adenosine is not a calcium channel blocker but is used to treat supraventricular tachycardia (p. 922).

53. a. Atropine would increase the heart rate and the work of the heart and make the patient's condition worse (p. 927).

54. b. Vistaril is often ordered concurrently to prevent this side effect (p. 943).

55. a. Haldol is a major tranquilizer (p. 937).

56. d (pp. 929, 945

ILLUSTRATION CREDITS AND ACKNOWLEDGEMENTS

Figs 10-2, 10-3, 10-11, 10-12A: Thibodeau: *Structure & function of the body*, ed 9, St Louis, 1992, Mosby (Illustrator E.W. Beck).

Figs 10-4, 10-6: Seeley-Stephens-Tate: *Anatomy & physiology*, ed 2, St Louis, 1992, Mosby (Illustrator David J. Mascaro & Associates).

Fig 10-16: Thibodeau: *Structure & function of the body*, ed 9, St Louis, 1992, Mosby (Illustrator David J. Mascaro & Associates).

Figs 10-8, 10-9: Thibodeau: *Structure & function of the body,* ed 9, St Louis, 1992, Mosby (Branislav Vidic).

Fig 10-12B: Thibodeau: *Structure & function of the body,* ed 9, St Louis, 1992, Mosby (Illustrator Christine Oleksyk).

Fig 10-13: Seeley: *Anatomy & physiology,* ed 2, St Louis, 1992, Mosby (Sims/Illustrator Jody L. Fulks).

Fig 10-14: Thibodeau: *Structure & function of the body,* ed 9, St Louis, 1992, Mosby (Illustrator Barbara Cousins).

Fig 10-15: Thibodeau: *Structure & function of the body,* ed 9, St Louis, 1992, Mosby (Illustrator William Ober).

Figs 18-1, 18-2, 18-2A: Cotton: *Mosby's paramedic study guide*, St. Louis, 1989, Mosby.

Figs 18-3, 18-11: Huszar: *Basic dysrhythmias*, ed 2, St Louis, 1994, Mosby.

NATIONAL REGISTRY OF EMT-PARAMEDIC EXAMINATION SKILL SHEETS

Courtesy the National Registry of Emergency Medical Technicians, Columbus, Ohio

National Registry of Emergency Medical Technicians
Advanced Level Practical Examination

PATIENT ASSESSMENT/MANAGEMENT

Candidate:_____ Examiner:_____

Date:_____ Signature:_____

Scenario #_____ Time Start:_____Time End:_____

PRIMARY SURVEY/RESUSCITATION

		Possible Points	Points Awarded
Takes or verbalizes infection control precautions		1	
Airway with C-Spine Control	Takes or directs manual in-line immobilization of head (1 point) Opens and assesses airway (1 point) Inserts adjunct (1 point)	3	
Breathing	Assesses breathing (1 point) Initiates appropriate oxygen therapy (1 point) Assures adequate ventilation of patient (1 point) Manages any injury which may compromise breathing/ventilation (1 point)	4	
Circulation	Checks pulse (1 point) Assesses peripheral perfusion (1 point) [checks either skin color, temperature, or capillary refill] Assesses for and controls major bleeding if present (1 point) Takes vital signs (1 point) Verbalizes application of or consideration for PASG (1 point) [candidate must assess body parts to be enclosed prior to application]	5	
	Volume replacement [usually deferred until patient loaded] - Initiates first IV line (1 point) - Initiates second IV line (1 point) - Selects appropriate catheters (1 point) - Selects appropriate IV solutions and administration sets (1 point) - Infuses at appropriate rate (1 point)	5	
Disability	Performs mini-neuro assessment: AVPU (1 point) Applies cervical collar (1 point)	2	
Expose	Removes clothing	1	
Status	Calls for immediate transport of the patient when indicated	1	

PRIMARY SURVEY/RESUSCITATION SUB-TOTAL 22 | |

SECONDARY SURVEY

NOTE: Areas denoted by "**" may be integrated within sequence of Primary Survey

Head	Inspects mouth**, nose**, and assesses facial area (1 point) Inspects and palpates scalp and ears (1 point) Checks eyes: PEARRL** (1 point)	3	
Neck**	Checks position of trachea (1 point) Checks jugular veins (1 point) Palpates cervical spine (1 point)	3	
Chest**	Inspects chest (1 point) Palpates chest (1 point) Auscultates chest (1 point)	3	
Abdomen/Pelvis**	Inspects and palpates abdomen (1 point) Assesses pelvis (1 point)	2	
Lower Extremities**	Inspects and palpates left leg (1 point) Inspects and palpates right leg (1 point) Checks motor, sensory, and distal circulation (1 point/leg)	4	
Upper Extremities	Inspects and palpates left arm (1 point) Inspects and palpates right arm (1 point) Checks motor, sensory, and distal circulation (1 point/arm)	4	
Posterior Thorax/Lumbar** and Buttocks	Inspects and palpates posterior thorax (1 point) Inspects and palpates lumbar and buttocks area (1 point)	2	
Identifies and treats minor wounds/fractures appropriately (1 point each)		2	

SECONDARY SURVEY SUB-TOTAL 23 | |

CRITICAL CRITERIA

____ Failure to initiate or call for transport of the patient within 10 minute time limit
____ Failure to take or verbalize infection control precautions
____ Failure to immediately establish and maintain spinal protection
____ Failure to provide high concentration of oxygen
____ Failure to evaluate and find all presented conditions of airway, breathing, and circulation (shock)
____ Failure to appropriately manage/provide airway, breathing, hemorrhage control or treatment for shock
____ Failure to differentiate patient's needing transportation versus continued on-scene survey
____ Does other detailed physical examination before assessing & treating threats to airway, breathing & circulation

You must factually document your rationale for checking any of the above critical items on the reverse side of this form.

P 201 11 93

National Registry of Emergency Medical Technicians
Advanced Level Practical Examination
PATIENT ASSESSMENT/MANAGEMENT

Candidate:_____ Examiner:_____

Date:_____ Signature:_____

Scenario #_____ Time Start:_____Time End:_____

		Possible Points	Points Awarded
PRIMARY SURVEY/RESUSCITATION			
Takes or verbalizes infection control precautions		1	
Airway with C-Spine Control	Takes or directs manual in-line immobilization of head (1 point) Opens and assesses airway (1 point) Inserts adjunct (1 point)	3	
Breathing	Assesses breathing (1 point) Initiates appropriate oxygen therapy (1 point) Assures adequate ventilation of patient (1 point) Manages any injury which may compromise breathing/ventilation (1 point)	4	

Circulation	Checks pulse (1 point)
	Assesses peripheral perfusion (1 point)
	  [checks either skin color, temperature, or capillary refill]
	Assesses for and controls major bleeding if present (1 point)
	Takes vital signs (1 point)
	Verbalizes application of or consideration for PASG (1 point)
	  [candidate must assess body parts to be enclosed prior to application]
		5	

	Volume replacement [usually deferred until patient loaded]
	  - Initiates first IV line (1 point)
	  - Initiates second IV line (1 point)
	  - Selects appropriate catheters (1 point)
	  - Selects appropriate IV solutions and administration sets (1 point)
	  - Infuses at appropriate rate (1 point)
		5	

Disability	Performs mini-neuro assessment: AVPU (1 point) Applies cervical collar (1 point)	2	
Expose	Removes clothing	1	
Status	Calls for immediate transport of the patient when indicated	1	

PRIMARY SURVEY/RESUSCITATION SUB-TOTAL   22

SECONDARY SURVEY

NOTE: Areas denoted by "**" may be integrated within sequence of Primary Survey

Head	Inspects mouth**, nose**, and assesses facial area (1 point) Inspects and palpates scalp and ears (1 point) Checks eyes: PEARRL** (1 point)	3	
Neck**	Checks position of trachea (1 point) Checks jugular veins (1 point) Palpates cervical spine (1 point)	3	
Chest**	Inspects chest (1 point) Palpates chest (1 point) Auscultates chest (1 point)	3	
Abdomen/Pelvis**	Inspects and palpates abdomen (1 point) Assesses pelvis (1 point)	2	
Lower Extremities**	Inspects and palpates left leg (1 point) Inspects and palpates right leg (1 point) Checks motor, sensory, and distal circulation (1 point/leg)	4	
Upper Extremities	Inspects and palpates left arm (1 point) Inspects and palpates right arm (1 point) Checks motor, sensory, and distal circulation (1 point/arm)	4	
Posterior Thorax/Lumbar** and Buttocks	Inspects and palpates posterior thorax (1 point) Inspects and palpates lumbar and buttocks area (1 point)	2	
Identifies and treats minor wounds/fractures appropriately (1 point each)		2	

SECONDARY SURVEY SUB-TOTAL   23

CRITICAL CRITERIA
____ Failure to initiate or call for transport of the patient within 10 minute time limit
____ Failure to take or verbalize infection control precautions
____ Failure to immediately establish and maintain spinal protection
____ Failure to provide high concentration of oxygen
____ Failure to evaluate and find all presented conditions of airway, breathing, and circulation (shock)
____ Failure to appropriately manage/provide airway, breathing, hemorrhage control or treatment for shock
____ Failure to differentiate patient's needing transportation versus continued on-scene survey
____ Does other detailed physical examination before assessing & treating threats to airway, breathing & circulation

You must factually document your rationale for checking any of the above critical items on the reverse side of this form.

P 201 11 93

National Registry of Emergency Medical Technicians
Intermediate Practical Examination

VENTILATORY MANAGEMENT (EOA)

Candidate: _____   Examiner: _____

Date: _____   Signature: _____

NOTE: If candidate elects to initially ventilate with BVM attached to reservoir and oxygen, full credit must be awarded for steps denoted by "**" so long as first ventilation is delivered within initial 30 seconds.

	Possible Points	Points Awarded
Takes or verbalizes infection control precautions	1	
Opens the airway manually	1	
Elevates tongue, inserts simple adjunct [either oropharyngeal or nasopharyngeal airway]	1	
NOTE: Examiner now informs candidate no gag reflex is present and patient accepts adjunct		
**Ventilates patient immediately with bag-valve-mask device unattached to oxygen	1	
**Hyperventilates patient with room air	1	
NOTE: Examiner now informs candidate that ventilation is being performed without difficulty		
Attaches oxygen reservoir to bag-valve-mask device and connects to high flow oxygen regulator [12-15 liters/min.]	1	
Ventilates patient at a rate of 10-20/min. and volumes of at least 800ml	1	
NOTE: After 30 seconds, examiner auscultates and reports breath sounds are present and equal bilaterally and medical control has ordered placement of an EOA. The examiner must now take over ventilation.		
Directs assistant to hyperventilate patient	1	
Identifies/selects proper equipment	1	
Assembles airway	1	
Tests cuff	1	
Inflates mask	1	
Lubricates tube [may be verbalized]	1	
NOTE: Examiner to remove OPA and move out of way when candidate is prepared to insert EOA		
Positions head properly with neck in neutral or slightly flexed position	1	
Grasps tongue and mandible and elevates	1	
Inserts tube in same direction as curvature of pharynx	1	
Advances tube until mask sealed against face	1	
Ventilates patient while maintaining tight mask seal	1	
Directs confirmation of proper placement by auscultation bilaterally and over epigastrium	1	
Inflates cuff to proper pressure and disconnects syringe	1	
Continues ventilation of patient	1	
NOTE: Examiner to ask "If you had proper placement, what would you expect to hear?"		

TOTAL 21

CRITICAL CRITERIA

____ Failure to initiate ventilations within 30 seconds after applying gloves or interrupts ventilations for greater than 30 seconds at any time

____ Failure to take or verbalize infection control precautions

____ Failure to voice and ultimately provide high oxygen concentrations [at least 85%]

____ Failure to ventilate patient at rate of at least 10/minute

____ Failure to provide adequate volumes per breath [maximum 2 errors/minute permissable]

____ Failure to hyperventilate patient prior to placement of the EOA

____ Failure to successfully place the EOA within 3 attempts

____ Failure to assure proper tube placement by auscultation bilaterally **and** over the epigastrium

____ Inserts any adjunct in a manner dangerous to patient

You must factually document your rationale for checking any of the above critical items on the reverse side of this form.

P-202B/4-93

National Registry of Emergency Medical Technicians
Paramedic Practical Examination
CARDIAC ARREST SKILLS STATION
DYNAMIC CARDIOLOGY

Candidate:_____   Examiner:_____

Date:_____   Signature:_____

Set #_____   Time Start:_____Time End:_____

	Possible Points	Points Awarded
Takes or verbalizes infection control precautions	1	
Checks level of responsiveness	1	
Checks ABC's	1	
Initiates CPR if appropriate [verbally]	1	
Performs "Quick Look" with paddles	1	
Correctly interprets initial rhythm	1	
Appropriately manages initial rhythm	2	
Notes change in rhythm	1	
Checks patient condition to include pulse and, if appropriate, BP	1	
Correctly interprets second rhythm	1	
Appropriately manages second rhythm	2	
Notes change in rhythm	1	
Checks patient condition to include pulse and, if appropriate, BP	1	
Correctly interprets third rhythm	1	
Appropriately manages third rhythm	2	
Notes change in rhythm	1	
Checks patient condition to include pulse and, if appropriate, BP	1	
Correctly interprets fourth rhythm	1	
Appropriately manages fourth rhythm	2	
Orders high percentages of supplemental oxygen at proper times	1	

CRITICAL CRITERIA   TOTAL 24 [ ]

____ Failure to deliver first shock in a timely manner due to operator delay in machine use or providing treatments other than CPR with simple adjuncts

____ Failure to deliver second or third shocks without delay other than the time required to reassess and recharge paddles

____ Failure to verify rhythm before delivering each shock

____ Failure to ensure the safety of self and others [verbalizes"All clear" and observes]

____ Inability to deliver DC shock [does not use machine properly]

____ Failure to demonstrate acceptable shock sequence

____ Failure to order initiation or resumption of CPR when appropriate

____ Failure to order correct management of airway [ET when appropriate]

____ Failure to order administration of appropriate oxygen at proper time

____ Failure to diagnose or treat 2 or more rhythms correctly

____ Orders administration of an inappropriate drug or lethal dosage

____ Failure to correctly diagnose or adequately treat v-fib, v-tach, or asystole

You must factually document your rationale for checking any of the above critical items on the reverse side of this form.

P203A

National Registry of Emergency Medical Technicians
Paramedic Practical Examination
CARDIAC ARREST SKILLS STATION
STATIC CARDIOLOGY

Candidate:_____   Examiner:_____

Date:_____   Signature:_____

Set #_____

NOTE: No points for treatment may be awarded if the diagnosis is incorrect.
Only document incorrect responses in spaces provided.

	Possible Points	Points Awarded
STRIP #1		
Diagnosis:	1	
Treatment:	2	
STRIP #2		
Diagnosis:	1	
Treatment:	2	
STRIP #3		
Diagnosis:	1	
Treatment:	2	
STRIP #4		
Diagnosis:	1	
Treatment:	2	
TOTAL	12	

P-203B 3/93

National Registry of Emergency Medical Technicians
Advanced Level Practical Examination
INTRAVENOUS THERAPY

Candidate:_____   Examiner:_____

Date:_____   Signature:_____

Time Start:_____Time End:_____

	Possible Points	Points Awarded

Checks selected IV fluid for:
    - Proper fluid (1 point)
    - Clarity (1 point)
	2	

Selects appropriate catheter	1	
Selects proper administration set	1	
Connects IV tubing to the IV bag	1	
Prepares administration set [fills drip chamber and flushes tubing]	1	
Cuts or tears tape [at any time before venipuncture]	1	
Takes/verbalizes infection control precautions [prior to venipuncture]	1	
Applies tourniquet	1	
Palpates suitable vein	1	
Cleanses site appropriately	1	

Performs venipuncture
 	
    - Inserts stylette (1 point)
    - Notes or verbalizes flashback (1 point)
    - Occludes vein proximal to catheter (1 point)
    - Removes stylette (1 point)
    - Connects IV tubing to catheter (1 point)
	5	

Releases tourniquet	1	
Runs IV for a brief period to assure patent line	1	
Secures catheter [tapes securely or verbalizes]	1	
Adjusts flow rate as appropriate	1	
Disposes/verbalizes disposal of needle in proper container	1	

TOTAL   21   [   ]

CRITICAL CRITERIA

____ Exceeded the 6 minute time limit in establishing a patent and properly adjusted IV

____ Failure to take or verbalize infection control precautions prior to performing venipuncture

____ Contaminates equipment or site without appropriately correcting situation

____ Any improper technique resulting in the potential for catheter shear or air embolism

____ Failure to successfully establish IV within 3 attempts during 6 minute time limit

____ Failure to dispose/verbalize disposal of needle in proper container

You must factually document your rationale for checking any of the above critical items on the reverse side of this form.

P-204A 3/93

National Registry of Emergency Medical Technicians
Paramedic Practical Examination
INTRAVENOUS BOLUS MEDICATIONS

Candidate:_____

Date:_____

Examiner:_____

Signature:_____

Time Start:_____ Time End:_____

NOTE: Check here (____) if candidate did not establish
a patent IV and do not evaluate these skills.

	Possible Points	Points Awarded
Asks patient for known allergies	1	
Selects correct medication	1	
Assures correct concentration of drug	1	
Assembles prefilled syringe correctly and dispels air	1	
Continues infection control precautions	1	
Cleanses injection site (Y-port or hub)	1	
Reaffirms medication	1	
Stops IV flow (pinches tubing)	1	
Administers correct dose at proper push rate	1	
Flushes tubing (runs wide open for a brief period)	1	
Adjusts drip rate to TKO (KVO)	1	
Voices proper disposal of syringe and needle	1	
Verbalizes need to observe patient for desired effect/adverse side effects	1	

CRITICAL CRITERIA   IV BOLUS SUB-TOTAL 13 [   ]

____Failure to begin administration of medication within 3 minute time limit

____Contaminates equipment or site without appropriately correcting situation

____Failure to adequately dispel air resulting in potential for air embolism

____Injects improper drug or dosage (wrong drug, incorrect amount, or pushes at inappropriate rate)

____Failure to flush IV tubing after injecting medication

____Recaps needle or failure to dispose/verbalize disposal of syringe and needle in proper container

INTRAVENOUS PIGGYBACK MEDICATIONS

	Possible Points	Points Awarded
Has confirmed allergies by now (award point if previously confirmed)	1	
Checks selected IV fluid for: - Proper fluid (1 point) - Clarity (1 point)	2	
Checks selected medication for: - Clarity (1 point) - Concentration of medication (1 point)	2	
Injects correct amount of medication into IV solution given scenario	1	
Connects appropriate administration set to medication solution	1	
Prepares administration set (fills drip chamber and flushes tubing)	1	
Attaches appropriate needle to administration set	1	
Continues infection control precautions	1	
Cleanses port of primary line	1	
Inserts needle into port without contamination	1	
Adjusts flow rate of secondary line as required	1	
Stops flow of primary line	1	
Securely tapes needle	1	
Verbalizes need to observe patient for desired effect/adverse side effects	1	
Labels medication/fluid bag	1	

CRITICAL CRITERIA   IV PIGGYBACK SUB-TOTAL 17 [   ]

____ Failure to begin administration of medication within 5 minute time limit

____ Contaminates equipment or site without appropriately correcting situation

____ Administers improper drug or dosage (wrong drug, incorrect amount, or infuses at inappropriate rate)

____ Failure to flush IV tubing of secondary line resulting in potential for air embolism

____ Failure to shut-off flow of primary line

You must factually document your rationale for checking any of the above critical items on the reverse side of this form.

P-204B 3/93

National Registry of Emergency Medical Technicians
Advanced Level Practical Examination
SPINAL IMMOBILIZATION
(SEATED PATIENT)

Candidate:_____   Examiner:_____

Date:_____   Signature:_____

Time Start:_____Time End:_____

	Possible Points	Points Awarded
Takes or verbalizes infection control precautions	1	
Directs assistant to place/maintain head in neutral, in-line position	1	
Directs assistant to maintain manual immobilization of head	1	
Assesses motor, sensory, and distal circulation in extremities	1	
Applies appropriately sized extrication collar	1	
Positions the immobilization device behind the patient	1	
Secures device to the patient's torso	1	
Evaluates torso fixation and adjusts as necessary	1	
Evaluates and pads behind the patient's head as necessary	1	
Secures patient's head to the device	1	
Reassesses motor, sensory, and distal circulation in extremities	1	
Verbalizes moving the patient to a long board properly	1	

TOTAL 12 [   ]

CRITICAL CRITERIA

___ Did not immediately direct or take manual immobilization of head

___Releases or orders release of manual immobilization before it was maintained mechanically

___Patient manipulated or moved excessively causing potential spinal compromise

___Did not complete immobilization of the torso prior to immobilizing the head

___Device moves excessively up, down, left, or right on patient's torso

___Torso fixation inhibits chest rise resulting in respiratory compromise

___Head immobilization allows for excessive movement

___Upon completion of immobilization, head is not in neutral, in-line position

You must factually document your rationale for checking any of the above critical items on the reverse side of this form.

P-205/6-93

National Registry of Emergency Medical Technicians
Advanced Level Practical Examination
RANDOM BASIC SKILLS
BLEEDING - WOUNDS - SHOCK

Candidate:_____   Examiner:_____

Date:_____   Signature:_____

Time Start:_____Time End:_____

	Possible Points	Points Awarded
Takes or verbalizes infection control precautions	1	
Applies direct pressure to the wound	1	
Elevates the extremity	1	
Applies pressure dressing to the wound	1	
Bandages wound	1	
NOTE: The examiner must now inform the candidate that the wound is still continuing to bleed. The second dressing does not control the bleeding.		
Locates and applies pressure to appropriate arterial pressure point	1	
NOTE: The examiner must indicate that the victim is in compensatory shock.		
Applies high concentration oxygen	1	
Properly positions patient (supine with legs elevated)	1	
Prevents heat loss (covers patient as appropriate)	1	
NOTE: The examiner must indicate that the victim is in profound shock. Medical control has ordered application and inflation of the Pneumatic Anti-shock Garment.		
Removes clothing or checks for sharp objects	1	
Quickly assesses areas that will be under the PASG	1	
Positions PASG with top of abdominal section at or below last set of ribs	1	
Secures PASG around patient	1	
Attaches hoses	1	
Begins inflation sequence (examiner to stop inflation at 15mm Hg)	1	
Checks blood pressure	1	
Verbalizes when to stop inflation sequence	1	
Operates PASG to maintain air pressure in device	1	
Reassesses vital signs	1	

TOTAL 19 [ ]

CRITICAL CRITERIA

____ Failure to take or verbalize infection control precautions

____ Did not apply high concentration of oxygen

____ Applies tourniquet before attempting other methods of hemorrhage control

____ Did not control hemorrhage or attempt to control hemorrhage in a timely manner

____ Inflates abdominal section of PASG before the legs

____ Did not reassess patient's vital signs after PASG inflation

____ Places PASG on inside-out

____ Allows deflation of PASG after inflation

____ Positions PASG above level of lowest rib

You must factually document your rationale for checking any of the above critical items on the reverse side of this form.

P-206A   11/93

National Registry of Emergency Medical Technicians
Advanced Level Practical Examination
RANDOM BASIC SKILLS
LONG BONE IMMOBILIZATION

Candidate_____   Examiner:_____

Date_____   Signature:_____

Time Start:_____Time End:_____

	Possible Points	Points Awarded
Takes or verbalizes infection control precautions	1	
Directs application of manual stabilization	1	
Assesses motor, sensory, and distal circulation	1	
NOTE: Examiner acknowledges present and normal		
Measures splint	1	
Applies splint	1	
Immobilizes joint above fracture	1	
Immobilizes joint below fracture	1	
Secures entire injured extremity	1	
Immobilizes hand/foot in position of function	1	
Reassesses motor, sensory, and distal circulation	1	
NOTE: Examiner acknowledges present and normal		

TOTAL   10   [   ]

CRITICAL CRITERIA

___ Grossly moves injured extremity

___ Did not immobilize adjacent joints, injury, or limb

___ Did not reassess motor, sensory, and distal circulation after splinting

You must factually document your rationale for checking any of the above critical items on the reverse side of this form.

P-206B

National Registry of Emergency Medical Technicians
Advanced Level Practical Examination
RANDOM BASIC SKILLS
TRACTION SPLINTING

Candidate:_____   Examiner:_____

Date:_____   Signature:_____

Time Start:_____Time End:_____

	Possible Points	Points Awarded
Takes or verbalizes infection control precautions	1	
Directs manual stabilization of injured leg	1	
Directs application of manual traction	1	
Assesses motor, sensory, and distal circulation	1	
NOTE: Examiner acknowledges present and normal		
Prepares/adjusts splint to proper length	1	
Positions splint at injured leg	1	
Applies proximal securing device (e.g. ischial strap)	1	
Applies distal securing device (e.g. ankle hitch)	1	
Applies mechanical traction	1	
Positions/secures support straps	1	
Re-evaluates proximal/distal securing devices	1	
Reassesses motor, sensory, and distal circulation	1	
NOTE: Examiner acknowledges present and normal		
NOTE: Examiner must ask candidate how he/she would prepare for transport		
Verbalizes securing torso to long board to immobilize hip	1	
Verbalizes securing splint to long board to prevent movement of splint	1	

TOTAL 14 [　]

CRITICAL CRITERIA

____ Loss of traction at any point after it is assumed

____ Did not reassess motor, sensory, and distal circulation **after** splinting

____ The foot is excessively rotated or extended after splinting

____ Did not secure ischial strap **before** taking traction

____ Final immobilization failed to support femur or prevent rotation of injured leg

NOTE: If Sagar is used without elevating the leg, application of manual traction is not necessary. Candidate will be awarded 1 point as if manual traction were applied.

NOTE: If the leg is elevated at all, manual traction must be applied before elevating the leg. The ankle hitch may be applied before elevating the leg and used to pull manual traction.

You must factually document your rationale for checking any of the above critical items on the reverse side of this form.

P-206C/4-93

National Registry of Emergency Medical Technicians
Advanced Level Practical Examination
RANDOM BASIC SKILLS
SPINAL IMMOBILIZATION
(LYING PATIENT)

Candidate:_____ Examiner:_____

Date:_____ Signature:_____

Time Start:_____Time End:_____

	Possible Points	Points Awarded
Takes or verbalizes infection control procedures	1	
Directs assistant to move patient's head to the neutral in-line position	1	
Directs assistant to maintain manual immobilization of head	1	
Evaluates motor, sensory, and distal circulation in extremities	1	
Applies cervical collar	1	
Positions immobilization device appropriately	1	
Moves patient onto device without compromising the integrity of the spine	1	
Applies padding to voids between the torso and the board as necessary	1	
Immobilizes torso to the device	1	
Evaluates and pads under the patient's head as necessary	1	
Immobilizes the patient's head to the device	1	
Secures legs to the device	1	
Secures patient's arms to the board	1	
Reassesses motor, sensory, and distal circulation	1	

TOTAL 14 [ ]

CRITICAL CRITERIA

____ Did not immediately direct manual immobilization of head

____ Orders release of manual immobilization before it was maintained mechanically

____ Did not complete immobilization of the torso prior to immobilizing the head

____ Device excessively moves up, down, left, or right on patient's torso

____ Head immobilization allows for excessive movement

____ Head is not immobilized in the neutral in-line position

____ Patient moved excessively causing potential spinal compromise

____ Did not reassess motor, sensory, and distal circulation **after** immobilization

You must factually document your rationale for checking any of the above critical items on the reverse side of this form.

P-206 D/6-93